D1611670

THE CHALLENGE
OF FACTS

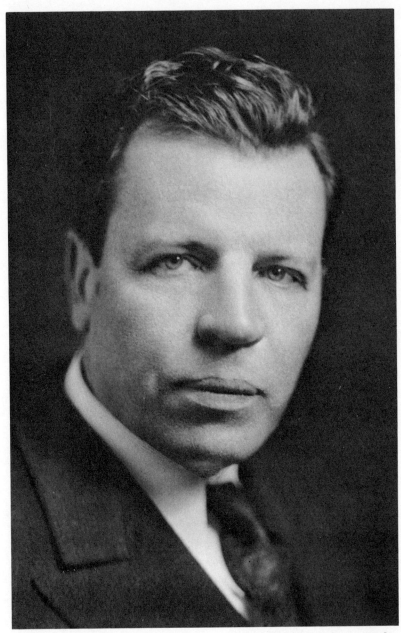

EDGAR SYDENSTRICKER
(1881–1936)

The
Challenge of Facts

Selected Public Health Papers of

EDGAR SYDENSTRICKER

Edited by Richard V. Kasius

Published for the Milbank Memorial Fund by

P R O D I S T

New York   1974

First published in the United States by
PRODIST
a division of Neale Watson Academic Publications, Inc.
156 Fifth Avenue
New York, N.Y. 10010
© 1974 Milbank Memorial Fund
Manufactured in the U.S.A.

Library of Congress Cataloging in Publication Data

Sydenstricker, Edgar, 1881 – 1936.
   The challenge of facts.

   CONTENTS: Wiehl, D. G. Edgar Sydenstricker: a
memoir. — Public health and evaluation: Greenberg, B. G.
Commentary. The measurements of results of public
health work. The statistician's place in public health
work. The changing concept of public health. Economy
in public health. [etc.]
   1. Hygiene, Public — United States. 2. Epidemiology. I. Title.
RA445.S78   362.1'0973   74-6072
ISBN 0 – 88202 – 056 – 0

Contributors

A memoir by Dorothy G. Wiehl,
and commentaries by Bernard G. Greenberg,
I. S. Falk, George W. Comstock, Robert F. Korns
and Peter Greenwald.

Contents

Preface

"I have confidence ... in the stimulating challenge of facts."
These words from Edgar Sydenstricker's De Lamar lecture of
1931 are an expression of a conviction that informed his multi-
faceted, productive, but relatively brief career as public health
statesman and advocate and particularly as public health statistician. Almost 40 years have passed since Sydenstricker's death and
he is now, even among many of his professional descendants, an
almost forgotten figure. Publication of this volume of selections
from the writings of a man whose public health career extended
from 1915 to 1936 is intended to acquaint the present generation
of workers in public health with his work and his contributions to
the development of our profession. It should serve to provide an
historical perspective on those issues in public health which
Sydenstricker addressed and which are still current and to illustrate the early development of concepts and methodology of public health research.

The idea for this collection originated with Robin F. Badgley,
while a member of the staff of the Milbank Memorial Fund. He
searched out and collected almost all of Sydenstricker's publications, but he did not have the opportunity of proceeding to the
next steps of reviewing and selecting the articles for publication.
Without Dr. Badgley's initial stimulus and preparation, this volume would not have appeared.

The 17 papers presented here were selected from among the more than 100 articles comprising Sydenstricker's bibliography. The criteria on which their selection was based included relevance to current issues, historical interest and significance, and a strong subjective weighting of personal interest. Preference was given to those papers expressive of Sydenstricker's continuing concern with program evaluation, and to articles of single, rather than multiple, authorship.

The review of this body of work was, if I may intrude a personal note, a provocative and informative experience, for Sydenstricker's writings, even four to six decades after, offer much to interest the reader of today. To be sure, some were of only immediate or transient substantive concern, but one is always engaged by the application of a rigorous and informed intellect to the issue at hand, and by a personal style of expression marked by clarity and force. Of interest in this regard is the opinion advanced by Pearl Buck, Sydenstricker's sister, who said in a letter in 1972 to a member of the staff of the Milbank Memorial Fund, "I have always felt that had he [Sydenstricker] chosen to be the writer, he would have been a much better writer than I."

Sydenstricker's interests ranged widely across the field of public health of his time and he wrote on topics as varied as the relation of wages to health and the lighting of post offices. The papers in this collection have been assembled in four categories, each representing a substantive area to which Sydenstricker made major contributions. These are: Public Health and Evaluation, Health Policy, Illness and Illness Surveys, and Epidemiological Studies. Each section is introduced by a commentary by a distinguished scholar, or scholars, and I wish to express my appreciation to George W. Comstock, I. S. Falk, Bernard G. Greenberg, Peter Greenwald, and Robert F. Korns for the thoughtful, critical assessments presented in these commentaries. Dorothy G. Wiehl, a colleague of Sydenstricker during much of his career in public health, has provided a memoir of his professional life. Her association with Sydenstricker from his early work in South Carolina to his years at the Milbank Memorial Fund gives her a unique capability for this task.

The graphs and figures were redrawn from the original publications by Mrs. Virginia Simon.

The Milbank Memorial Fund is grateful to the following organizations for their agreement to the publication of articles originally appearing in their journals: U.S. Department of Health, Education and Welfare; American Statistical Association; Academy of Political Science; American Lung Association; and the University of Chicago.

RICHARD V. KASIUS

New York, New York
February 1, 1974

1

EDGAR SYDENSTRICKER: A MEMOIR

DOROTHY G. WIEHL

Shortly before his death, Sydenstricker wrote in a paper included in this collection:

"Society has a basic responsibility for assuring, to all its members, healthful conditions of housing and living, a reasonable degree of economic security, proper facilities for curative and preventive medicine and adequate medical care—in fact the control, so far as means are known to science, of all of the environmental factors that affect physical and mental well being." (page 76)

In this concept of social responsibility, Sydenstricker expressed the culmination of his many years of studying environmental conditions, broadly defined, and their effect on health. A review of his professional career reveals a continuous series of activities which contributed to the development of this concept, although, at times, they seem to be unrelated. The successive activities could not have been planned, but throughout his career he was motivated to seek the facts needed to further the means by which more healthful living could be assured.

It was characteristic of the man that the philosophy expressed may seem idealistic, but his approach to solutions was very practical and called for an increase in scientific knowledge. To this end, during most of his career, he was engaged in investigations of morbidity and its associated environmental factors, and in evaluation of the efficacy and efficiency of public health practice.

3

Sydenstricker was born to missionary parents in Shanghai, China, on July 15, 1881. His father was Absalom Sydenstricker, D.D., a Presbyterian minister, and his mother was Caroline Stulting Sydenstricker, both from West Virginia. He was the only son and an only child until the age of 11 when the older of two sisters was born. In China, he had little companionship of children, and was educated at home by his parents until age 15, when he was sent to the United States. He attended Fredericksburg College in Virginia where he received an A.B. degree in 1900. After two years at Washington and Lee University, he received a Master's degree with honors in sociology and economics. There followed three years as principal of the high school at Onancock, Va., and two years as editor of the Lynchburg, Va., *Daily Advance*. The academic year, 1907–1908, was spent at the University of Chicago, where he was a post-graduate fellow in political economy. In the years following he was associated with the U.S. Immigration Commission and made extensive surveys of wages, working conditions and standards of living of industrial workers, especially of the foreign born. In 1914–1915 he was a member of the staff of the U.S. Commission on Industrial Relations, writing reports on collective bargaining in the anthracite industry and on conditions of labor.

His missionary background and contact with poverty in his early years probably influenced his life-long interest in finding ways to improve conditions for the underprivileged, an interest that was reinforced by his experience with his investigations of the living conditions of the foreign-born industrial workers.

Sydenstricker's professional career in public health began in 1915 and continued to his death in 1936. Educated as an economist with no formal education or experience in medical or health related fields, he was appointed the first public health statistician in the U.S. Public Health Service. With his training in statistics and experience with surveys of immigrant workers, the transition to studying illness in the family and community was easily accomplished. In fact, over the years his reputation became increasingly identified with his contribution to an understanding of the interrelationships between public health and economic and social conditions.

In the 20 years following 1915, health services in the United States expanded from a concern with sanitation, pure water and control of a few communicable diseases to the development of programs for promoting personal health by education on healthful living, by providing preventive health measures and by increasing the availability of adequate medical care. During these 20 years, Sydenstricker was a leader in public health research and an active participant in planning, promoting and evaluating health measures. The articles in this volume can suggest the range of his interests and his contribution to accumulating basic facts and to shaping public health policies, but his influence, as with any individual, cannot be isolated nor fully measured.

Shortly after Sydenstricker's death in 1936, his work in public health was appraised by Dr. Wade H. Frost in this personal communication:

"Sydenstricker has consistently followed one clear purpose, namely, to collect as exactly as possible the kind of facts which are needed to show in a perfectly dispassionate objective way what conditions affecting public health exist in this country and what is being done to meet them. He was inevitably impressed with the need for better distribution of medical care and was a rather strong advocate of some kind of system of sickness insurance. However, he was in no sense a propagandist. . . . It is my honest belief that in the last 20 years . . . he has done more than any other man in the U.S. to provide the kind of *facts* which *must* be known and heeded in planning the future development of public health."

The reports of his studies are of interest to students today because many of the problems are still current, the methodology is still applicable, and they express clearly many principles essential to developing public health science.

The professional activities of Sydenstricker in public health were carried out under the auspices of three agencies: the U.S. Public Health Service, the League of Nations, and the Milbank Memorial Fund. In each of these he was responsible for building a new service for organizing and directing statistical and research programs; and each provided excellent opportunities to study the epidemiology of diseases, to conduct research on public health and to cooperate with those engaged in promoting health programs.

Upon his initial appointment in the U.S. Public Health Service in 1915, he was assigned to assist Dr. B. S. Warren in a study of the organization and administration of sickness insurance in European countries. He co-authored several reports with Dr. Warren, but was soon transferred to South Carolina to work with Dr. Joseph Goldberger on his investigations of pellagra. Here, he conducted a series of house-to-house canvasses of families living in cotton mill villages to study their diets, illnesses, housing and sanitary conditions, and economic status. For these field surveys in 1916, 1917 and 1918, Sydenstricker organized and directed a staff of physicians, field investigators and office assistants to carry out a most intensive epidemiological study of pellagra.

The contribution of Sydenstricker to Goldberger's classic epidemiological study of pellagra has been summarized by Terris[1] as follows:

"The pellagra studies provide a brilliant example of the use of epidemiologic reasoning—that is, reasoning based on the behavior of a disease in the population—to develop an etiologic hypothesis. . . . Finally, the whole epidemiologic picture is presented: attention is focused not only on the dietary causes of pellagra but also on the underlying reasons for the dietary deficiencies. There emerges a thorough analysis of the economic and social basis of pellagra in the South. . . .

"This last achievement was undoubtedly due in large measure to the work of the economist Edgar Sydenstricker, whose investigations in the cotton mill villages of South Carolina led in a direct line to his pioneer morbidity studies in Hagerstown; he was later to become one of the great figures in public health and the author of the first American textbook of social medicine.[2] Sydenstricker's contributions to the pellagra studies are notable for their realism, comprehensiveness, and methodologic rigor; they represent an outstanding example of the effective collaboration of medical and social scientists."

The influenza epidemic in 1918 temporarily interrupted the completion of reports on the pellagra studies, as Sydenstricker was called to Washington to collaborate with Dr. Wade H. Frost in establishing a national center for information on the incidence of influenza. Frost was the senior Public Health Service officer in charge of the influenza studies, but the responsibility for building a staff and giving it technical direction was left to Sydenstricker. It was soon evident that physicians in different areas were not reporting cases with equal completeness and that mortality could not be used as an accurate measure of the incidence of the disease. In order to study its epidemiology, Sydenstricker and Frost set up surveys in eighteen localities where detailed data were collected by house-to-house canvassers. Thus, the method of household surveys used so successfully in studying pellagra was adapted to investigations of influenza. This method of studying illness was used in many later investigations and, in fact, was characteristic of much of Sydenstricker's research. A little more than a year after the influenza studies were started, Frost left the U.S. Public Health Service to become professor of epidemiology at the Johns Hopkins School of Hygiene and Public Health. However, he continued as a consultant to the Public Health Service and with Sydenstricker, contributed to the preparation of at least 25 papers on the history of influenza from 1910 to 1930.

Frost and Sydenstricker continued their collaboration on studies of other respiratory diseases. Frost recognized and respected Sydenstricker's technical competence and his imaginative, farsighted social outlook, and until Sydenstricker's death they shared a warm friendship and continued to have a close professional relationship.

In 1920, Sydenstricker's activities took on a new dimension in the Public Health Service with his appointment as Chief of the Office of Statistical Investigations which developed from the organization that had been assembled to service the influenza studies. New research units, staffed by statisticians and medical officers, were set up within the Office, and their programs were under Sydenstricker's direction. These were in addition to the continuing studies of influenza and pellagra. The many papers of which he was co-author during the 1920's were an expression of the research which he stimulated or guided as Chief of the Statistical Office.

A review of the projects of the Statistical Office at this time indicates a determined effort to expand the knowledge of illness in population groups by utilizing different data sources. One major source was the records of absenteeism of industrial workers which were studied by Dean K. Brundage. An intensive study of the health of school children was made in collaboration with Dr. Taliaferro Clark and Selwyn D. Collins in which more than 30,000 school children were examined by medical officers of the Public Health Service. The validity of height and weight measurements as an index of health or nutrition of the child was evaluated and doubt was thrown on the value of the widely used classification of "underweight" as an indication of poor general nutrition or poor health. Studies were made of venereal diseases based upon the case reports from cities and states. Unpublished tables of mortality were obtained from the U.S. Bureau of the Census and death rates from tuberculosis were intensively analyzed.

The internationally known Hagerstown Morbidity Survey was begun soon after the Statistical Office was established. This followed the method employed by Goldberger and Sydenstricker in South Carolina of continuous observation of a population to record the incidence of illness. This survey, discussed in more detail by Comstock in this volume, was the first attempt to record on so large a scale all illnesses in a typical population. To Sydenstricker, morbidity was the key to understanding the health of a population and he wrote: "Statistics of illness afford an indication of vitality that is not less significant and is more illuminating than that obtained through mortality statistics. They portray the condition of public health far more subtly than do death rates, and reveal the prevalence and incidence of disease upon a people in a manner that is as useful to the student of society as is clinical observation of the patient to the physician."[3] The series of publications on the Hagerstown survey are recognized as classics in their field. This survey is notable not only for the comprehensive data on morbidity that it provided but also, and of equal significance, for demonstrating the feasibility of and the important in-

formation to be gained from morbidity surveys of general populations. Studies of the Hagerstown population were extended to
problems other than incidence of illness and this community has
continued as a population laboratory for epidemiological investigations.

In the 15 years following the initial Hagerstown study, the
method of continuous observation of a population to obtain health
data was used in several more extensive investigations in which
Sydenstricker collaborated. One such study was made in
1928–1931 by the Committee on the Costs of Medical Care in
cooperation with the U.S. Public Health Service and state and
local health departments. In 1935–1936, the National Health Survey conducted by the Public Health Service with assistance from
the Works Progress Administration studied illness in approximately 750,000 families. The desirability of a continuing study to
obtain data on illness and disability resulting from chronic
diseases was discussed by Frost and Sydenstricker before the
latter's death. This objective was fulfilled by the five-year study of
sickness in the Eastern Health District of Baltimore (1938–1943),
which was directed by Jean Downes of the Milbank Memorial
Fund and by Selwyn D. Collins, the successor to Sydenstricker in
the Public Health Service.

Records of medical examinations collected by the Life Extension Institute were utilized by Sydenstricker to supplement the
picture of ill health provided by mortality data and morbidity
surveys. He described the value of health examinations as follows: "Morbidity and clinical records, although they indicate
reactions to disease and environment that the death certificate or
the autopsy protocol never mentions, fail to disclose those impairments and conditions which do not manifest themselves immediately in illness or in death."[4] Examinations had been begun
at the Life Extension Institute in 1921, and were offered by life
insurance companies to their policy holders in the belief that
knowledge of physical impairments would lead to early care and
the prevention of illness. Sydenstricker, in collaboration with
Rollo H. Britten of the Public Health Service, made an extensive
analysis of over 100,000 examinations, reported upon in several

papers. Britten followed these with further analyses of data from this and other related sources. These were the first data on a very large cross section of a general population. Examinations had been made by many doctors in many different communities. An important finding was that examiners varied greatly in their evaluation of physical defects and impairments, making the absolute rates of prevalence for different groups unreliable. However, relative prevalence rates could be used to show variations according to sex, age and occupation. Also, significant interrelationships of conditions were disclosed, such as the association between obesity and high blood pressure. In addition to the factual data provided, these analyses of physical impairments were important for their stimulation of a continuing interest in the use of such data for epidemiological investigations.

In 1923, Sydenstricker was granted a year's leave of absence to organize a statistical and epidemiological service in the Health Service of the League of Nations. This epidemiological intelligence service initially met a need to receive and disseminate data on cases of plague, cholera, typhus and other serious communicable diseases. Reports of cases anywhere in the world were published in a weekly bulletin. Available vital statistics for all member nations were assembled also in monthly and annual reports. It was evident to Sydenstricker that the comparability of these statistics needed to be investigated. Since infant mortality was used as a major index of health conditions, the Health Section began a series of studies on procedures for recording live births, stillbirths and infant deaths in different countries. Although Sydenstricker stayed in Geneva only one year, he set in motion a program for the preparation of handbooks describing the vital statistics in various countries and for international cooperation to improve comparability of mortality data for the different countries.

When the Milbank Memorial Fund looked for someone to appraise the health services in the three geographic areas in which the Fund was supporting demonstration programs, its Statistical Advisory Committee turned to Sydenstricker. In 1925, he was asked to review the Demonstration services and especially to advise on a program for evaluating their effectiveness. This led to his appointment as a part-time consultant on loan from the U.S. Public Health Service and to his writing "The Measurement of Results of Public Health Work" which is included in this volume. In 1928, he accepted the position of Director of Research with the Milbank Fund and was retained as a consultant to the Service. In 1935, he became the administrative head of the Fund with the title of Scientific Director.

The program of measurement proposed for the demonstrations was unique at this stage in the development of health departments. Communities had been urged by social agencies and socially minded citizens to increase health services, especially to provide preventive care for infants and school children and to control the spread of diseases such as tuberculosis and diphtheria, in addition to the conventional sanitary measures for the community. The American Public Health Association had prepared an "Appraisal Form" which relied on a count of individuals served and amount of services given to serve as a standard for health services. The standards were necessarily based on a consensus of "expert" opinion. The effect on the health of the community was judged by changes in mortality with attention given chiefly to infant and tuberculosis mortality. Sydenstricker viewed the measurement of results of specific health measures as necessary in the development of public health as a science. He wrote: "Our purpose . . . is *to find out whether or not, or how far, a specific social effort, which seeks to attain a specific objective by a specific method, actually accomplishes the result it is designed to accomplish.* [Emphasis in original]. If an objective is essentially not measurable by any quantitative method, let us recognize the fact. If it is, let us so plan that the measurement of the results of the social effort to attain it be an essential part of the process of its enactment."[5]

The research projected by Sydenstricker for the Milbank Memorial Fund was designed to continue the study of social data on factors affecting the health of human populations as well as to evaluate effectiveness of specific health measures. The first annual report of the Fund's Division of Research lists the projects under four general headings, as follows:

    I. Studies on the Accuracy of Vital Statistics.
    II. The Measurement of Results of Public Health Activities.
    III. Diseases and Impairments of Adult Life.
    IV. Differential Birth Rates in the United States.

Studies on accuracy of vital statistics were necessary because tabulations of births and deaths for communities were available only by place of occurrence. The increasing numbers of non-residents using urban hospitals made it essential to correct rates by allocating births and deaths to place of residence.

The relationship of differential birth rates to problems of public health may not be obvious. However, trends in birth rates for different socio-economic groups and differential infant mortality affect the composition of the population and a knowledge of such changes is complementary to an understanding of future health problems. Investigations in later years were extended to all aspects of the population problem, and included evaluation of methods of family limitation. The program has been described fully in "Forty Years of Research in Human Fertility."[6] Sydenstricker was one of very few who foresaw the significance of the population problem.

The program of the research division until 1936 was developed almost entirely on the ideas, plans and methods elaborated by Sydenstricker. Although he followed closely the conduct of the studies and analysis of data, he was co-author of only a few of the many articles published by members of the staff and collaborators.[7] His reputation among public health workers had steadily increased, and after 1930 he was called on to give more and more time to special activities outside the Fund's program of research.

During 1930 and 1931, he wrote "Health and Environment"[8] for the President's Research Committee on Social Trends.[9] The major portion of the data for this volume was provided by the studies of morbidity, mortality and physical impairments which had emanated from the Office of Statistical Investigations. It was "a frank attempt to review very briefly, in a dispassionate manner, the more important evidence bearing upon environment and health, without, however, losing sight of the established laws of heredity."[10] In this book, he gave scholarly interpretation of available facts indicating associations between environmental conditions and health. The evidence that unfavorable environment affected mortality rates and sickness pointed to the need for more information on causative factors on ill health, but also gave support for the improvement of social and environmental conditions for the betterment of the people's health.

He had actively participated in the work of the Committee on Costs of Medical Care from 1928 to 1931. He put much effort into collecting and analyzing data for this Committee and expressed his great disappointment with the Committee's report, which he would not sign because he said it failed to answer the questions for which the Committee had been created. His interest in the problem of how medical care would be financed and made available to all the people continued and became greater as the economic depression deepened.

When public health officials became concerned about the efforts of the economic depression on the health of the people in the years following 1930, the Surgeon General of the U.S. Public Health Service requested Sydenstricker and the Milbank Memorial Fund to investigate. Sydenstricker took direct action and in 1933 arranged for surveys to be made of sample populations that were known to be seriously affected by unemployment. Home visits were made to families in eight cities, in several cotton mill villages in the south and to several mining villages in West Virginia. For about 12,000 wage earners' families, a record was obtained of their economic history and mortality in 1929–1932 and of any illness that occurred in a three-month period just prior to the visit. Records of family diets for a one-week period were obtained from about 1,000 families and about 1,000 school children in two cities were given special examinations. The findings from this investigation gave evidence that rates of disabling illness were relatively high among the unemployed, that public health facilities were being cut back and increased numbers of persons were unable to pay for medical care.

In 1934, President Roosevelt asked his Cabinet Committee on Economic Security to study, among other subjects, the risks to economic security which arise out of ill health. Sydenstricker was appointed to head a technical staff which was asked, at first, to study only health insurance. The staff, however, suggested that such a study would be incomplete and the Committee's studies were expanded to deal, first, with measures to prevent illness, and, second, with measures to deal with economic consequences which follow in the wake of illness.[11]

In December 1934, the Committee was given a report prepared by Sydenstricker and I. S. Falk, whose commentary to Section 3 of this volume presents a more extended review of these actions. Assisting in the preparation of this report were consultants representing the public health profession, the dental profession and the Bureau of Medical Economics of the American Medical Association. At Sydenstricker's request, typical of his statesmanship and judgment, the Committee had appointed a Medical Advisory Board, and Advisory Committees to represent the public health, medical, dental, hospital and nursing professions which met with and counseled the technical staff.[12] This report was the principal basis for a report by the Committee for Economic Security to the President and for the specific recommendations included in the Economic Security Bill referred to the Congress in the spring of 1935.

Years of research and critical evaluation of the factual knowledge on illness in families, of time lost from work because of disability, and of costs to families of medical care and loss of wages made Sydenstricker the most informed and best prepared person in the nation to advise on a national program to reduce the impact of illness on economic security. He could interpret for the Committee the interrelationships between public health and economic and social conditions. In fact, working with the Cabinet Committee gave him the opportunity to bring to practical results a lifetime of studies concerned with the concept that the health of the people was fundamental to its economic welfare and was, therefore, a social responsibility.

As finally passed, the Economic Security Bill called for the Federal Government to increase substantially its appropriations to the Public Health Service and the Children's Bureau for aid to state and local governments in their public health programs. The Children's Bureau was given funds also to provide medical care and other services to crippled children. After his death, Katherine Lenroot, Chief of the Children's Bureau, said of the Social Security Program, "if it becomes a really effective measure for promoting the economic and social and health welfare of our people, [it] will be in part a memorial to Mr. Sydenstricker's scientific attainments and to his statesmanship."[13] Health insurance was not included in the Social Security Act, which provided increased funding for the expansion of the usual activities of official agencies to promote community health and provide preventive medical services. The technical staff continued to work on a report with recommendations for some type of insurance to budget against medical costs. Sydenstricker's studies during the previous 20 years of the experience of European countries with various forms of health insurance provided the background data on which a program was developed and submitted to the several advisory committees for discussion. The Medical Advisory Board recommended that any action on an insurance program should await the accumulation of experience with programs for limited groups and with various methods of making care available. Although no Federal program of health insurance was adopted, this was the beginning of an aroused public interest in the subject, and also, a greater awareness on the part of the medical profession of their responsibility to make medical care available to all groups in the population.

On March 19, 1936, at age 54 years, Sydenstricker died suddenly as the result of a cerebral hemorrhage. At this time, his influence clearly had extended beyond the field of research in which his reputation was firmly established, into the area of health policy and application of medical knowledge for betterment of the health of individuals. His knowledge of health problems, coupled with a sincere concern for the less fortunate, and a modest, friendly personality made him an effective spokesman for public health. If there had been no depression and no service with

the Committee on Economic Security, his research contribution
would have given him an outstanding place in the history of
public health. Through his work with the Committee, he is remembered for his role in establishing the concept of health care as
a public, and especially as a Federal responsibility, to maintain
the public welfare.

Notes and References

1. Terris, M. (Editor), Goldberger on Pellagra. Baton Rouge: Louisiana State
   University Press. 1964, p. 15.
2. Sydenstricker, E. Health and Environment. New York: McGraw-Hill Book
   Company, Inc. 1933.
3. Sydenstricker, E. "Morbidity," in Encyclopaedia of the Social Sciences, Vol.
   11. New York: The Macmillan Co. 1933, pp. 3–4.
4. Sydenstricker, E. and Britten, R. H. "The Physical Impairments of Adult Life.
   General Results of a Statistical Study of Medical Examinations by the Life
   Extension Institute of 100,924 White Male Life Insurance Policy Holders
   Since 1921," The American Journal of Hygiene 11: 73–94. Jan. 1930.
5. Sydenstricker, E. "Methods of Measuring Results of Public Health Work with
   Especial Reference to the Prevention of Diphtheria." Unpublished mss., no
   date.
6. Kiser, C. V. "The Work of the Milbank Memorial Fund in Population since
   1928," The Milbank Memorial Fund Quarterly 49: 15–62. Oct. 1971, Part 2.
7. The findings on studies of health services provided much of the basic data for
   the books describing the health demonstration programs. The following vol-
   umes reported on the programs in Cattaraugus County, Syracuse and New
   York City:
   a. Winslow, C.-E. A., Health on the Farm and in the Village. New York: The
      Macmillan Co. 1931.
   b. Winslow, C.-E. A., A City Set on a Hill. Garden City: Doubleday, Doran
      and Co. 1934.
   c. Winslow, C.-E. A., and Zimand, S., Health Under the "el." New York:
      Harper and Brothers. 1937.
8. op cit.
9. The Committee was named by President Hoover in 1929 to survey social
   changes in order to throw light on emerging problems.
10. op cit. p. 3
11. Roche, J., "Economic Security and Health," in Policies and Procedures in
    Public Health. New York: Milbank Memorial Fund. 1935.
12. Ibid.

13. The Next Steps in Public Health. New York: Milbank Memorial Fund. 1936,
    p. 45.

Dorothy G. Wiehl
Formerly, Senior Member,
Technical Staff
Milbank Memorial Fund

2
PUBLIC HEALTH
AND EVALUATION

COMMENTARY

BERNARD G. GREENBERG

In assessing the scientific writings of a pioneer such as Edgar Sydenstricker, a reviewer is faced with several alternatives. One extreme is to adopt the stance of hero-worshipper and ascribe the genesis of all modern knowledge and practices in a specialty field to the creativity and genius of the person himself. An antipodal posture for the reviewer is to be highly critical and disparaging by portraying the earlier figure as naive in not recognizing the trend of developments occurring around him or in not anticipating the progress that would subsequently take place.

Examination of the four papers published in this section has caused me to take a somewhat medial position between the two extremes, but with a strong leaning in the direction of the first approach. Sydenstricker leaves no alternative, because rereading the first article has made me realize how much of my own thinking and philosophy were shaped by his writings fifty years ago and the impact which these ideas must have had upon his colleagues.

Turning to the first paper, "The Measurement of Results of Public Health Work, An Introductory Discussion," I must confess regret in not having known about its existence when my initial crude attempts in evaluation research started in the early 1950s.[1,2] Although I was unaware of the paper, its influence must have been through intermediaries because the probability is zero that I would have rediscovered independently all of his definitions, advisory rules, procedures and basic tenets. In fact, earlier direct knowledge of this paper would have saved me a lot of unnecessarily long and complex thought about the problems of evaluation.

Although the popular term we use today is *evaluation*, that word itself does not appear in the title or any section headings in this article and, in fact, does not occur until the mid-point of the paper (p. 51). Nevertheless, his thinking on the subject is still current. He wrote in the very first paragraph about "ascertaining the effectiveness of certain measures for the prevention and control of disease and for the promotion of individual and community health." Substitute "evaluating" for "ascertaining" and we have in this classic paper a definition superior to any currently in existence.

Sydenstricker anticipated the confusion to be created later in the concept of evaluation when it would be used as a measurement of effort or as a synonym for the use of yardsticks. He pointed out that "measurement of public health work by yardsticks" (p. 41) developed by expert opinion is a possible interpretation of evaluation but not as good as what he had in mind. This reviewer is ambivalent on this point because a comparison with established yardsticks or accepted standards is certainly desirable and not necessarily "pseudo-evaluation." I have sometimes referred to that procedure as "quasi-evaluation."[3] A new term for this same idea which is gaining currency is *value system analysis*.[4]

Sydenstricker also pointed out that the body of service statistics or the amount of work done is helpful but inadequate. Again, I take a more compromising stand and say that "services performed" may not give *true evaluation* but such statistics are worthwhile evaluative tools when the service properly applied is known to be effective. For instance, I see no problem in counting the insertion of intra-uterine devices among new contraceptors as a quasi-evaluative tool to measure effectiveness of a family planning program without having to wait three or five years to observe the eventual decline in the birth and fertility rates; or, in studying the number of persons inoculated with an established vaccine without having to wait for conclusive proof that an epidemic was averted.

On one point regarding definitions Sydenstricker and I absolutely agree. Evaluation is neither another word for, nor synonymous with, community diagnosis and a study of needs.

The objects of Sydenstricker's attention in this paper were two health demonstrations under way in New York State at the time. He used "demonstration" almost equivalently with the idea of an experimental program whose results of effectiveness were yet to be proved. But Sydenstricker was a scientist as well as public health missionary. He pointed out that a demonstration program must also have methodological implications, namely that a primary purpose is also "to contribute ... to developing methods of measurement which are practicable and sound and which might be useful elsewhere" (p. 39).

Currently, I think we would add to the goals of *demonstration* the purpose of showing to others the details of how to operate a program successfully (that is, a training mission) as well as an accounting function of measuring benefits vis-à-vis costs. He was not ignorant of the cost factors, however; early in the paper he distinguished between efficacy of the programs (i.e., accomplishment of objectives) and efficiency of the methods (i.e., benefits in relation to costs).

His criterion of success is an interesting point worth stressing. He placed all of his emphasis on the final test of success — accomplishment of long-range goals by preventing sickness and death. In his era, when acute infectious disease constituted the crucial health problems, and infant and maternal mortality rates were what we now consider phenomenally high, his reliance on the ultimate goal was understandable. He did not foresee the day of chronic diseases when the accomplishment of an intermediate or immediate goal might be the more reasonable, or the only feasible, criterion of success. For instance, today we might be content with measuring an increase in knowledge, a change in attitude, or an alteration in patterns of behavior. Thus, in a program to prevent coronary artery disease, we should not frown upon use of data such as the number of persons giving up smoking or modifying their dietary habits. There is no question, however, that Sydenstricker was correct in insisting upon fulfillment of eventual goals. He believed fully in establishing such goals, and in subsequent measurement of their accomplishment as a sine qua non in studying a program's worthwhileness.

Sydenstricker anticipated the whole field of operations research by pointing out that measurement of the efficacy of different administrative methods was absolutely essential in public health at the local level. He did not foresee, however, the possibility of actual experiments in the community such as the controlled clinical or field trial. For instance, the 1954 test of the Salk poliomyelitis vaccine[5] would be something he might not have imagined possible. He suggested instead, and wisely so, at least the use of statistical controls to adjust for factors not otherwise manipulable.

He felt that there were almost insurmountable problems in incorporating scientific principles of experimentation in order to evaluate a demonstration project. Thus, he pointed out that heredity could never be matched equally (other than perhaps in homozygous twins) in community health programs. He was aware of the fact that ethnic differences needed to be allowed for in any interpretation of results. Similarly, he stressed the influence of socioeconomic differences as an obstacle to valid measurements and unbiased comparisons. All of these raise the question as to whether there are ever two equivalent communities for a true experiment.

In this respect, he excelled in warning program administrators in public health not to take credit for all health improvements observed over time. He wrote that the influence of other activities in the community, advances in medical educational practice, and the whole spectrum of other symbiotic forces should constitute a basis for warning to, say, tuberculosis workers to be on guard for this pitfall in observing a reduction in the incidence or mortality of the disease.

As indicated earlier, he felt that a true experiment such as a controlled clinical trial in the community would be impossible to conduct or to analyze unequivocally. We have learned that this is not always so. Moreover, we have developed improvements in statistical procedures, such as "balancing" in the allocation of subjects to treatments, regression techniques and covariance analysis for adjustment of measurable differences that overcome the limitation that was of concern to him.[6,7] Our armamentarium of statistical tools useful in the analysis of contingency tables[8,9] has also minimized many of the difficulties envisioned by Sydenstricker.

Controls are also sometimes omitted today in the study of cure or management of disease whose epidemiology is well known. As an obvious illustration, one would be on more than fairly safe ground to omit the use of placebo controls in the case of rabies, a disease whose case-fatality ratio is invariably unity.

Speaking of case-fatality rates (or ratios), Sydenstricker wisely warned against their use from year to year to measure progress in treatment because the "changes in virulence of the pathogenic organisms may result in change in its morbific or lethal effect upon the human host" (p. 45). He did not mention but undoubtedly recognized that case-fatality rates were also improper tools to measure progress in the treatment of chronic diseases, such as tuberculosis.

The foregoing paragraphs might create the impression that Sydenstricker was a statistical or epidemiological purist and not very practical. Such an impression would indeed be misleading because he tempered the previous advice by a sage example where longitudinal comparisons over time can, and did, serve an evaluative function without the use of rigid controls. He called it "definite efforts that are being carried on under our eyes" (p. 45). The illustration cited, however, was not a single preventative intervention but a whole program carried out by a part-time public health physician over a period of thirteen or more years.

One might still fault Sydenstricker and his exemplar physician for not having investigated whether the same changes had occurred in neighboring communities without a comparable public health program. Also, whether the part-time physician might have been seeing a different class of patients later on in his private practice when commenting upon the apparent disappearance of malaria, typhoid fever, and infantile cholera. In other words, any evaluator, including Sydenstricker and this reviewer, should never leave any possible openings for criticism even if the observed changes are dramatic and occurring under our very eyes.

To this reviewer, the most valuable part of this article occurs in Part III where underlying principles for evaluative methodology are enumerated and discussed. These include the following:

1) Define the specific programs to be evaluated rather than attempt an assessment of all programs simultaneously being carried out in the health department.

2) Select the parameters to be measured for the criteria of success and be specific in the program's objectives on a time basis (immediate versus long-term goals.) Also, define indices of results as narrowly as possible. For instance, if a program is supposed to reduce infant deaths from respiratory diseases, all infant mortality would be too broad and insensitive as the response variable of interest.

3) Attempt to conduct the demonstration program by incorporating into the design as many principles of experimentation as possible. (Sydenstricker did not enumerate in this article which principles of experimentation he had in mind other than the use of controls). Evaluation is necessary, he pointed out, whenever the program has new procedures, new given conditions (locale, personnel, or environment), or there is need to quantify how much can be accomplished under a given set of conditions.

4) Use control groups or areas whenever possible. If not, past events must be analyzed by using appropriate statistical methods of adjustment. He clarified the use of controls by indicating that they can be simultaneous in the observed area (by use of sub-areas or sub-populations), or contemporary in other areas. If self-controls are relied upon, as in "before-after" experiments, care must be exercised to ascertain that the condition would have been expected to continue at the same rate. If sub-areas within a health jurisdiction are utilized for comparative purposes, the health program under scrutiny is deliberately withheld until observed data are available to make the comparisons. If differing sub-populations are utilized, the groups must be essentially comparable or adjustments possi-

ble by statistical methods. Sydenstricker commented that
sub-areas are more difficult to implement in evaluative studies
because measurement of the results on a small area basis is not
ordinarily available to a health administrator unless costly,
special arrangements are made for monitoring changes.

5) Observe results at periodic intervals to time their appearance
and to adjust for changing conditions of associated relevant
factors in the community, especially population changes.

The final section of this manuscript is entitled simply "Some
Applications," and it contains an elaborate listing of practical
considerations in dealing with selected illustrations. The author
takes the reader step-wise through a web of logical reasoning to
show how to make some of the early decisions about goals and the
parameters to measure. In his first example for the control of
measles, he points out that the age distribution of the incidence of
cases during the control period can be compared to prior eras by
making adjustment for reporting errors, seasonal influence, virulence and population changes. Mortality rates as well as case-
fatality rates can be used in the analysis of changes in age-specific
groups.

In the second example, involving anti-tuberculosis work, he
warned against the use of mortality as an index. Deaths may be
high because of increased incidence, prevalence, or lethality.
Furthermore, in 1925 the tuberculosis death rate had declined to a
relatively small figure and sampling fluctuations might constitute
a real hazard to interpretation. Inasmuch as an individual's death
may have resulted from a disease process started many years
earlier, Sydenstricker recommended that more stress be placed
upon prevention of new cases. Here again, however, he warned
against using only one criterion, such as incidence, when the
anti-tuberculosis worker really has multiple objectives in mind
for his activities.

The penultimate example involves the health of pre-school
children. This was (and still is) difficult to study because various
health programs for them are not well defined, they are carried out
by many different agencies, and it is extremely difficult to keep
the children under continuous observation. Since mortality de-

clines rapidly after the second and third years of age, he recommended that mortality was not a sensitive parameter. Instead, he thought that one might use the end of the pre-school period for stock-taking when the child receives a physical examination upon entering school. A comparison of the physical and mental condition of each cohort of children entering school is possible provided care is taken to ascertain "why any children reaching school age do not enter school" (p. 61). Also, care must be taken to use the same diagnostic standards from year to year. Unfortunately, this latter is more easily said than done.

Finally, the author examined the problems in studying the value of school hygiene activities. This group offers wonderful opportunities for evaluation studies because the children are under constant surveillance, frequent records are made and remain readily accessible, efforts are made to prevent deleterious conditions, and the services provided are known and measurable. As a suggested index of health for school children, the author wisely discarded gross mortality because its rate is miniscule. The weight of the child (adjusted for age, sex, height, and sometimes race and build) is similarly discounted by the author because it can not be considered a delicate general index of individual health. He did mention, however, that weight sometimes can be very useful for group comparisons.

He omitted the use of attained stature as an index which, when adjusted for the other variables, can be an excellent measure of health.[10] This is surprising in light of his publications with Clark and Collins, in 1922 and 1924, on height and weight as indices of nutrition among school children. Instead, he recommended the sickness or absence record, and some index termed "nutrition" based upon a well-defined scale. He also predicted that eventually we will construct a general index of health status combining weight (height is probably better), nutrition, sickness, and the absence or presence of certain conditions. In this respect, he anticipated the development of multivariate statistical techniques and discriminant functions.

In observing the absence or presence of certain conditions, such as diseased tonsils, poor posture, or defective hearing, he cautioned against observer error. In some respects, this situation may still be true today but the development of audiometry has tended to minimize this problem in the case of hearing.

In the concluding paragraph the author stated that "measurement of results of public health work is not something that can be done by one who is wholly detached from the work" (p. 64). This is probably a correct statement, but it is also true that evaluation is not something that can be done by one who is too closely involved with the responsibility of providing the service. A compromise needs to be reached. Methods for doing this are discussed in an article by the reviewer.[3]

Sydenstricker claimed this article was only a brief outline and rough condensation of a longer treatment which he was preparing for subsequent publication. Unfortunately, the latter appears never to have been accomplished before his untimely death.

The second paper of this section on "The Statistician's Place in Public Health Work" is a short, somewhat pedestrian piece with a few general truisms and assorted observations on the public health statistician, his or her role, qualifications, and training. Sydenstricker began this article with his credo that the public health statistician is a scientist with "trained brains" who understands his data and their limitations, and who has sufficiently trained himself so as to be equipped with mathematical techniques.

Interestingly enough, the first general qualification the author demanded in the public health statistician was that he have a social viewpoint. Owing to the fact that public health had a social objective, Sydenstricker felt that the public health statistician must appreciate that his employer was the public, and that he should have a responsibility and perspective that is social in origin. This reviewer happens to be partially sympathetic with Sydenstricker's philosophy, but it certainly cannot be easily validated or substantiated.

Must every obstetrician be a female, every penologist have a prior criminal record? Certainly not. Must he or she be sympathetic to the subject for effective performance? Perhaps, but assessment is dubious. In fact, if the first condition applies, namely, the public health statistician is a scientist with "trained brains," then it is unnecessary for the holder of the title of public health statistician to be socially sympathetic. A person with "trained brains" will be impartial.

The second general qualification is that the public health statistician should experience formal scholastic education in public health at a university. Sydenstricker, who was trained as a political economist, perhaps was lamenting a void in his own background, cautioning others not to repeat the same omission, or excusing himself because of wide experience and some kind of grandfather provision.

Sydenstricker proceeded to distinguish between two fields of application for the public health statistician, viz., administration and research. In the former category, he enumerated the following five functions.

1) Vital registration and record keeping.
2) Enumeration, tabulation and presentation of data.
3) Interpretation of vital statistics for current administrative purposes.
4) Economic studies involving the money cost of services provided.
5) Evaluative studies including input-output studies.

He rightly indicated that the last function (i.e., evaluation) at that period of time had overlap with the role of the research statistician. As new methods of measurement became practical, he believed that evaluation would become the province more of the administrative type rather than of the research methodologist. In the opinion of this reviewer, the administrative type will play a larger role in evaluation but there will always be new challenges for the research type. I am surprised that Sydenstricker did not see more of a role for the research statistician in the third function: interpretation of vital statistics.

In Sydenstricker's judgment, the statistician was always a principal investigator and never a statistical consultant. It is in this connection that the reviewer feels that Sydenstricker failed badly to foresee the growth of public health statistics as a specialty in itself. On page 70, he viewed the statistician as an epidemiologist, nutrition worker, industrial hygienist, etc., "who has the statistical technique necessary for handling his facts in the mass." In this connection, he reverts almost like a palindrome to the opening remark (that a statistician is a scientist) by saying *"the scientist must be a statistician"* (italics in the original). What he meant, of course, was that the public health scientist should be his own statistician by understanding experimentation and the rules of scientific procedure. So does a statistician understand these rules, and in that sense a scientist is a statistician. This reviewer would hope that a statistician was more than that, however, and should have mathematical expertise to be a specialist in probability.

On one score, this reviewer and Sydenstricker concur completely, namely, that the public health statistician must understand his subject thoroughly and why he is undertaking the analysis at hand. In setting up standards for training statisticians, Sydenstricker prefers to use the elusive and hard-to-define quality of creating the ability to *think scientifically*.

In judging the role of the public health statistician in the health department, Sydenstricker was not as clairvoyant as in other areas. The duties of the statistician, currently and for the past twenty-five years, have fallen into three main categories: registration activities; tabulation and data processing with electronic machines and computers; and statistical consulting services for a wide variety of applications. The reader is encouraged to read Swinney[11,12], Whiteman[13], Puffer[14], Mattison[15], Reed[16], Tayback[17], Velz[18], and others. More recent developments in medical care areas have been described by Deardoff[19], Taback and Williams[20], and others. The latest development is in the direction of the public health statistician who organizes a state center of health statistics, or a state health information system, based upon the model of the National Center for Health Statistics.[21,22]

If Sydenstricker failed to foresee the growth of public health statistics in terms of its volume, or the breadth and scope of its activities, or even its training requirements, he more than made up for this failing in his view of public health itself. In "The Changing Concept of Public Health," all one need do is to change a few disease names here and there, and the result is an article more timely for the present than 1935. In brief, Sydenstricker foresaw the changing role of public health in chronic diseases, geriatrics, medical care, health insurance, and the inevitable role of the federal government. He anticipated Medicare and Medicaid as absolutely necessary for the special groups involved. In fact, he probably helped to establish the axiom that the health of the community is as much a responsibility of government as education or roads. His approach was that of the political economist who visualized economic insecurity arising out of ill health, and vice versa. His concept of public health on page 76 can be viewed as the genesis of the WHO definition of health adopted over a decade later.

"Society has a basic responsibility for assuring, to all of its members, healthful conditions of housing and living, a reasonable degree of economic security, proper facilities for curative and preventive medicine and adequate medical care—in fact the control, so far as means are known to science, of all of the environmental factors that affect physical and mental well-being."

It is possible that the thread of continuity between Sydenstricker's notions and the WHO definition can be traced through the era of Franklin D. Roosevelt. Sydenstricker indicated that political leaders from Disraeli to Roosevelt have enunciated the concept that the health of the public must be the first concern of the State at all times and not merely during catastrophic emergencies.

In viewing the community as a whole organism whose health was to be protected and enhanced, the author pointed out that Americans were not as healthy as they would be if current knowledge were applied appropriately. In the mid-1930s he was mentioning the need for the complete elimination of diphtheria, typhoid fever, and smallpox, a large reduction in tuberculosis and infant mortality, an even larger decline in maternal deaths, and the avoidance of many crippling conditions that were preventable. Today in the mid-1970s, we are still faced with Americans who are not as healthy as current knowledge makes possible; we are challenged with reducing infant and maternal mortality in special high-risk groups, preventing many lung cancers by discontinuing smoking, reducing cardiovascular episodes by refraining from smoking, improper diet, or failure to treat early signs of hypertension. We have not yet found the way to control drug abuse, to minimize incapacitation from mental illness, and to reduce the heavy toll of life caused by accidents.

To focus the reader's interest on problems of adult life and degenerative diseases, the author pointed out that life expectancy at age 40 was about the same in 1935 as it was in 1850 or 1900. In proposing a greater role for the federal government, he indicated that it need not be a kind of "state medicine" or "regimentation of physicians." He simply sought some sensible plan for coordination to reach a social and economic objective, and encouraged the use of experimentation to attain this goal. Specifically, Sydenstricker called attention to the following measures to attack the problem.

1) Greater economic measures (unemployment insurance, old age pensions, relief for the disabled) to break the cycle of association between poverty and ill health.
2) Greater financial appropriations for public health purposes.
3) Slum clearance and better housing for persons of low income.
4) Better nutrition through education and greater use of supplementary foods.
5) Development of programs of physical training, recreation, and hygiene education in public schools at all levels.
6) More information and education about family planning methods.
7) Social work efforts to coordinate social and welfare services with health services.
8) Readily available medical care not only for curative purposes but immunizations and physical examinations for preventive purposes.

He concluded with a plea for experimentation with some forms of health insurance based upon the experience of certain

European nations and Japan. In adopting any or all of these measures, he warned against expecting any one of them to be a panacea or sufficient in itself. Different problems require varying modes of attack, and they involve different groups, interests and individuals.

How appropriate these words of caution are today! National health insurance schemes are still under consideration by the Congress at the present time but the decisions are being left to politicians under the lobbying influence of the private practice of medicine. Nobody has been delegated to speak for the general public and the consumer of health services.

In the fourth article of this section, "Economy in Public Health," Sydenstricker reasserted his concern for public health measures from an economist's point of view. At the very outset, he differentiated false economy from the true meaning of economy which calls for expenditure of funds so as to gain the greatest advantage, that is, a kind of cost-benefit approach. False economy is the reduction of spending for no valid reason other than to cut down on appropriations.

The occasion for this paper was passage by Congress of the Social Security Act of 1935 followed by its failure to appropriate the authorized funds. The legislation authorized federal support for health services at local and state levels, and Sydenstricker was, in essence, trying to mount a drive to persuade the Congress to appropriate funds in 1936. He was also making a plea that the money should be spent wisely (economically) if and when funds were made available.

The national Committee on Economic Security had recommended a strong program to prevent ill health and economic insecurity. The Committee's report indicated that much preventable illness and premature death still occurred unnecessarily. Part of the explanation for this, and the justification for federal intervention, was that state and local fiscal support for public health had been niggardly and was actually shrinking during the depression. The report also maintained that there was ample precedent to establish federal responsibility for health of the public because of the many governmental health agencies already in existence at that time. Moreover, the concept of federal grants-

in-aid to promote public health facilities had also been established earlier. The justification for all of this support could be
made on economic grounds without need to fall back upon any
humanitarian motives.

Sydenstricker urged all persons interested in public health to
contact their governmental representatives at all levels to plead
against false economy. He predicted that federal appropriations
for health services would reach 50¢ to $1.00 per capita within a
decade. With this support to bolster state and local funds, he urged
health administrators who had responsibility to spend these funds
to do so wisely according to his definition of economy.

This point of view allowed him to restate his 1925–26 ideas on
evaluation. Interestingly enough, in 1936 he continued to refer to
the process as measuring the results of public health programs,
but he clearly uses the words "scientific evaluation" in a modern
usage. On page 88 he wrote "The necessity for scientific evaluation of each specific health procedure is greater now than ever
before." By stressing the need then (1936) more than previously,
he had in mind the standardization of procedures that had developed during the previous decade. He feared that the process of
standardization may not have been critical enough in establishing
the validity of most procedures in common use. For instance, he
challenged the notion that the public health nurse must make 8
visits to each and every case of whooping cough. He wondered
whether 4, 2, or 1 visit(s) would not have accomplished as much in
terms of spread of the disease or the complications to the case
itself.

In general, this manuscript pleaded for a tone of healthy skepticism about procedures commonly used in health agencies. In
line with this philosophy, he urged that the federal government
use evaluative procedures in connection with the allocation of
grants-in-aid to the states. He claimed that $2,000,000 of the au-
thorized $13,800,000 was intended to carry out such evaluative
research by the Division of Research of the National Institute of
Health in collaboration with universities and other institutions.

A final plea was made that Congress appropriate funds no
lower than the authorized amount. This must have been one of the
early papers concerned with what has turned out to be an annual

drama—appropriation of funds vis-à-vis the amounts authorized The relevancy of this problem is still of current applicability, except that the additional obstacle of executive impoundment of funds has now been added to the mix. There is also current relevance in the 1973 proposals for revenue sharing at local and state levels. As Sydenstricker pointed out, when financial hardships occur, one cannot depend upon local and state authorities to place a high enough priority on support of public health. His argument was that public health should be primary in national priorities and that such expenditures constituted a sound economic investment.

In summary, this last article and the preceding one on the changing concept of public health establish Sydenstricker as a political, public health economist. His training in political economy shines through with brilliance.

His understanding of the role of the public health statistician was not nearly as brilliant. Although he was the first statistician appointed in the U.S. Public Health Service, his contributions were in the concept of evaluation and in the application of statistical methods for administrative purposes. He was a superb user of statistics, and thus an important innovator of practice even though not a great contributor to new statistical methodology.

References

1. Greenberg, B. G., Harris, M. E., MacKinnon, C., and Chipman, S., "A Method for Evaluating the Effectiveness of Health Education Literature." American Journal of Public Health 43:1147–55. September, 1953.
2. Greenberg, B. G., and Mattison, B. F., "The Whys and Wherefores of Program Evaluation." Canadian Journal of Public Health 46: 293–99. July, 1955.
3. Greenberg, B. G., "Evaluation of Social Programs," Review of the International Statistical Institute 36 (1968): 260–78. Reprinted in Francis G. Caro, Readings in Evaluation Research, New York, Russell Sage Foundation, 1971, 155–75.
4. Zukin, P., Gurfield, R. M., and Klein, W., "Evaluating a Primary Care Clinic in a Local Health Department," Health Services Reports 88: 65–76. January, 1973.
5. Francis, T. Jr., et al., "An Evaluation of the 1954 Poliomyelitis Vaccine Trials,

Summary Report," American Journal of Public Health 45: Part II: 1–51 and Appendix. May, 1955.

6. Cochran, W. G., "Matching in Analytical Studies," American Journal of Public Health 43: 684–91. June, 1953.

7. Greenberg, B. G., "The Use of Analysis of Covariance and Balancing in Analytical Surveys," American Journal of Public Health 43: 692–99. June, 1953.

8. Grizzle, J. E., Starmer, C. F., Koch, G. G., "Analysis of Categorical Data by Linear Models," Biometrics 25: 489–504. September, 1969.

9. Goodman, L. A., "The Analysis of Multidimensional Contingency Tables: Stepwise Procedures and Direct Estimation Methods for Building Models for Multiple Classifications," Technometrics 13: 33–61. February, 1971.

10. Greenberg, B. G., and Bryan, A. H., "Methodology in the Study of Physical Measurements of School Children, Part I," Human Biology 23: 1–20. May, 1951.

11. Swinney, D. D., "Current Organizational Patterns of Statistical Activities in State Health Departments," Public Health Reports 64: 621–41. May 20, 1949.

12. Swinney, D. D., "Distribution and Salaries of Directors of Vital Statistics and Statisticians in State Health Departments as of August 1948," Public Health Reports 64: 1133–47. September 9, 1949.

13. Whiteman, E. B., "Uses of Statistical Data in State Health Departments," American Journal of Public Health 37: 1267–72. October, 1947.

14. Puffer, R. R., "Application of Statistical Analysis in a Health Program," Public Health Reports 67: 729–36. August, 1952.

15. Mattison, B. F., "The Administrative Value of Statistics to a Local Health Officer," Public Health Reports 67: 747–54. August, 1952.

16. Reed, L. J., "The Role of Vital Statistician in the Community as Evolved by W. Thurber Fales," American Journal of Public Health 45: 11–20. January, 1955.

17. Tayback, M., "The Biostatistician and Health Administration," American Journal of Public Health 54: 603–8. April, 1964.

18. Velz, C. J., "Vistas in Public Health Statistics," Public Health Reports 67: 725–8. August, 1952.

19. Deardorff, N. R., "The 1948 Experiences of the Health Insurance Plan of Greater New York with the Utilization of Physician Services by the Enrollers in Each Age-Sex Group," American Journal of Public Health 40: 1536–45. December, 1950.

20. Taback, M., and Williams, H., "Statistics in a Health Department Medical Care Plan," Public Health Reports 68: 157–66. February, 1953.

21. Ervin, T. R., "The Art of Relevance in the Development of Health Information Systems," Proceedings of the Public Health Conference on Records and Statistics, 12th National Meeting, June 1968, Department of Health, Education and Welfare, Washington, D.C.

22. Ervin, T. R., "Funding Opportunities for State Centers for Health Statistics," Proceedings of the Public Health Conference on Records and Statistics, 13th

National Meeting, June 1970, Department of Health, Education and Welfare, Washington, D.C.

Bernard G. Greenberg, Ph.D.
Kenan Professor of Biostatistics and Dean
School of Public Health
The University of North Carolina at Chapel Hill

1

The Measurement of Results
of Public Health Work
An Introductory Discussion
EDGAR SYDENSTRICKER

With the development of two of the New York Health Demonstrations† to a stage where the more important activities are well under way, it is now pertinent to consider, in a preliminary manner at least, means for "ascertaining the effectiveness of certain measures for the prevention and control of disease and for the promotion of individual and community health"* that have been put into operation in these two American communities.

The measurement of results has been regarded from the outset as an essential step in the program of the demonstrations. It is not merely to satisfy a natural curiosity as to what may have been accomplished that an attempt will be made to evaluate the work of the demonstrations. The primary purposes are, rather, to make available, in as definite terms as possible and from a reasonably dispassionate point of view, the experience which will have been gained; and to contribute in some degree to developing methods of measurement which are practicable and sound and which might be useful elsewhere. The proposal is not a novel one, of course; nor will the principles and methods that may be employed be essentially new. On the contrary, it is in line with the increasingly critical attitude on the part of sanitarians in appraising the effectiveness of their work. For as public health develops into a

†[In Cattaraugus County and Syracuse. ED.]
*Annual Report 1925, p. 17.

39

science itself, it is being realized that the modes of science must be employed. As the objectives of a social program, such as the improvement of public health, become more clearly defined, and as the methods of carrying out a program are improved, the more rigid must the standards and the more accurate must be the means by which we must measure the efficacy of the program and the efficiency of the methods. No longer can the mere "putting over" of a project be regarded as the final test of success; for while undoubtedly it is an essential step in the accomplishment of a specific project, the final criterion is the ultimate result—the prevention of a given disease, the lessening of sickness and death from specific and related causes, and the promotion of health to a discernible degree.

The fact must be faced that the measurement of the results of public health efforts is no easy task. The confusion which has characterized some recent discussions of what public health work has accomplished has served a useful purpose in revealing in some degree the intricacy of any inquiry as to the general benefits of such work or as to the specific results of a specific effort. Methods of measuring public work, or any activity directed toward a social effect, will undergo gradual development just as the technique of every science has been developed. They cannot be formulated by any one person or set forth completely in any one exposition. But there are some things which can and ought to be done at the outset. We can define clearly just what we conceive the objects of "measurement of results" to be. We can take stock of the various factors that are involved and of the difficulties that are inherent in the undertaking. The application to the particular problems in hand of underlying principles common to all scientific inquiry ought to be considered. The most practicable approach to the task can be sought. Attempts already made to measure results can be scrutinized and tentative suggestions for further attempts may be made.

It is thought advisable at this time to consider the question from these general points of view, and in the following pages a very brief summary is given of a preliminary survey of the problem. In doing this, the primary purposes in mind are not only to set forth what seem to be some fundamental considerations of the subject, in the full realization that later experience probably will modify any statement that can be made now, but also to submit them for suggestions and criticism.

I. What is Meant by Measurement?

Since there is some danger of confusion when one speaks of the "measurement" of public health efforts, it is worth the time and the space to consider first some of the uses to which the word has been put, in order that the particular interpretation with which we are concerned may be differentiated from other interpretations and the term may be clearly defined for our own purposes.

1) The measurement of public health work by *yardsticks* is a current phrase. By it we mean that a public health activity or an administration is judged by some standard that has become conventional or that has been set up deliberately. The "appraisal forms" which are being developed under the auspices of the American Public Health Association are the most conspicuous example of this mode of measurement. In a real and important sense the "yardstick" method is a way of measuring public health work, since the yardstick itself is assumed to represent the best opinion of the time.

2) Again, we may apply a measure to public health activities in terms of the *amount of work done.* So many children are weighed and re-weighed, so many home visits are made by nurses, so many clinics are held. Undoubtedly these also are modes of measuring public health work; and they are by no means to be belittled, because they are predicated upon a logically sound reasoning. Thus, we measure the effectiveness of a campaign against caries by the number of individuals known to have this defect who have received the necessary treatment, because we know that the treatment itself is effective when applied.

3) In the third place, we seek to measure the effectiveness of a particular *method of applying* such knowledge as we have of how

to relieve, cure, or prevent a disease or condition. Thus we may test the efficacy of different administrative methods of bringing about treatment of caries in a group of school children. We may find that there are, or we may deliberately select, several groups of children of comparable age, race, social and economic status, whose teeth can be examined according to a standard method at approximately the same time, the groups being differentiated as to the administrative methods to be used in bringing about corrections. The success of these different methods of bringing about corrections can be ascertained for each of these groups, and the effectiveness of the various administrative methods can thus be compared and measured. This approaches the experimental method of measurement. It is purely inductive. When it is impracticable to stage an actual experiment a statistical analysis of records may be made, eliminating the major irrelevant factors, provided suitable data are available or can be obtained.

4) Finally, we may seek, and we do seek constantly, to measure the effectiveness of our activities *by changes or contrasts in the state or condition of public health itself.* Here we set up but one standard, and that is the health of the population, or of a specific population group, denoted adequately by some expression, preferably in numerical form. In other words, the state of health, or of freedom from a given disease or defective condition, is the ultimate measure of our success in trying to prevent disease and to promote health. We ask ourselves whether or not public health activities during a given time in a given population have had the net result of a greater reduction in the death rate than might have been brought about by other factors. We apply the crucial test of the expectation of lengthened lives. Thus we have contrasted the morbidity and the mortality from small-pox in populations where vaccination is compulsory with those in populations where it is voluntary, and the facts speak for themselves. We have observed the fall of the typhoid rate in places where efficient sewage and water systems have been put into operation, and compared it with the rate in places where these modern necessities have come tardily, or in the same localities before they were in general use. We have seen the effects of measures against the hookworm and malaria, of the war against yellow fever and the

bubonic plague, reflected in a decline in their prevalence which is proportionate to the effort expended. Such are the terms of measurement of efforts with which a public health administration is concerned primarily. It is the last two modes of measurement that we propose to discuss in the following pages.

II. The Nature of the Task

When we come to consider the obstacles in the way of applying scientifically correct methods of measurement, the basic difficulty that presents itself is the fact that even the most ordinary of human beings is one of many extremely intricate and delicate, similar yet different, organisms; living in an environment complicated beyond comprehension; and possessing an inheritance unknowable.

In the bundle of conditions that must be taken into account heredity must be recognized as one of the factors to be considered. Of the phases of heredity that bear directly upon our problem we know very little. There are unmistakable indications of racial differences in susceptibility to certain diseases and to the effects of certain diseases. There is indubitable evidence that resistance to certain diseases "runs in" families. It is probable that resistance to some diseases has been bred into an appreciable portion of our population. Apparently, because of a natural adjustment of individuals to occupation and climate, some localities may have a larger proportion of certain kinds of susceptibles than others. When we compare groups of persons, differentiating inheritances should be determined as accurately as possible and taken into account; but in attempting to measure the results of a public health activity, the question may be legitimately raised whether or not the period for which records of health or disease are available is too short for any biologic changes of this kind to have exerted significant effects.

Furthermore, we are faced with economic and social changes that ought to be evaluated for their effect upon the population and upon the prevalence of a given disease before the results of public health activities can be measured accurately. Evolution in mechanical processes, transformations in commerce that affect not only the volume and the profits of industry but also its seasonal activity, improvements in banking and credit facilities which modify cyclical variations in the demand for labor, the steady increase in wages and stabilization of family income, limitation of the labor supply by restrictive immigration laws, shifting of industrial populations from locality to locality—these are some of the more important developments that cannot have failed to affect the well-being of the population. They should not be overlooked in any attempt to appraise the net result of public health efforts.

Closely allied to factors such as these are the general effects of the public health movement itself as distinguished from any specific result of a specific activity. There is a curious symbiosis of the influences which are put into force. The antituberculosis activities undoubtedly have influenced the public's attitude toward other diseases and developed its conception of health. Changes in ways of living undoubtedly have been brought about partly by education in personal hygiene, partly by improvements in architecture, developments in ideals of physical beauty, and other influences; and these changes are disseminated the more widely and rapidly by modern standardization in life. Add to these factors the tremendous advances in medical education, equipment, and practice, and we have a group of conditions whose combined force or whose influence on any one activity is extremely difficult to evaluate.

All these obstacles are enhanced by the impossibility of treating human beings as laboratory animals. We cannot segregate them easily into two homogeneous groups for any purpose and treat one group as an experimental population and the other as a control. The factors to which brief allusion has been made are so many and so interrelated that it is extremely difficult to employ the statistical methods of manifold classification or of partial correlation. While statistical methods are necessarily the tools best adapted to our purpose, they are badly dulled by indirect and unsuitable observations and records of disease and by indefinite indices of the factors which we wish to hold constant in our analysis.

Any particular disease in question invariably presents difficulties. There are only a few diseases whose natural history we may be confident we have mastered; yet no intelligent evaluation of the real success or failure of an effort to control a disease can be made without a knowledge of its behavior independent of any attempt to control it. We should know the character and magnitude of its trend, its periodic and seasonal variations. Even with this knowledge we are faced with changes in virulence of the pathogenic organism that may result in changes in its morbific or lethal effect upon the human host, and with the appearance of new strains that are unexpected, unaccounted for, and disconcerting. Each disease possesses epidemiological characteristics that must be taken into account before the influence of any new factor, deliberately introduced, can possibly be correctly observed. Ignorance of the simplest facts of epidemiology probably accounts for the common and ridiculous mistake of comparing the death rate in a non-epidemic year with that in the preceding epidemic year and crediting the "decrease" wholly to the work of a vigilant health administration.

Yet the task is not quite so formidable in all its phases as the foregoing considerations imply. It is possible to draw a distinction between the attempt to measure the net result of public health efforts over a considerable period of time, for which our information is usually vague and fragmentary, and the measurement of specific, definite efforts that are being carried on under our eyes, as it were, where we have the opportunity to observe and record events as they occur, and make our analyses of the data with a fairly intimate understanding of influencing conditions.

Let us use an illustration. In 1909 Dr. B. B. Bagby went to West Point, Virginia, to engage in the practice of medicine. At that time, so he recalls, the city fathers of West Point boasted of having the healthiest town in Virginia. It may have been then, although every home had an old-fashioned privy, the water supply was inadequate, the town scavenger was also the dairyman, not a dwelling was completely screened, and no attempt had been made to drain the marshes and get rid of the malarial mosquitoes which plagued the population.

In the years between 1909 and 1922, some marked changes

were brought about by Dr. Bagby, the State Board of Health, and an awakened public interest. By 1922, 80 per cent of the milk was being produced and sold under sanitary conditions. Even the poorest negro tenements had good window and door screens. The town and State had drained the marshes. A complete sewage system had been installed. An adequate water supply had been secured, and every house was compelled to connect with it.

Dr. Bagby is a physician who practices preventive as well as curative medicine, and among his other professional accomplishments he keeps a careful record of all his patients. At the fifty-third annual meeting of the Medical Society of Virginia he read a paper entitled "Changes in a Small Town Brought About by the Health Department"* which is a human document of scientific value. In it he said:

"During the five summer months of 1909 I saw 158 town patients. During the same period of 1922 I saw 202 town patients. Of the 158 patients seen in 1909, 96 had well-defined cases of malaria, with chills, fever, sweats, etc.: 15 had cholera infantum, ileocolitis, or dysentery, with two deaths, and 7 had typhoid fever, making a total of 108 cases out of 158 that should have been prevented.

"During the five summer months of 1922 I did not have in town a single typical case of malaria, typhoid fever, or cholera infantum. I had one—a typical case—of malaria that was most probably contracted out of town; I had only one case of ileocolitis that lasted over five days, and this was the only case of dysentery or infectious diarrhea in town this summer. There has not been a case of typhoid fever in West Point since February, 1919. Dr. A. S. Hudson, the other physician in West Point, says he has not had a case of malaria, cholera infantum or typhoid fever this summer. So malaria, typhoid, and infantile diarrhea have about disappeared in West Point.

"We work so hard and accomplish so little from day to day for the betterment of humanity," remarks Dr. Bagby in commenting on his experience, "that all of us at times get discouraged in our

*Virginia Medical Monthly, December, 1922, Vol. 49, No. 9. Reprinted in the U.S. Public Health Reports, March 9, 1923, 38:456.

work. But after looking over my records of 13 years I am made to feel that our work has not been in vain but rather a great blessing to humanity. And I am sure that ours has been the experience of many other physicians and towns in Virginia."

This simple account puts into words, more succinctly and vividly than otherwise may be possible, the purpose, the basic principles, and the fundamental method of measuring what we actually are accomplishing in public health. For the measurement of some results more detailed information is necessary and more refined statistical methods of statements and analysis are desirable; but the essential requirements are illustrated in Dr. Bagby's plain story of what the situation was in 1909, what specific measures were taken during the period 1909–1922, and what the situation was in 1922, and in his comparison of the two years with respect to the prevalence of the specific diseases concerned.

In accordance with this general conception—the measurement of the results of current health activities or, at the most, of public health work during its period of adequately recorded history—we may review in more detail some of the ways in which some of the underlying principles of scientific procedure may be applied to our problem.

III. Some Underlying Principles

1. Specific Activities, Rather than the Program as a Whole, Should Be Measured First

The great number of activities that constitute modern public health administration and the multitude of quasi-public and professional enterprises that form an important part of our effort to relieve, cure, and prevent disease, at once suggest that the promotion of public health is characterized by 1) a manifold and interrelated variety of *objectives*, and 2) a wide differentiation in the *methods* employed to attain these objectives. This is so obvious an observation that its reiteration here would be unnecessary were it not for the especial significance which it has for our particular problem.

Now it is possible and entirely proper to regard the modern health program as a single factor and to attempt to measure its influence upon the health of a population by the use of one or more general indices of health, such as the mortality rate or some life-table expression. But of greater practical importance is the application of a principle which underlies not only the procedure in public health work but also method of measurement. This principle in its application here, may be expressed in the following terms:

A general health demonstration or a public health administration should not be regarded primarily as a single undertaking or experiment, but rather as a group of experiments, each of which has a definite objective; and the results of each should be measured by the most sensitive index that it is possible to employ.

For the more *specifically* the objectives are outlined and followed, and the more *definite* the indices of results, the more satisfactory will be the results themselves, whether they are positive or negative. It will be discovered, too, that some objectives can be attained more quickly than others, and some will require even more years to show results than we can have time to observe.

Yet, although what will be said in the following pages will be upon this general principle, it should not be understood as implying that, *after* we have attempted to measure the results in a specific way, we should fail to state the net results in such general terms as we can. The point to be emphasized is that if we confine ourselves to an attempt to measure the results of a health demonstration as a whole in general terms only, we shall not be certain ourselves, and we cannot satisfy others, *how* it was done. Justice cannot be given to the work of a health administration unless the influence of conditions impossible to control, or subject to relatively light control, is recognized and taken into account and unless the results of specific objectives are measured as definitely as possible. Our contribution will be immeasurably greater— whether the gross result is positive or negative—if it is capable of being analyzed into its component elements.

2. The Objectives and Methods of a Public Health Effort
Should Be Clearly Defined

A second consideration of basic importance follows from what already has been said: namely, that the objectives of each activity, of each phase of public health work, must be defined in unmistakable terms before any satisfactory attempt can be made to measure it. In fact, it might well be said that if a clear definition of each objective were insisted upon before any public health activity were undertaken, we would be working along many lines with a degree of intelligence in perspective and direction that would be more nearly commensurate with our enthusiasm in effort. And, knowing exactly and specifically what we want to accomplish, our choice of method and devising of ways would be more precisely suited to the task. Certainly, if any definite measurement of results is to be attempted, it is absolutely necessary to have the objective definitely set forth; otherwise we shall not know whether the objective has been reached nor can we measure the extent to which it has been attained.

While the statement just made may seem to be a platitude, its implications are not always fully realized. They have a practical application that is of undoubted importance. Let us take a very simple example. The prevention of mortality among infants is one of the major aims of public health work, and, on the face of it, appears to be an objective that is definite enough. Yet when we consider the causes of infant deaths we find that they may be classified broadly as is shown in the accompanying table.

Distribution of deaths under one year of age in the United States birth registration area during 1923, according to cause

Cause	Per Cent
Epidemic and infectious diseases	9.29
Tuberculosis	1.97
Respiratory diseases	15.14
Diarrhea and enteritis	15.97
Congenital malformation and debility	13.27
Premature birth and injuries at birth	29.10
All other causes	15.26

**A comparison of infant death rates from
certain diseases and conditions in two American cities**

Diseases and Conditions	DEATH RATE PER 1,000 LIVE BIRTHS, 1922-1924		Ratio of rate for Fall River to rate for Seattle
	Seattle, Washington	Fall River, Massachusetts	
Total	**48.46**	**103.79**	**2.14**
Epidemic and infectious	3.74	8.27	2.21
Tuberculosis	.81	1.11	1.37
Respiratory	5.30	18.57	3.50
Diarrhea and enteritis	2.56	27.48	10.73
Congenital malformations and debility	7.92	9.94	1.25
Premature birth and injuries at birth	17.46	26.73	1.53
All other causes	10.80	11.69	1.08

Of the total deaths, 42 per cent were due to congenital defects and conditions at birth, for the prevention of which the necessary activities are entirely different from the activities against communicable diseases and tuberculosis, which caused 11 per cent of the deaths, or against respiratory diseases, which caused 15 per cent of the deaths, or against intestinal disorders and diseases, which caused 16 per cent of the deaths. The measurement of results of efforts to prevent infant mortality would be far more definite if expressed in the terms of their specific objectives. A comparison of the infant mortality of two cities is made in the table shown above.

Although all the specific rates given above are higher for Fall River than for Seattle, it is quite clear that the greatest differences in favor of Seattle are for the communicable, respiratory, and diarrheal diseases, which are the very diseases which have been the principal objectives of infant mortality work. Let us suppose that as the result of an intensive campaign along these lines in Fall River the Seattle rates would be reached within a certain period of years, and let us substitute the Seattle rates as having been attained at the end of that period in Fall River for these three groups of diseases. The gross infant mortality rate would have been brought down to 61, a reduction of 43 per cent, which, if the annual number of births were constant, would mean the prevention of 155 infant deaths a year. More nearly accurate and far more expressive of the results of our efforts, however, would be the following statement: a reduction of 76 per cent in the death rate from these three causes, or, better still, of 27 per cent for tuberculosis, 55 per cent for communicable diseases, 72 per cent for respiratory diseases, and 91 per cent for diarrheal diseases.

3. Principles of Experimentation Should Be Applied

A third consideration is that the essential principles underlying a demonstration are those of *scientific experimentation*. We cannot deviate from that basic requirement if we are to succeed in measuring the effectiveness of our efforts. It does not matter what degree of simplicity of terms we may choose to employ in describing our methods or in proclaiming our results. By all means let us use words of one syllable whenever we can. But, whether we call it the use of "common sense" or the application of the accumulated wisdom of generations of technicians, whether it be evaluating the effect of a single cause or determining the resultant influence of several factors among the complex inter-relations of many conditions, whether we state our conclusions for the laity or for the erudite, the fundamental postulate is the same for all demonstrations: the rules of experimentation must be rigidly followed.

The modern health demonstration is more than merely the repetition of an experiment for purposes of education; it is in an important sense a new experiment, since we are trying to measure the results of a modern health program. To put this fundamental conception a little more clearly, let us attempt to restate some of the purposes of experimentation:

1) To find out whether or not a *hypothesized* procedure can accomplish a result under given conditions; or,

2) To show that an *accepted* or *proven* procedure will accomplish a specified result under given conditions; or,

3) To *ascertain how much of a result* can be accomplished under given conditions by the application of procedures that have already been proven or are accepted as effective.

By "under given conditions" we may connote, on the one hand, those conditions comprised under the general terms of the situation to be dealt with, including the population and its environment; and, on the other hand, those conditions set by the limitations of operation, such as a maximum per capita cost.

Now it is obvious that in a demonstration such as a general

health demonstration, or even a demonstration of a program against a single condition or disease, more than one of these objectives may be involved, since nearly all demonstrations are quite complex in their character.

To illustrate:

It is already a proven fact that the use of toxin-antitoxin according to prescribed procedure will immunize practically all susceptible individuals against diphtheria. We are not concerned primarily with the mere repetition of this experiment but with two essentially *new* experiments: 1) the testing of the methods we adopt to bring about the immunization of certain age groups of a population; and 2) since we know that, for practical reasons, in all probability we cannot immunize all of this group, our problem is to find out *how much* reduction in the diphtheria rate will result from the immunization of varying proportions of the population groups concerned under varying conditions.

4. The Use of "Experimental" and "Control" Groups or Areas

In the fourth place, experimentation, whether it be the analysis of past events by statistical methods in order to discover their relationships or the influence of a given factor, or the deliberate manipulation of conditions, postulates *a comparison* of events that follow when the specific factor is present or introduced in varying degrees, with events that follow when that factor is not present. When such a comparison is made possible, we say we have a "controlled" experiment. It is often easy, in the maze of conditions encountered in practical work, for even the most clearheaded of us to overlook the dictum that an experiment or an experimental analysis cannot be conducted successfully without applying this control principle in some form.

It is easy to set up "controls" in some form or other. The difficult thing is so to plan our comparison that the "control" groups or areas shall be in all essential and *relevant* respects the same as the experimental group or area, save in the one respect

which constitutes the thing to be tested or measured. It is sometimes more difficult, when we cannot so set up our conditions
deliberately, to evaluate the effect of differences in actual conditions other than the factor that we wish to test or measure. Yet
obviously this comparability—whether it can be planned deliberately or attained by statistical methods—is the very essence not
only of a successful demonstration but also of any approach to
accurate measurement.

The practical difficulties will be considered in more detail in
later reports when we come to take up the specific items in the
health program, but the application of the principle of "control"
may be discussed briefly and in general terms.

Theoretically at least, it is possible to consider the two general
kinds of "control," which are based on well-known principles of
experimentation:

1) The use of control areas or population groups for comparison with the area or population group in which a health program or
activity is carried on, in the observation and evaluation of results;

2) The observation of results within the area or population
group in which the experimental health program is carried on, at
successive intervals of time. The fundamental assumption here is
that the condition prevailing before and at the time the demonstration was begun *is what might be expected* to continue unless
some new factor is introduced or unless some existing factor or
factors are bringing about changes independently of the factor
deliberately introduced. It is realized, of course, that this method
can be applied only after very careful analysis of the possible
influence of factors already involved, as evidenced in past variations.

The use of control areas or populations groups.—Such areas
or groups may be either *outside* the field of demonstration or
inside. The essential requirements, it will be recognized, are: 1)
that the observation of results must be comparable for the control
and the experimental areas or groups; 2) that the health program in
the control area must be actually different from that in the demonstration area, and that the nature of these differences must be def-

initely ascertained and understood; 3) and that the other conditions in the two areas or groups shall be in all relevant respects similar or shall be capable of evaluation and statistical adjustment.

The application of this method is, of course, over a given period of time. This will again necessitate, obviously, a determination of the *trend* before the demonstration is begun, in both the control and experimental groups, in order to eliminate as far as possible differences in the changes which might be expected without the introduction of the experimental factor. In some cases other types of time variables must be taken into account.

The use of control area outside the field of demonstration, if feasible, has the advantage of results that are more impressive and convincing to the lay mind, but the obviously necessary requirements for proper comparisons are extremely difficult to meet. In the first place, the indices by which we can measure differences that may appear in the health of the two areas are limited and are often susceptible of conflicting interpretations. To refine these indices or to obtain more accurate indices is a large and expensive undertaking. Secondly, the evaluation of differences in the health program and its execution in two areas, particularly cities, is a delicate task, and differences in opinion, even on relatively unimportant details, may confuse the acceptance of justifiable conclusions. Even if we are convinced as to these differences, it is difficult to demonstrate, to the satisfaction of persons not conversant with the situation, that relevant conditions in the two areas are similar or that differences are statistically evaluated and taken into account.

While at this juncture the use of control counties or cities should not be condemned, the grave difficulties presented by this method of measurement should be realized. On the other hand, the following general propositions suggest themselves: 1) that comparison with "control" areas be made upon the principles outlined above, but that these should not be relied upon as the *sole* basis of measuring the results of the demonstration; 2) that "control" areas be utilized rather as an indication of the general trend, measured by such indices of health as are common to all, an indication which will be of service in a study of the events as they occur in the demonstration areas.

If control areas or groups inside the field of demonstration are used, two fairly well defined methods suggest themselves: 1) the comparison of results in two sub-areas, in one of which a general hygiene program or a specific activity is carried on, while in the other no effort along this line, or a measurably less or different effort, is made; 2) the comparison of results in two groups of persons, one a group which is successfully reached by the activity or activities in question, and the other a group not so reached for one reason or another.

In either case, the observations may be made for a single trial within a definite period of time or at successive intervals. In either case also, the condition is postulated that the health program is to be instituted in certain sub-areas or population groups but is deliberately or otherwise held in abeyance for a long period to warrant satisfactory comparisons in other sub-areas or groups. Furthermore, as in the case of control areas outside the field of demonstration, it is essential that, whatever index of health is used, the observations on the health of the population in both the experimental and the control areas shall be comparable as to character, accuracy, and completeness, and that the population groups concerned shall be essentially comparable.

Now it is evident that the conditions for comparison of sub-areas are not met with under ordinary circumstances. *The indices of health or of disease would be limited to those which are not ordinarily available to the average health administration,* unless special observation areas could be set up for control—a difficult and expensive undertaking. On the other hand, the opportunities for comparison of results in groups of individuals are ordinarily more frequent and involve fewer difficulties than the comparison of sub-areas. The essential principles may be stated thus:

The comparison for determining the results of a given activity is between individuals who are successfully reached and actually treated and similar individuals (i.e., similar as to sex, age, race, general physical condition, economic status, occupation, and general environment) who are not successfully reached and treated. This, if based on a sufficiently large experience, should afford a measure of the result in a sample of the population; and this, if we have the data as to the incidence of the condition in the entire population, should present a fair basis for estimating the size of the result.

The observation of results at successive time intervals.— Whatever index of health or of a given condition may be selected, it is evident that in many instances serious difficulties must be solved in employing it for this purpose. One is the effect of factors favorably or unfavorably influencing the health of the population that conceivably might be wholly unrelated to the health program. This we ordinarily attempt to summate by determining the trend of health from the experience of preceding years. Our general indices of this trend are limited usually to records which do *not* accompany a health program, and we must rely upon the mortality rate and the incidence of communicable diseases. Another difficulty is met in some areas where the population itself changes materially. Assuming that a given period for observation is selected, our proposed method postulates that the population which is the subject of hygiene work shall be the *same* population, or at least population of the same sex, age, and race stock, throughout the period; otherwise we would be in the position of continually introducing new and unknown elements into the experiment. Still other difficulties are opposed by changing industrial conditions, variations in the virulence of the disease under observation, and other changes to which reference already has been made. In the case of a disease like tuberculosis, such factors as these must be taken into account, and it becomes evident to the analyst of the course of tuberculosis mortality that he cannot rely upon the crude rate, but that rates specific for sex and age and other relevant categories of the population must be used, with as specific correlation as possible with influencing conditions as well as with the various efforts to prevent deaths from the disease.

Some Applications

It is not to be expected in a brief essay upon so broad a subject that the detailed procedure in the measurement of the results of even a single major public health activity can be set forth, discussed, and applied fully. Such treatment would require a mono-graph in itself. But a somewhat more specific discussion of a few applications of the underlying principles and methods which have been summarized in very general terms is demanded.

Let us take a communicable disease as our first illustration. In the first place, it is assumed that the analyst who attempts to measure the results of efforts to control a communicable disease has at his command the known etiological and epidemiological facts relating to the disease; that he knows precisely what method or methods are being employed to control it in the particular instance; that he has at hand adequate records of what is being done; and that he intends to measure as definitely as he can the results of the *specific* effort in the specific etiological and epidemiological situation.

Now, since in public health administration and especially in a public health "demonstration" we are not so much concerned with showing that any of these methods are capable of producing results as with ascertaining *how much* of a result can be accom-plished by the specific application of a method *under practical conditions*, obviously the most definite measure of the result is to be found in the specific terms of the given method of control. Thus if the method is to eliminate the infecting organism, as in yellow fever, or to render the population immune, as in small-pox and diphtheria, the most direct measure of the effect is to be found in the subsequent incidence of the disease in the same population or in its incidence in another population in which the disease is prevalent and not interfered with. Or if the control is by elimina-tion of contact, the best measure is the subsequent incidence of cases resulting from the specific contact or contacts against which control efforts have been directed: for example, the pasteurization of milk supplies and the incidence of milk-borne scarlet fever and typhoid. Or, again, the prompt isolation and quarantine of all cases, suspects, and contacts of a disease that has appeared in a school. Or if the method of control is to prevent infection at those ages when the disease occurs in most serious form or with serious sequelae, as in measles, clearly the most definite measure is the subsequent actual or relative incidence of the disease at these ages as compared with its incidence in periods prior to the effort and in areas in which no special effort was made.

The most effective method of controlling measles, as Dr. Godfrey* has emphasized in a recent illuminating paper, that we are now certain of is the prevention of cases among infants and very young children, in whom the disease is most frequently attended by serious sequelae and fatal results. It seems probable that soon we can also immunize children in these ages who have been exposed. What is the best measure of the success of our efforts along these lines? Obviously, they are:

1) A comparison of the age-distribution of cases of the disease during the epidemic in which control was exerted with that of prior epidemics of comparable season, size, and virulence. Care must be taken, of course, to keep separate the records of cases reported by physicians and those found by special inquiry, and to correct the figures for changes in the age and racial distribution of the population concerned, in order that the records for the two periods may be more comparable.

Further refinements may be necessary when marked changes have taken place rapidly in the amount of opportunity for ordinary contact.

2) A comparison of the mortality and the fatality of the disease at different ages or at all ages in the control period with that in prior epidemics or in epidemics in other localities, due consideration being given of the possibility of unusual occurrences of virulent or mild strains.

The efficacy of immunization against measles is a subject for a different sort of experimental test, with which we are not immediately concerned here.

In sharp contrast to the method of measuring the efficacy of an anti-measles campaign is that for the measurement of anti-tuberculosis work. We are accustomed to evaluate the effects of the latter in terms of mortality, although we realize, or ought to realize, that a death is a poor index of what we are trying to measure. It is a faulty statistic for the reason that it may indicate on

*Godfrey, Edward S., Jr., M.D.: The Administrative Control of Measles. *American Journal of Public Health*, xvi: 571, June, 1926.

the one hand the prevalence or incidence of the disease, and on the other hand its fatality. It measures neither the one nor the other accurately. Furthermore, the death rate from tuberculosis has already reached such a low level in many American communities that the annual number of deaths is so small as to be subject to wide variation from fortuitous circumstances. Again, it is a poor measure in this instance because our greatest emphasis is on preventing tuberculosis, and on arresting the disease in those in whom the tubercle has been activated; and the tuberculosis death rate can therefore measure only a fraction of the full force of the campaign. Furthermore, in the measurement of anti-tuberculosis efforts we are attempting to observe the effects of various preventive and curative activities upon a stream composed of many continuous cases, each of which has its own course over a period of time. We have come to describe the changes in the course of a case by repeated classification according to "stage" of the disease. From this point of view the measurement of anti-tuberculosis work in adolescent and adult ages must be upon different principles from those upon which we measure an effort to prevent a definite event, such as a case of diphtheria or a death from measles. It is also necessary to keep in mind that an anti-tuberculosis campaign is not an effort directed toward a single objective; its objectives are several, each calling for a different kind of activity. It includes the attempt to prevent incipient tuberculosis; to prevent the development of incipient cases into more serious stages; to arrest advanced cases and to prolong the lives of such cases; to relieve cases in very advanced stages and so far as possible to prolong their lives also. Obviously any single measure is inadequate, and case records, rather than death records, must be relied upon to satisfy the requirement for proper statistical analysis and conclusions.

The measurement of infant welfare work by infant mortality rates has already been touched upon in the preceding pages from one point of view. Space does not permit of a complete discussion here, and rather than go into any details of this broad field, we may take as another example the possibility of measuring the results of health activities among pre-school children.

This offers, for several reasons, an illustration of a problem in measuring results quite different from that encountered in appraising the effectiveness of work for the prevention of communicable diseases. Health activities in the pre-school population, even in our best health administrations, are not always well defined. In the typical American city they are not usually concentrated in or co-ordinated under central control, since they are carried on by a number of agencies, both public and semi-public. Children of these ages, except those who are in day nurseries and kindergartens, are not as continuously or as completely under observation as children in the grades, and the opportunity for recording their physical condition is correspondingly less. No satisfactory general index of results of public health work in terms of their health has been worked out. Public health administrators, generally speaking, have so far dealt with the pre-school child almost entirely upon the case basis and with more or less scatter-gun methods. Individuals pass in and out of observation; "contacts" with cases are subject to fortuitous or special circumstances; and it appears impracticable under ordinary conditions to apply the principle of controlled experiment, or of experimentative observation, in the same way as in judging of the effectiveness of an immunization campaign. To keep under continuous observation a group of pre-school children large enough to determine the effectiveness of various health activities would be an expensive undertaking for the average community, although it will be agreed that well planned and carefully made observations of this kind would be a great contribution to the child hygiene work of the future. Mortality is not a satisfactory general index of health, since the death rate rapidly decreases after the second and third years of age and represents relatively few causes.

It is clear, therefore, that we must rely upon some other index of health and some other method of measuring results than those afforded by the mortality, the records of communicable disease, and the more or less casual records of cases treated by nurses, clinics, and other agencies. One practicable method would be to "take stock" of the health of pre-school children at the end of the pre-school period. The opportunity for this stock-taking is presented in the physical examination given to every child upon entering school. This suggestion is based on the assumption that the physical examination of children entering school will reflect both in a general way and in specific ways the effects of the various health activities as they develop over a period of years. That is, as successive generations of pre-school children are "exposed" to the influence of hygiene work, we should expect a favorable reaction to be manifested to an increasing degree in successive years or semesters, in the physical and mental condition of the groups of children as they enter school.

Obviously there are certain conditions and requirements which must be followed. Data relating to sex, age, race, and other facts should be recorded, in order that the successive comparisons may be made of groups of children similar in these respects. For the same purpose a record should be made of the reasons why any children reaching school age do not enter school, since it is conceivable that the amount of elimination of unhealthy children might change. For the same purpose also the incidence of communicable diseases during pre-school ages should be recorded, since one group of children may be affected by a given epidemic to a greater extent than a preceding or succeeding group. Finally, it is of the utmost importance that the index of health, or the record of physical and mental conditions, should not vary from year to year. This postulates the use of the same diagnostic standards throughout the period, the uniform application of diagnostic standards by the various examiners, and the selection of symptoms, indications, and indices of health which are least subject to personal judgment.

Under certain conditions this method may be adapted also to the observation of experimental and control areas or population groups, especially when conditions that might be expected to exert an influence on health exist in one group and not in the other, or when the school hygiene program or a specific program differs in important respects in the areas or population groups.

An illustration of a still different kind will be found in measuring results of school hygiene activities. In one sense school children offer the best opportunity for observing the results of public health program. For nine months of the year they are potentially under constant observation by teachers, nurses, and specialists in health work. More frequent and complete records are made of their health and of efforts to prevent deleterious conditions among them than in any other population group. For the most part the objectives of school hygiene are quite definite and the methods employed are fairly specific. Since the development of school hygiene has come to bear upon all phases of the individual's physical and mental condition, the space at our disposal will not permit a complete discussion of the measurement of all or any of the activities involved. We may use it, however, as a basis for discussing briefly the question of adequate *indices* of health, which are essential to any measurement of health work.

We are accustomed to speak of school hygiene as a whole. Is it possible to measure its results in terms of a single index of health? Let us consider some indices that suggest themselves.

The first, of course, is the gross mortality rate, but for practical purposes that may be discarded, since only from two to five deaths per thousand annually among individuals of school age may be expected, and relatively small groups of children are dealt with by a health administration. The weight of the child, after taking into consideration sex, age, height, and sometimes race and build, is the most commonly used index of health. Yet we know that among normal and healthy children the variations in weight, even after holding constant the factors named, are so great that weight cannot be considered a very delicate general index of the health of an individual child. For group purposes it is useful within reasonable limitations. A decrease, for example, in the proportion of children in successive school generations who are fifteen to twenty per cent under an average (assuming that this average is based on comparable experience) may be a significant indication of improvement in health. Probably as accurate as weight, and for some purposes a better index of health, is that which we connote by the term "nutrition," provided the estimate of nutrition is based on fairly specific signs, such as in the use of the Dunfermline scale* or some reasonable modification of it. The sickness

*[A four-point scale of childhood nutritional status, developed in 1914 by Dr. Alister McKenzie of the Carnegie Dunfermline Trust, Scotland. Four nutritional grades were defined: excellent, good, requiring supervision and requiring medical treatment. ED.]

record during school sessions is an index of health which has not been developed sufficiently for practical administrative purposes, and it is a practicable index, especially when the causes of sickness are recorded in some detail.

It is not improbable that a general index of the health of the school child will be constructed from the various diagnostic observations that are ordinarily made, including weight, nutrition, incidence of sickness, and the presence or absence of certain conditions, which will be, in a sense, an appraisal of the child's health. In principle it is already employed in certain phases of school work for educational purposes, and it is not unreasonable to consider the possibility that it might be adapted in a more scientific way for purposes of individual appraisal as well as of group appraisal.

Of more importance as indices, perhaps, are the records of specific conditions which we may seek to measure the results of specific health activities among school children. The task has the appearance of being extremely simple. For what could be a more adequate and accurate index by which to measure the effectiveness of a campaign to improve tonsil conditions, or posture, or hearing, than the prevalence of diseased tonsils, or of faulty posture, or of defective hearing? Yet to those who have attempted to analyze the observations of trained medical observers it has been painfully apparent that the diagnosis of a tonsil condition as "3x" by one physician may be and often is not comparable with a "3x" diagnosis by another physician, and that the standard of diagnosis even by the same physician varies from time to time. No term could be more vague than "faulty posture," since it involves different esthetic ideals as well as different hypotheses of the unknown relation of posture to health. Until improved mechanical apparatus was devised very recently for testing hearing, it has been extremely difficult to compare results of tests in one group of children with those made in another.

It is essential, therefore, that before attempting to evaluate the effects of specific activities for the prevention of many defective conditions, a standardization of diagnosis and a greater uniformity of observation shall be established, as well as continuity in the standard and uniformity. Comparatively little effort has been made in American cities to refine diagnostic standards from these points of view. The setting up of a classification such as "no defect" and "1x," "2x," "3x" defects, even though accompanied by careful instructions, does not solve the difficulty by any means. The way in which the classification is used is also an essential determinant of comparability.

Reference has been made to school hygiene activities from only one point of view, in order to illustrate the importance of selecting, or constructing, accurate indices of the results which are to be evaluated. The measurement of hygiene work among the population at school, in itself a broad field, will be discussed later, when reports are made upon various phases of school health activities.

It has been impossible, in the foregoing pages, to do more than suggest, in rather general terms and with very sketchy applications, some of the more important considerations and methods in the measurement of public health efforts, including the New York Health Demonstrations and similar undertakings. In fact, this brief, unfinished outline is a rough condensation of a much longer but only partly completed treatment of a broad topic.

Measurement of results of public health work is not something that can be done by one who is wholly detached from the work, or after the work has progressed to the point when an evaluation is desirable. The principles underlying measurement and the methods by which it is to be accomplished partake of the very essence of the work itself. They are the basis of inductive reasoning, of scientific procedure, of efficient practice. Upon them and by them clarity in objective is made possible, the ways and means of doing what we set out to do are rendered sound, and results are made satisfying. This is but another way of saying that if we plan and execute our work well, we shall have at hand the basic data and the conditions for proper measurement.

Milbank Memorial Fund Annual Report
December, 1926

2

The Statistician's Place
in Public Health Work
EDGAR SYDENSTRICKER

"What we want," said Karl Pearson, "are trained brains, and not a knowledge of facts and processes crammed into a wider range of untrained minds."

It would be difficult to find a more incisive or more comprehensive answer to the two questions recently discussed at a meeting of the American Statistical Association "What is expected of statisticians by employers?" and "How shall statisticians be trained?" than this sentence from the notable lecture in which a distinguished statistician and scientist summed up his own rich experience. The present paper in presenting the point of view of public health, medicine and biology, takes for its text this quotation because it expresses one of the fundamental requirements for all scientific work, whether the work be in research or in the application of results. It applies with peculiar insistence to the statistician; for, what is statistical method unless it is orderly reasoning by induction? So, in an unusual sense, we assert that the statistician must be a scientist. It is demanded of him not only that he shall understand the data with which he deals, not only that he be equipped with mathematical technique, but also that he shall have a trained mind, the sort of mind which old Francis Bacon described as "nimble and versatile enough to catch the resemblance of things (which is the chief point), and at the same time steady enough to fix and distinguish their subtler differences," and as possessed by a man who "hates every kind of imposture."

With this rather high standard in mind, we may consider briefly, first, certain general qualifications which should be possessed by the statistician in the field of public health, and then, more specifically some requirements for the statistician in public health administration and in the various contributory lines of research as well as in public health research itself. Medicine, for the purposes of our discussion at least, may be regarded as synonymous with public health, since we limit ourselves in this discussion to its social and preventive aspects. It is proper also to qualify the sense in which we shall consider biology by suggesting that we are concerned here with the contributions to public health from human biology, more particularly with "that branch of biologic science," as Pearl puts it, which deals with the "quantitative aspects of vital phenomena," now recognized as biometry.

The first of two general qualifications to which attention is invited arises out of the fact that public health has a social objective. The sanitarian—by whom is meant anyone who is engaged in public health activities—of necessity must have a perspective and a responsibility that are *social*. To employ the terminology of our program, we may say that in the field of public health, and in medicine and biology as well, the "employer" is the public. Only in a very narrow administrative sense is the employer in public health personified. The sanitarian, be he laboratory technician or field investigator, visiting nurse or sanitary inspector, school physician or administrative statistician, must satisfy not merely his administrative chief, who frequently has a shorter term of office than himself, but also the local public, as well as meet the scrutiny of other workers in his own field. All of his work flows directly into the current of public activity. Just what specific training for getting this social viewpoint and for realizing this social responsibility can be afforded by the colleges and universities must be left to our pedagogical associates. The suggestion is not impertinent, however, that no one who is deliberately equipping himself for the work of a sanitarian, statistical or other, should omit adequate courses in the social sciences.

The second general qualification arises out of the fact that public health has become a profession and, I may assert, a science in itself. The various contributing sciences are being knit together, their results are being amalgamated, and a new methodology is being evolved, to constitute a body of facts and a scheme of procedure that can be learned up to a certain point more advantageously by means of formal training than by the fortunes of experience. Already a number of the large universities have begun to supply this training. The statistician in public health work cannot stand aloof as a detached worker. He should make this scholastic training in public health a part of his necessary equipment.

We come now to consider the requirements which relate more specifically to the *statistician* in public health work. Here it is necessary to distinguish roughly between two rather definite fields, namely,

    I. Administration, and

    II. Research,

but in suggesting this distinction I do not mean to imply in any whit that the administrative statistician needs the basic qualifications less than the research worker. For the research statistician the general qualifications and training that have been emphasized are obviously essential; but without them the administrative statistician is a mere bureaucratic functionary than which I can imagine no more lamentable fate for himself or no more unfortunate thing for the public.

I. In public health administration, statistics and statistical technique are occupying more important places as the organization of record keeping is developed and as a greater dependence is placed upon accumulated experience. The functions of the statistician in this field may be outlined roughly as follows:

1) The registration of vital statistics, which include births, deaths, marriages, cases of diseases notifiable under laws or regulations, and to which may be added the enumeration and estimation of population.

2) The tabulation and publication of current vital data in forms suitable for biometrical and epidemiological analysis.

3) The interpretation of vital statistics for current administrative purposes, which implies the use of proper technique for the

analysis of time variables in order to distinguish between endemic conditions and the occurrence of unusual or epidemic
conditions.

4) The determination of the money cost of administrative,
preventive, and control activities.

5) To these should be added a fifth activity in which statistical
procedure is fundamental, namely, the measurement of the effectiveness of preventive and control work in terms of changes in the
health of the population. This is still in the research stage because
few of the available methods of measurement are delicate and
practical enough to afford satisfactory results. As adequate
methods are devised, however, it will be expected of the administrative statistician in public health that he shall know how to
employ them in order to guide the executive along lines of
greatest efficiency.

To perform these duties efficiently the statistician needs a
sound and broad training. Dr. W. H. Davis,[1] the Chief Statistician
for vital statistics in the Bureau of the Census, has likened the
public health adminstrative statistician to the general practitioner
in medicine who must "if special problems arise which require
knowledge beyond his own . . . recognize his own limitations and
call upon the specialist—whether it be a specialist in medicine,
mathematics, sociology, law, epidemiology, or a specialist in
some other line," but who in his own education "should not
confine himself to mathematics but should acquire as broad training as possible, medical, sociological, mathematical, etc." These
are undoubtedly sound statements. It appears reasonable to say
that the administrative statistician in public health should include
in his professional education thorough courses in certain
branches of medicine and law, in public health, biology, and the
social sciences, upon which should be based a training in statistical technique, particularly in administrative statistical procedure
in public health. Whether he is called a sanitarian with statistical
training or a statistician with a sanitarian's education does not
much matter. The important thing is that he be adequately trained
both in his field and in his particular functions.

[1]*American Journal of Public Health*, December, 1925, pp. 1081–1082.

II. Finally, we may consider the place of the statistician in public health research.

If there is or can be a science of public health, then here is a specialized field for workers of a high order of research ability. For as we observe the conditions that affect the physical and mental well-being of the population, as we analyze and generalize from them according to logical rules in the search for underlying laws and in the quest for formulae by which public health can be improved, and as we plan and conduct experiments in public health and interpret results, we are in fact postulating a science. In such a science the methodology is essentially statistical for the reasons that the materials are mass data and the processes are inductive. Again, many sciences contribute to public health in each of which statistical technique occupies a place of basic importance. There is epidemiology, dealing with the manifold and interrelated conditions in nature and society that influence the prevalence of disease; physiology, which is beginning to take adequate account of the variations in individuals and groups of individuals; human biology, as well as the biology of lower forms of life which are concerned in the incidence of human disease, such as parasitology and bacteriology; the study of the reactions of individuals and groups of individuals to disease, as revealed in immunology and by accumulated clinical observations and hospital records; economics and sociology, since industrial and social conditions often must be taken into account; genetics; anthropology—the list could be extended were it necessary, but it is sufficient to give emphasis to a point which I would like to offer as inherently important. It is this:

Each of these contributing sciences, as well as the science of public health itself, is a *specialty*. There is no room in any of them for dabblers. There is little room even for pure technicians or mechanicians, except in a subordinate capacity or as consultants in mere technique. Every worker must understand what he is doing and why he is doing it. The man or woman trained in statistical technique alone cannot walk into one of these workshops or laboratories and play with figures if he has any fear of consequences or any real sense of responsibility beyond that of an exaggerated ego; he must first understand the subject matter thoroughly and broadly, be the particular "ologist" in question, and then, if he possesses that originality and resourcefulness and humility which are indispensable to scientific work, he may apply his statistical ability to great advantage.

If this is true, where, then, does the statistician *per se* find his place in scientific research? Who, may we ask, *is* the "statistician"? I speak from the field of public health only when I say that I cannot visualize him except as the epidemiologist, the biologist, the physicist, the chemist, the researchist in nutrition, industrial hygiene, infant welfare, *who has the statistical technique necessary for handling his facts in the mass*. The statistician in biology is essentially a biologist who knows how to generalize from, and apply the principles of experimental analysis to, biological data; in other words, he is a biometrician. And so with the other sciences, including that of public health itself. In short, since statistical method is the orderly process of inductive reasoning in any science, the *scientist must be a statistician*. To postulate less is to limit our definition of statistician on the one hand to the expert in pure statistical technique who, despite his preëminence in the field of mathematical reasoning, is a dangerous person to be let loose in fields of facts with which he is unacquainted; or, on the other hand and even more unjustly, to the mechanical assistant and statistical clerk.

On the contrary, if we are to recognize a place for the statistical method in scientific research, it would seem that our demands upon the "statistician" must be even greater and that we must require of him that, in addition to an intimate knowledge of the data in his particular field and an adequate training in statistical technique, he must understand thoroughly the principles of scientific procedure. I refer especially to those governing experimentation and experimental analysis. Unless he is so equipped it is to be doubted that he really can apply statistical methods properly. If the essential principle of experimentation is the observation of events under controlled conditions in order to measure the influence of specific factors, it must be evident that this principle is postulated in well established statistical procedures, of which the following are only a few examples:

1) In the preliminary elimination of such complicating factors as may be possible by *selection* of groups that are similar in all pertinent respects save that which is to be the subject of inquiry;

2) In the establishment of *"controls"* that are essentially homogeneous with the group observed in all respects save the specific condition to be studied;

3) In analysis by means of *manifold classification*, since in effect we are holding constant conditions *a, b, c, d* in order to observe and measure changes in *x* and *y*;

4) In *partial correlation*, by holding constant certain variables believed to represent influencing factors in order to observe the association of *x and y*;

5) In the use of the calculus of *probability* in taking into account the effect of unknown conditions that do not have a constant or correlated influence upon our series of variables.

The thing not to be lost sight of in setting up standards of training in statistics, is that methods such as these are more than mere technique. Their proper use postulates the ability to *think* scientifically. Something more than courses in technique is necessary—a *quality* of training that Professor J. A. Thompson had in mind in one of his essays where, in referring to "the pernicious fallacy, which has deceived many, that science can be pruned of its theoretical developments and yet continue to bear fruit," he pointed out that "one of the deleterious results of the fallacy is that it has suggested to students and directors of studies—at all levels—the mistaken policy of trying to secure a 'technical education' without an adequately substantial scientific training."

Journal of the American Statistical Association
June, 1928

3

The Changing
Concept of Public Health[1]
EDGAR SYDENSTRICKER

Various historians have pointed out that the modern public health movement has undergone marked and fundamental changes. Some of these changes were precipitated by epoch-making scientific discoveries; others came through the evolution of social objectives and methods. The early days of the movement were dominated by the "filth" theory, that public health could be achieved by community cleanliness and sanitation. Then came the period initiated by the epoch-making work of Pasteur and Koch and their followers. This was an era of bacteriology in which the dominant idea was that public health could be achieved by medical measures. The campaign against tuberculosis gradually ushered in the third period during which it was realized that a disease such as tuberculosis could not be conquered by community sanitation and medical measures alone, because its prevalence was so bound up with many other environmental factors. Since then the concept of the scope of public health necessarily has broadened with attacks on such problems as infant mortality, dietary deficiency diseases, industrial hygiene, and mental hygiene.

Although considerable specialization (which so often narrows the view) has taken place, a further broadening of the concept of

[1]A portion of this paper was contained in an address read at the Institute of Public Affairs, University of Virginia, July 5, 1935.

public health is evident. "Public health is not hygiene or preventive medicine," as the late and beloved Dr. Linsly R. Williams
once said.[2] "It is a concept of the condition of health of the
community. Efforts to conserve the public health include both
those which affect the health of the community as a whole, and
those which seek to prevent any individual or group of persons
affecting adversely the health of others." Recently, in the consideration of ways and means whereby economic security of the great
mass of the population may be enhanced, the current concept of
the term "public health" has come in for renewed scrutiny since
so much economic insecurity arises out of ill health. Public health
is being looked upon more as a major social objective, not as
merely sewage disposal, or the prevention of infectious diseases,
or popular instruction in hygiene. This is the natural result of a
keener appraisal of all of the things yet to be done and a clearer
realization of the fact that many forces, although apparently directed toward widely different objectives, have a common basic
aim.

I

It is worth a few minutes' time to take stock of some of the
things that need to be done and that can be done in the further
promotion of public health. Readers of Dr. Bolduan's brief but
illuminating article in the last issue of the *Quarterly* will recall his
impressive exhibit on the conquest of pestilence in New York
City. But, as he comments, "while the course of the City's death
rate during the last eighty years as here recorded is most gratifying, there is danger that it may make us too complacent, and
inclined to believe that there is little left for health officers to do."
Moreover, the task should be measured not merely in terms of the
mortality rate. It has been pointed out[3] that among an average

[2]Williams, Linsly R. "The Rôle of the Practitioner in Modern Public Health
Work." Preventive Medicine and Public Health. New York: Thomas Nelson &
Sons.

[3]Report to the President by the Committee on Economic Security, January 15,
1935, pp. 38–39.

million persons in the United States, there will occur annually between 800,000 and 900,000 cases of illness. It may be predicted for this average million persons that, though 470,000 will not be sick during a normal year, 460,000 will be sick once or twice, and 70,000 will suffer three or more illnesses. Of those who become ill, one-fourth will be disabled for periods varying from one week to the entire year. The gigantic annual money loss in wages caused by sickness in families with small and modest incomes in the United States is estimated to be not less than nine hundred million dollars, and the still larger expenses of medical care probably are not less than one and a half billion dollars. These are only the direct costs. The much larger costs of depreciation in capital values of human life are incalculable. Even the direct costs could be borne if they were distributed equally, but they are not.

Science has not yet given us the means with which to prevent all of this sickness or to enable everyone to live healthfully until the end of the natural span is reached. But, as I have tried to emphasize in an earlier paper,[4] the plain fact must be faced that notwithstanding great advances in medicine and public health protection, the American people are not so healthy as they have a right to be. Millions of them are suffering from diseases and over a hundred thousand die annually from causes that are preventable through the use of existing scientific knowledge and the application of common social sense.

Ample evidence exists to support this sweeping statement. The ravages of typhoid fever, diphtheria, and smallpox have been enormously lessened; they ought to be and can be eradicated. The infant death rate has been cut in half in the last quarter century, but it can again be cut in half. Mortality from tuberculosis has been reduced by 60 per cent since 1900, and could be halved again. Two-thirds of the annual thirteen thousand maternal deaths are unnecessary. At least three-fourths of a million cases of syphilis are clinically recognized annually; but more than half of these do not obtain treatment at that stage of the disease when the possibility of cure is greatest. We have been rather vociferous in

[4]"Health in the New Deal." Annals of the American Academy of Political and Social Science, November, 1934.

recent years over the health and welfare of children; yet it is estimated that 300,000 are crippled, a million or more are tuberculous, and nearly half a million have heart damages or defects.

The mortality of adults of middle or older ages has not appreciably diminished. The expectation of length of life at forty is about the same now as it was in 1850, 1890, or 1900. The mortality of adults who should be in their physical prime—20–44 years of age—is almost as great as that of the younger group, which includes babies and children. The mortality of persons who ought to be in full mental vigor and still capable of many kinds of physical work is over three times that of the younger adults. In the young adult ages, 20–34 years, tuberculosis still tops the list as a disease; accidents and homicides snuff out about one life in a thousand annually; organic heart disease appears in even this young age period as the third most important cause of death. All careful studies of illness and physical impairments corroborate these ghastly records; in fact, they reveal even more impressively than mortality statistics the extent to which the vitality of the population is damaged in the most efficient period of life. This disconcerting evidence of impaired efficiency among our adult population takes on a graver significance in view of the changing age of our adult population. We can no longer squander the vitality of our grown men and women. The task of health conservation in the future must be broadened to include adults as well as children.

II

Such a situation need not exist if public health be made, as political leaders from Disraeli to Roosevelt have pronounced, the first concern of the State. Public health never has been the *first* concern of the State except in catastrophic situations. We are somewhat accustomed to accuse the politicians of lack of understanding, the medical profession of failure to cooperate, employers of unenlightened selfishness, trade unions of insistence upon measures not directly related but even inimical to health, and so on. If there is any blame to be attached to any one group, the professional sanitarian should come in for his share since the

public looks to him to define the scope of public health. The
trouble lies deeper. The prevailing concept of public health responsibilities has been and is too narrow. It is restricted to a few
activities such as community sanitation, water supplies and food
inspection, control of infectious diseases, education in hygiene,
the medical care of the tuberculous and mentally diseased, and
the medical care of the indigent. A newer concept which many
sanitarians are coming to accept is much broader and far more
sound. It may be stated in terms somewhat as follows:

> Society has a basic responsibility for assuring, to all of its
> members, healthful conditions of housing and living, a reason-
> able degree of economic security, proper facilities for curative
> and preventive medicine and adequate medical care—in fact
> the control, so far as means are known to science, of all of the
> environmental factors that affect physical and mental well-
> being.

Such a concept in no way postulates any particular form of
government. There is no reason why society cannot discharge this
responsibility under any form of government through which it can
express its will. Nor does this concept postulate "state medicine,"
"regimentation of physicians," or Sovietized control of those who
render health services. It is the expression of a social objective.
The public health of the future demands some sensible coordination of public health functions with private medical practice,
some solution of the economic problems that are involved in
obtaining preventive and curative medicine, some set of procedures by which the physician, sanitarian, and social worker can do
their best work in preventing disease, in the care of the sick, and in
the rehabilitation of the unfortunate. To what avail, for example, is
the instruction of an expectant mother by a health department
nurse if she cannot pay for the services of a competent obstetrician
and afford the special services needed if her case is a difficult one?
I do not propose that there should be a uniform national plan or set
of procedures, because, in a country so large and diversified as
ours, methods and procedures necessarily must vary according to
states and communities. The interrelationship of the essential

environmental conditions involved demand, however, a concept of society's responsibility for the health of its members that rises above the petty jealousies and bickerings that too frequently impede honest attempts to find satisfactory methods and procedures. It will not always be so. Some day the basic criterion of any condition or any practice or any proposal will be the effect it may have upon the public health.

III

In the light of these considerations, some of the more direct modes of attack on the general problem of public health may be referred to briefly. Science and experience have taught us some methods by which specific approaches can be made. Other methods, which may or may not be practical, are being proposed and need to be considered dispassionately and experimented with.

1. Greater economic security for families of modest and low incomes, whether attained by unemployment compensation, old age annuities, wage increases, or other methods, is, in itself, a preventive measure against ill health. This conclusion follows inevitably from the long-known association of poverty and disease and the vicious circle which this association contains. The fact that the American people have not suffered to a greater extent from ill health than might have been expected during a severe economic depression is due, I believe, in large measure to the sharing of savings by related persons, to private philanthropy, and later, to the provision of relief and employment by the State and Federal Governments on an extraordinary scale.

2. The prevention of ill health through the extension and development of direct public health measures of proved value is essential. In the past, expenditures for this purpose, except in comparatively few areas, have been niggardly, and the policy of placing the responsibility for preventive measures upon communities and states has failed ignominiously. The average expenditure out of tax funds for public health purposes in American cities in 1929 was only $1.00 per capita, less than half the sum

which competent experts have estimated is necessary. Only about one-fifth of the rural population of the United States has the benefits of organized health machinery and in nearly all the 500-odd counties having some sort of health services, the budget and personnel are regarded as far below any reasonable standard of efficiency. Up until the recent passage by Congress of the Economic Security Act, efforts to get the Federal Government to do for public health what it has done for education, agriculture, and roads, had been unsuccessful. It is exceedingly gratifying that for the first time in the history of the United States, the President has recommended to the Congress a very considerable increase in appropriations for public health purposes, and that the authorization of these specific measures was not opposed in the Congress.

3. The precise relationship of housing to health is not fully known but there is no question that certain types of housing are conducive to the spread of infectious diseases and tend to break down the resistance of inmates to other diseases. Slum clearance in our cities and better housing for persons of low incomes wherever they may live are clearly preventive measures which are in the category of public health functions.

4. The application of the newer knowledge of nutrition through education and through better distribution of the so-called supplementary foods, constitutes another preventive attack upon the general problem of ill health. In his presidential address before the American Medical Association last June, Dr. James S. McLester gave an illuminating exposition of the possibilities in this direction. He pointed out that "it is difficult to estimate how many persons in this country are so poor that they are unable to purchase the food necessary to keep them in health," but he ventured to say that, "something like twenty million American people are living near or below the threshold of nutritive safety."

5. Physical training, recreation, and education in hygiene and community health are matters about which we "confer" at length but do very little except in a few localities. We lag far behind some other countries in providing adequate facilities for training and recreation and in properly correlating health education with other

subjects in our curricula. One may say that our public school system is so vast and so routinized that it cannot easily be altered; yet in education lies a powerful means toward public health.

6. The new interest in population questions in this country gives some promise that limitation of size of family, redistribution of population, and other methods of population "control" will be considered more scientifically than before. These possible measures obviously have real significance from the viewpoint of health conservation.

7. Social work has so long been coordinated with health services that it is perhaps unnecessary to do more than mention it as a definite public health measure. The policy of relief on a gigantic scale during the past few years has given greater emphasis to the need for an even closer and more efficient coordination of social work and health services, including medical care.

8. Medical care is an essential health service, but the people do not get enough of it. It is not fully applied. It has been thoroughly established that under existing conditions, even in normal economic periods, thousands upon thousands of families are unable to purchase medical care when sickness occurs. Less than 10 per cent of the population have had even a partial physical examination; less than 5 per cent are immunized against any disease. These conditions persist in spite of the fact that there are enough doctors, nurses, and others who render or assist in rendering medical services—about a million persons all told—to take care of all sicknesses and do nearly all of the preventive work for individual patients that we now know how to do.

The subject of medical care recently has come to the fore in discussions of public health and the economic security of the patient and the physician. Opinion is divided as to the best methods of obtaining a better distribution of medical care. But there seems to be no dissent from the proposition that care of the indigent sick and crippled and otherwise unemployable persons should be a responsibility of the government; that the diagnosis and treatment of persons affected with certain types of disease (such as tuberculosis, cancer, syphilis, and gonorrhea) should be a

tax-supported function; and that federal, state, and local governments should join in providing general hospital facilities in areas
unable to support them locally. But beyond this, wide divergence
exists in the views of those who are studying other ways of distributing medical care. There are still a few who are satisfied with
the *status quo*. Others take the view that before any statewide and
national plan is considered, local experimentation with various
ways of paying for medical care should be carried on. Some of
these experiments have been in operation for some time and new
ones are being started. This is an encouraging sign of a growing
consciousness of the situation on the part of the medical profession and of the public. Other proposals involve programs on a
larger scale. Only recently the distinguished commissioner of
health of New York State, Dr. Thomas Parran, Jr., proposed that all
persons participating in the old age annuity plan and unemployment compensation under the Economic Security Act and all
others having annual incomes of less than $2,500 should be given
"public care for costly illness." He suggested that the types of
medical care which might be provided at public expense, in
whole or in part, for the lower-income groups of the population,
might be facilities for accurate diagnosis, obstetrical care, hospital
care, home nursing, and the treatment of chronic diseases. Then
there are the much debated proposals of various kinds for health
insurance among individuals who, though not dependent, lack
sufficient income to budget against the costs of needed medical
care, especially the more costly medical services. These proposals are of two general types. One is insurance against the loss of
wages resulting from illness, and the other is insurance against the
costs of medical care. Many proposals for variations within each of
these two general types are being considered. The experience of
European nations as well as of Great Britain and Japan with health
insurance of some form or other has, of course, suggested to many
the possibility of health insurance in the United States, provided
its administration can be so safeguarded as to preserve the advantages of the private practice of medicine and to prevent the inter-
ference of politicians.

IV

All of these should be considered as possible strategic approaches in the attack upon ill health and its consequences. No one of them is sufficient by itself. There is no single panacea, for the obvious reason that all of man's environment is involved. Different modes of attack involve different interests, groups, and individuals. Conditions, social and physical, which affect health vary according to locality and climate. Whether in the future some coordination of all these efforts in a comprehensive plan under central control in the community or the state or the country will appear advisable is another question. But the concept of public health as a major social objective should be broadened to a degree where the importance of each effort, each measure, each method gradually may be seen in its true perspective.

Milbank Memorial Fund Quarterly
October, 1935

4

Economy in Public Health
EDGAR SYDENSTRICKER

Economy in public health is a phrase which is given two entirely opposite meanings. In this respect, public health shares with many other fields the ambiguity which attaches to the word "economy." Some interpret economy to mean the reduction of appropriations (by federal, state, or local governments) for the support of specific public health procedures of proven value for no other reason than that appropriations for less vital purposes are being reduced. The other interpretation of economy calls for expenditure of appropriations to the end that the money should be used to the greatest possible advantage. The one is as surely false as the other is true. If economical appropriations are to be made, it is necessary to understand fully (1) the existing need for public health protection, and (2) the degree in which this protection actually can be afforded by effective public health administration and public health methods.

The questions of false and true economy in public health take on a national significance because of the Social Security Act of August 14, 1935. "For the first time," said Dr. E. L. Bishop in his presidential address at the 1935 meeting of the American Public Health Association, "the importance of public health protection as an element in national security has been fully recognized by expression of a national policy for the strengthening of state and local health agencies. Passage of the Social Security Act by the last

Congress presents the public health profession of this country with the greatest opportunity to establish constructive programs of health service that has been given to any group in our history." In another connection in the same address, Dr. Bishop pointed out that, "The establishment of a national health policy through passage of the Social Security Act, together with the existence of at least the elementary facilities for the application of knowledge, today places the public health profession of this country at the cross-roads of opportunity. If its fullest possibilities are to be realized, this turning point in our history must be met in the spirit of highest idealism."

Under the Social Security Act, authorization was made for federal appropriations totaling $13,800,000[1] for federal public health services and grants-in-aid to the states for their public health activities. But, since the Congress was balked in the closing hours of its last session, by the filibuster of one Senator,* in its intention to appropriate money under this Act, the size of appropriations under the Act will come up again for consideration at the session which begins in January, 1936. The Act itself authorizes but does not make appropriations. It may become an acute issue because of the pressure to reduce federal expenditures generally along horizontal lines. In view of the general approval expressed

[1]This total includes $8,000,000 for grants-in-aid to states through the United States Public Health Service, $3,800,000 through the Federal Children's Bureau for maternal and child health, and $2,000,000 to the Public Health Service for research and additional personnel. This is exclusive of the $2,850,000 authorized in the Act for crippled children, including services and facilities for children suffering from conditions which lead to crippling, and $1,500,000 for child welfare in predominantly rural areas, although the public health values, both direct and indirect, of these services are clear and unequivocal. Sound provisions for unemployment compensation and old-age security may be regarded as indirect measures for health maintenance, but the question of the soundness of the provisions for these purposes which were embodied in the Act is not germane to the subject under discussion here.

*[Huey P. Long of Louisiana. Long filibustered through the final hours of the Senate session ending on August 26, 1935, in opposition to an agricultural provision in a Deficiency Bill which also included authorization for the public health appropriations. Long was assassinated on September 8, 1935 and this was his last speech in the Senate. ED.]

for the public health provisions of the Act last summer, it may be assumed that the intended appropriations will be made and it is not unlikely that the increase in federal appropriations will be followed in many instances by increases in state and local appropriations for public health. This possibility raises the question of how this additional money can be expended most effectively and therefore most economically.

I

The necessity for increased federal appropriations for public health was fully realized by the Committee on Economic Security, by the President and by the Congress, as evidenced in the Committee's report, the President's message, and the action of the Congress itself. The members of the Committee's staff to whom the subject of "Risks on Economic Security Arising Out of Ill Health," was assigned, had proposed as a fundamental consideration that no program of dealing with these risks could be regarded in any sense as complete or effective without adequate provision of measures for the prevention of ill health. In presenting this view to the Committee, it was pointed out that the application of the sound principle of prevention in this instance should be viewed in the light of four broad considerations which may be stated briefly as follows:

1) Although one-third of the burden of preventable illness and premature death has been lifted in progressive communities since modern public health procedures were introduced, there is recognized opportunity for continued progress and wider application. Only a fraction of the population has benefitted to the fullest extent from the application of existing knowledge of disease prevention through public health procedures of proven effectiveness.

2) The policy of leaving to localities and states the entire responsibility for providing even minimal public health facilities and services has failed in large measure. Only 21 per cent (75 counties and 102 cities) of counties and cities have thus far developed a personnel and service which can be rated as even a satisfactory minimum for the population and the

existing problems. Only 540 out of 2,500 rural counties have even a skeleton health administration.[2] Yet the federal government has a definite constitutional responsibility for the protection of all of the nation's population against disease or other causes harmful to the public health. The responsibility of the federal government for national health is well established in the United States Public Health Service and in several other federal agencies such as the Children's Bureau, the Bureau of the Census, the Office of Education, the Food and Drug Administration, the Bureau of Home Economics, and the Bureau of Animal Industry.

3) The precedent of federal aid to states for state health administration and local public health facilities has been established in various laws for grants-in-aid and in loans of technical personnel to states and localities.

4) Public health has been demonstrated as a sound economic investment. Public health authorities estimate on good evidence that our annual national economic loss in wage-earnings and in other items incident to preventable sickness directly attributable to lack of reasonably efficient rural health service alone is over one billion dollars. On the other hand where reasonably effective health programs have been developed, it has been demonstrated that expenditures for carefully planned health programs executed by trained workers yield large dividends.

The necessity for federal aid in expanding existing health services throughout the country is further emphasized by the fact that the formerly inadequate appropriations by local, state, and national governments had been further reduced drastically in

Number of counties, townships, or districts having whole-time health services

	Jan. 1 1931	Jan. 1 1932	Dec. 31 1932	Dec. 31 1933	Dec. 31 1934
Number	557	616	581	530	540
Increase or decrease		+59	−35	+51	+10

[2]As of December 31, 1934. The following figures are from the United States *Public Health Reports* for November 1, 1935, p. 1553:

many localities during the depression. The experience of cities in 1934 showed that health budgets have been reduced on the average about 20 per cent since 1931, reductions varying from one and two per cent to as high as 50 per cent. Where this reduction amounted to 30 per cent or more, practically complete breakdowns of the public health protective facilities have resulted. The proposals for annual appropriations under the Social Security Act were purposely made modest for the reason that the Committee's staff and its advisers recognized the necessity for slow and gradual, rather than hurried or sudden, expansion. Sufficient trained personnel, for example, are not available to warrant the expenditure immediately of larger sums. In the interest of sound economy, the amount proposed for additional direct health work is therefore almost infinitesimally small in comparison with the tremendous sums which have been expended for more indirect methods of health conservation through relief, housing, and the like. Certainly the proposed public health expenditures are insignificant when compared with many other federal expenditures for purposes less vital to the well-being of the population.

It was anticipated by the Committee's staff that this proposed sum should not be curtailed by the kind of false economy already referred to. On the contrary, increasing appropriations on the part of the federal government for aiding the states and localities and providing health services were regarded as inevitable. If one may express a personal opinion or venture an estimate, I would say that within the next decade or so, federal appropriations for health services and health facilities should reach the sum of not less than 50 cents per capita and perhaps as much as $1.00 per capita, in addition to state and local funds. Even this—say a minimum of $65,000,000—would be a relatively small investment in so priceless a thing as improved physical and mental health of the people who compose the nation.

II

Each health officer and individual interested in health should exert every influence he possesses to encourage adequate appropriations on the part of federal, state, and local governments. It should be realized, however, that appropriations of public funds for public health place upon health authorities a very definite responsibility for the effective use of the money. This responsibility has not always been adequately discharged in the past. For example, many years ago Dr. Charles V. Chapin, in Providence, Rhode Island, showed that the disinfection and fumigation of houses in which cases of communicable disease had resided was a useless expenditure of public funds. Yet, in spite of this, the practice of indiscriminate disinfection and fumigation was kept on, long after its worthlessness had been demonstrated. Over ten years ago, in an illuminating address on "Rendering Account in Public Health,"[3] Dr. W. H. Frost pointed out:

> As various lines of activity are suggested to him (the health officer) by contemporary practice or urged upon him by special propagandists it is his duty to consider what returns are to be expected from each one and to decide how much of his capital he will put into each one. Since his capital comes entirely from the public, it is reasonable to expect that he will be prepared to explain to the public his reasons for making each investment, and to give them some estimate of the returns which he expects. Nor can he consider it unreasonable if the public should wish to have an accounting from time to time, to know what returns are actually being received and how they check with the advance estimates which he has given them. Certainly any fiscal agent would expect to have his judgment thus checked and to gain or lose his clients' confidence in proportion as his estimates were verified or not.

The present writer, at about the same time, in an attempt to discuss methods of measuring results of public health work, observed that the necessity for rendering an account "is in line with the increasingly critical attitude on the part of sanitarians in appraising the effectiveness of their work." I venture to quote the following from an earlier paper:[4]

> As the objectives of a social program such as the improvement of public health become more clearly defined, and as the

[3]Frost, W. H.. "Rendering Account in Public Health." *American Journal of Public Health*, May, 1925, xv, No. 5, pp. 394–398.
[4]Sydenstricker, Edgar. "The Measurement of Public Health Work." Annual Report of the Milbank Memorial Fund for 1926.

methods of carrying out a program are improved, the more
rigid must be the standards and the more accurate must be the
means by which we must measure the efficacy of the program
and the efficiency of the methods. No longer can the mere
"putting over" of a project be regarded as the final test of
success; for while undoubtedly it is an essential step in the
accomplishment of a specific project, the final criterion is the
ultimate result—the prevention of a given disease, the lessening of sickness and death from specific and related causes, and
the promotion of health to a discernible degree.

The necessity for the scientific evaluation of each specific
public health procedure is greater now than ever before. This is
true not merely because of the probability of increased appropriations for public health but also because a great deal of public
health work has undergone a process of standardization. The more
it becomes standardized, the more easily and, at the same time,
the more rapidly can it be put into wider operation when the
necessary financial support is available. If a given standard procedure is not a scientifically tested procedure, a definite and grave
danger is involved. An uneconomical or ineffective procedure, for
example, may, by the very process of standardization, be adopted
by many communities with the result that its improvement or its
eradication would be all the more difficult for no other reason than
its routinized application on a large scale. The appraisal form, for
example, which has been developed carefully through many
years of earnest and hard work, has undoubtedly rendered a service of tremendous value. It is a "yardstick" method for measuring
public health work. The yardsticks it contains have not always
been altogether accurately calibrated, however. Such a statement
does not in any way place any blame upon those who have devised
the yardsticks since the yardsticks represent the best opinion and
experience at the time. But unless the public health procedures
such as are set forth in the appraisal form, or in textbooks on public
health administration, or in standards set forth by official or non-
official agencies, are continually put to the test of actual efficiency
in accomplishing their specific objectives, we cannot be sure that
all of our present appropriations for public health are used to the

best possible advantage. The Committee on Administrative Practice of the American Public Health Association has, itself, recognized these dangers inherent in the establishment of standards, and has periodically reviewed the standards. Unfortunately, they have not always had available data by which they could evaluate the accomplishments of a procedure as much as the extent of its application.

This is not idle nor destructively critical comment. By way of illustration, one may properly ask: What are the scientific bases or the actual experience upon which are based some of our public health standards? We call for eight visits of a public health nurse to each and every case of whooping cough. This standard, as is well known, is rarely measured up to and more than one health officer has asked himself the question: What evidence is there of prevention of mortality from or reduction in incidence of whooping cough by eight visits rather than by four or two or one? Or again, school medical examinations have become so wide-spread and so routinized that they involve a not inconsiderable portion of the health budget. The health officer properly may have reasonable doubts as to the efficacy of school medical examinations as they are now carried out in practice. And so the entire list of public health procedures might well be viewed in the light of a healthy skepticism, not for the purpose of tearing down what has been so carefully set up, but for the purpose of improving the procedure itself.

In the scheme of public health, therefore, it seems clear that this healthy skepticism should be met by providing facilities for scientific testing of most procedures now in operation and of each new procedure before it is put into operation on a wide scale, and of each standard by which the application of procedures is measured. A beginning has been made along these lines by some of the foundations interested in public health, by individual health officers here and there who have the point of view which actuated Dr. Chapin for many years, and by the United States Public Health Service through the newly created Office of Studies of Public Health Methods as well as in the laboratories of the National Institute of Health.

Since the Federal Public Health Service and the Federal

Children's Bureau are primarily charged with the responsibility (within certain prescribed limits) for allocating grants-in-aid to states, it is obviously necessary that these agencies should possess the facilities for the evaluation of the public health procedures for which the grants are to be made. The staff of the Committee on Economic Security had this function in mind when it proposed to the Committee that $2,000,000 additional should be appropriated to the Public Health Service for research and for additional personnel in order that the Service, through its own Division of Research, the National Institute of Health, and in cooperation with universities and other institutions, might undertake and encourage the task of testing public health methods. If this relatively modest sum of $2,000,000 is seriously curtailed by the policy of horizontal cuts in appropriations, without regard to the importance of the purposes for which the appropriations should be made, one of the primary objectives of true economy in public health work will be hampered. Doubtless other agencies including foundations, universities, and local health departments, will continue to contribute to the scientific evaluation of public health procedures but the leadership and aid of the federal health agencies are greatly needed.

III

Thus the public health profession and the Congress and the Administration have before them a problem of vital importance. It is a question of whether that type of false economy which has prevailed so long in federal expenditures for health shall be persisted in, or whether true economy shall prevail at this time when, as Dr. Bishop has said, public health is "at the cross-roads of opportunity." The appropriations authorized in the Social Security Act are extremely modest. In the framing of this Act, careful consideration was given to the principles of true economy. The members of the staff of the Committee on Economic Security, to whom was assigned the general subject of health, estimated that not $14,000,000 but a minimum of $24,000,000 was needed to assist states and localities in providing even minimal health services of proven value. But in view of the lack of facilities and personnel and the time required to train personnel and provide facilities, the total amount proposed was scaled down by over 40 per cent in the interests of true economy. In other words, to use a phrase familiar in the making of budgets, there was no "padding" in the final estimate. A further reduction in the appropriations authorized would seriously curtail the very modest and practical program proposed. Furthermore, it was intended by the Committee's staff and its advisers that this program should be limited to federal aid for public health procedures of *proven* value. It was anticipated that larger appropriations would be made in succeeding years, as new procedures are found to be effective by scientific tests and by experience.

Economy in public health, therefore, demands adequate appropriations for providing health services of proven effectiveness in every locality according to its needs. It places a definite responsibility upon health authorities for efficient administration of funds appropriated. Efficient administration requires competent personnel for carrying on such public health procedures as have been proven to be effective and adequate facilities for discovering, through research and experimentation, new procedures as well as improving existing ones by scientific methods.

Milbank Memorial Fund Quarterly
January, 1936

3

HEALTH POLICY

COMMENTARY

I. S. FALK

I. Background for Evolution of Social Policy

The health services have long been in a troubled state in the United States, because it has not been feasible for the nation to have clear, unambiguous or durable social policy for health. The persistent dichotomy of what among the health services is in the public sector and what in the private sector has traditionally been resolved—more or less—by allocating the "community-wide services" to the public and the "personal health services" to the private domains. But such a division has been easier to make in principle than in practice because the boundaries for the dichotomy have not always been susceptible of sharp delineation. Indeed they have been confused: first, by colonial inheritance of the doctrines and dogmas of Elizabethan poor laws and the responsibilities for health services that flowed from them; second, by the growing obligations of government to provide or to pay for various institutional and non-institutional categories of personal health services (as for mental health or tuberculosis) that could not be actually available through non-governmental resources; third, by the need to systematize governmental provisions for the availability of personal health services for the near-poor as well as for the poor; and, finally, by the changing nature of health care needs, the increasing complexity of health service technology and the rising costs of the services.

95

Social policy for health—applicable at one point in time and
not at another, or for some kinds of communities and not for others,
or for some kinds of services and some groups in the population
and not for others—has therefore had to be complex and respon-
sive to the evolving societal scene. Changing needs and problems
have ever been in search of policies as the bases for programs
—new policies and new programs for old. But new policies in
general and new programs in particular meet resistance from
those in our society who are content with the old and the accustomed, and from those who are fearful of the new and the unknown. A consequence is lag between changing needs on the one
hand and, on the other, adoption of adequate policies and development of useful programs for meeting them. In the last half
century that lag has been augmented by an unprecedented increase in the complexity and in the costs of health services.

Edgar Sydenstricker became concerned about the emerging
need for new and better health policies in the United States from
his studies on the importance of health in a society which was
rapidly urbanizing and industrializing in the early decades of this
century. He saw the need for protection of the worker who is
dependent on wages against the loss of his earnings and his
earning capacity in periods of illness and disability; and he saw
the need for protection of the family against variable and rising
costs of medical care that were creating higher and higher barriers
to the actual availability of the services and larger and more
frequent financial burdens after their receipt. He also saw, more
clearly than most, that the social insurance patterns already developed in European countries for protection against these sequelae of illness were inadequate because they focused principally on care in episodes of illness, to the substantial neglect of
prevention of illness. He proposed that in the United States we
should have a true *health* insurance and not merely a *sickness*
insurance. He advocated this concept and undertook the design of
measures to implement "health insurance as a health measure,"
and not merely as a measure of "insurance" or "relief," by providing for strengthened services to prevent illness and to encourage
diagnostic and therapeutic services early in disease that is not
prevented. And this became—for the two decades from 1915 to his

untimely death in 1936—a persistent theme in his studies and writings and in his counseling among those with influence in the formulation and adoption of health policy for the nation.

When the U.S. Public Health Service published in 1916 the classic *Public Health Bulletin*[1] which Sydenstricker wrote with Dr. B. S. Warren, the focus for the development of new and better health policy was on the several states and their local governments. The principal responsibilities for both the community-wide health services and the licensures and other regulations applicable to the personal health services of the civilian population were lodged under the "police" powers of the several states. This was to persist until 1933 when the focus changed. The near-collapse of the national economy in a deepening economic depression led to a rush to Washington for help on many fronts soon after Franklin D. Roosevelt assumed the Presidency—since state and local government, private industry and commerce and the voluntary community agencies could not cope with the disasters that were overwhelming our society. The measures that were instituted by Congress and the Administration, while concentrated on the emergency needs of the economy, had also to deal with the health services which were in danger of collapsing. And the Federal Government became involved, perforce, through emergency provisions to support various aspects of essential health services and medical care. The focus for health policy began to shift—from the 48 states and their responsibilities under their "police" powers, to Washington and its as yet ill-defined authorities and responsibilities under the "general welfare" clause of our Constitution, with its limited delegations of powers from the states.

A year later, President Roosevelt announced his intention to develop a long-term program of "economic security" to provide protections against future recurrences of the kinds then confronting the country and to obviate the need to rely on emergency measures. His Executive Order No. 6757, signed June 29, 1934, created a (Cabinet) Committee on Economic Security and gave it the far-reaching assignment to deal with all the major common risks to economic security, including "the risks arising out of ill health." Sydenstricker was asked to take charge of the studies and the development of protections with respect to illness, and I was to serve as his associate, the Milbank Memorial Fund agreeing that we could be available to the Cabinet Committee. The initial intent was that we should tackle the problems of (a) loss of earnings from illness and incapacity and the design of disability insurance, and (b) the costs of medical care and the design of health insurance.

Sydenstricker and I were not content with this formulation of the undertaking. We therefore proposed a broader perspective to the Cabinet Committee, embracing not only the traditional elements in the European models of social insurance, but also all major elements required for an adequate health program —extending to the resources needed for preventive as well as curative medicine and for protections against their costs. The Cabinet Committee knew that we were pursuing the major elements in the program design that had resulted from the five-year studies of the Committee on the Costs of Medical Care, 1927–32; and they knew of the controversies that had been precipitated by that Committee's final report. Nevertheless, the Cabinet Committee accepted our proposals, and we proceeded in accordance with broadened terms of reference. Thus, Sydenstricker's theme of "health insurance as a health measure" became embraced within a still larger framework, and we were launched on what was to become a program for national health policy, with the focus not on the several states but on the nation. The primary locus for formulation and development of social policy for health had shifted to Washington—where it remains to this day.

Our studies for the Cabinet Committee, in which various colleagues joined us as adjunctive members of the staff, bore only limited fruit in 1935 and in the enactment of the Social Security Act, August 14, 1935. Intense controversy had been precipitated over the possibility of including "health insurance;" and the Cabinet Committee's chairman (the Secretary of Labor) persuaded the President that this controversy might endanger the enactment of *any* social security legislation in that Congress. Accordingly, when reporting to Congress on January 17, 1935, the President's message and the accompanying report of January 15, 1935, from the Cabinet Committee recommended only certain limited proposals (for public health and for maternal and child health) from among our staff recommendations. With respect to the need to develop public medical services and insurances against wage-losses and the costs of medical care, the transmittal presented only "guidelines" from our preliminary reports to the Cabinet Committee and promised further recommendations later. But our Final Report of March, 1935, presenting the comprehensive health policy and national health program, was not subsequently transmitted to the Congress, and it was never released. The major elements of the program were not to become public until three years later when, in somewhat adapted and further developed form, they would appear as the agenda of the National Health Conference of July 18–20, 1938, and, in further adapted form, as the first explicit legislative proposal toward a comprehensive national health program in a bill (S. 1620) introduced by Senator Robert F. Wagner of New York on February 28, 1939, intended to be the "National Health Act of 1939."

Sydenstricker's writings selected for reprinting in this volume illustrate his activities in three periods in the course of evolution toward the formulation and adoption of social policy for health. The first, represented by his 1917 paper with Warren, concerns his participation in the early campaign for health insurance and their efforts to give the movement breadth and perspective toward emphasis on health measures and especially on the prevention of disease. The second involves the proposals developed by the Committee on the Costs of Medical Care and his efforts to overcome the stultification which flowed from the controversy precipitated by the Committee's Final Report of late 1932. The third focuses on the new chapter which began with President Roosevelt's initiation in 1934 of the studies that were to lead to the Social Security Act, including concern for protections against the risks arising out of ill health.

II. The Early Campaign for Health Insurance

The paper by Warren and Sydenstricker reprinted here, to be fully understood, must be viewed in the context of the times. The United States was engaged in a bitterly fought movement for health insurance which had been launched in 1914 by the American Association for Labor Legislation. This was intended to achieve the "next step" in the development of social insurance following the successful war to win initial enactments of workmen's compensation. This health insurance campaign was to end in complete disaster in 1920, when the American Medical Association, deciding to repudiate earlier limited endorsements, joined large elements of the insurance industry and many other groups to oppose and condemn health insurance. The discussions and debates of that period were intense and highly political, fought with weapons and slogans both fair and foul—not unlike those that had occurred before on related subjects and were to recur between the 1930's and the 1960's—and such as we are witnessing again today. The Warren-Sydenstricker paper, presented in 1917 and finally published two years later when the campaign was already in trouble, was therefore an act of professional scholars who believed in the role of temperate and reasoned marshalling of fact and argument—an act of statesmanship and of faith and courage.

The paper had been preceded by one of the most notable treatments of health insurance in the publication of a fuller discourse by the same authors—"Health Insurance: Its Relation to the Public Health,"[2] published by the United States Public Health Service in March, 1916. This appeared (in two editions) in a period of intense interest in this issue when some 20 states were in the process of establishing official commissions for study of legislative proposals for health insurance. The commissions' recommendations emerged—variously—for and against, and with proposals for further study, but in no state was there full enactment.

The Warren-Sydenstricker *Bulletin*, the paper reprinted here and other papers from one or both authors set a standard for rational and scientific discussion which was matched by few other publications of the time and exceeded by none. Their special distinction was in the undertaking to build into the design of health insurance the specifications and measures that would make it a public health program with emphasis on prevention of disease and control of illness and disability. Sydenstricker was to pursue the studies of morbidity and mortality, foreign as well as domestic, presented in these writings through his numerous later publications on these subjects illustrated elsewhere in this volume and finally presented at length in his book "Health and Environment" in 1933.[3] He was to pursue his quest for insurance or prepayment continuously and persistently to deal with the financial problems of illness and medical care, and for system improvements to modernize the organization and delivery of medical care.

III. The CCMC Period

The Committee on the Costs of Medical Care (CCMC) was a self-constituted private organization of nearly fifty knowledgeable persons which came into being in 1927 "to study the economic aspects of the care and prevention of illness." Its primary focus was on the economics of medical care; but to deal adequately with the economics its scope of interest had to be broad, extending to the resources for health services generally, to organization for availability and delivery of care, and to preparation for the health care needs of the future. The Committee had come into being with strong support from the Milbank Memorial Fund, and Sydenstricker was an active member throughout its five-year engagement in studies and in program formulations. Some of its main technical studies drew heavily on his experience and skills in research design and performance; and the Committee's family and community surveys borrowed heavily from his pioneering work in these fields—as from his South Carolina and Hagerstown studies presented in this volume.

The Committee's staff studies were generally well-received, but its own Final Report in October, 1932,[4] failed to achieve unanimity among the Committee members. Indeed, some of its recommendations precipitated a national controversy which became intense with the formal endorsement of the dissenting Minority Report No. 1 by the American Medical Association.

Principally at issue were the majority's recommendations for the financing of medical care through voluntary "group payment" and for the increasing provision of medical care through voluntarily developed "group practice." The minority opposed societal intrusion into the medical profession's control of either how medicine should be practiced or how people should pay for it. And controversy was heightened because even some of the medical leaders of the time who favored encouragement of group practice feared that health insurance, voluntary or compulsory, would embed "solo practice" and should therefore wait on the extensive development of group practice. Much of the public discussion, therefore, focused not only on *what* needed to be done but also in what sequence.

Sydenstricker's paper of April, 1934, reprinted here, was directed specifically to the question: Which comes first, group payment or group practice? Since it reflected discussions he and I were pursuing and which led to several substantially simultaneous public papers, it should be read as the first of three related documents. His paper included in this volume was presented in late December, 1933, a year after the CCMC Final Report, though published in June of the following year. It was complementary to a paper of mine, published almost simultaneously, on the general question of societal involvement in organization for the availability and delivery of medical care, in which I distinguished the *content* of medical practice (what a physician does) from the *form* (how the services are organized and how paid for).[5] And Sydenstricker's paper was followed shortly by his next paper—on standards for a health insurance system and its essential economics, utilizing formulations and analyses we were pursuing in our staff studies at the Milbank Memorial Fund.[6] It is worth noting that in this paper, Sydenstricker italicized his view that "a health insurance system, to be effective, must be at least state-wide and must rest upon a compulsory basis."

Which comes first? Sydenstricker in effect expressed the conclusion that society has no real choice. If it would have group practice in the discernible future—as it must for technologic, quality and economic reasons—"the reorganization of medical practice which is badly needed will not come of itself, the product of *laissez faire*. It will come—if at all—only as the fruit of strong and directed labors, the product of compelling forces" (p. 133). Development of group practice and of group payment, he argued, are not contrasting courses of social action; they are not antithetical but, on the contrary, they are complementary; and, in order to effect improvement in the organization of service, we must first provide for payment and use "the power of the purse" to implement a program of medical reformation.

It is a tragic irony that this prescience was not heeded. We proceeded in the United States for the next quarter century with private voluntary insurance that did not engage in systems improvement and which, indeed, developed a new and massive financial bulwark for the organizational *status quo*. Thus, as I remarked in a recent paper, "private insurance effected precisely what had been feared from national insurance and what had been used as an argument when advising against the institution of national financing." Now, when medical care is nationally in crisis, that debate is ended and there is "a near-consensus that national financing and system improvement are inseparable needs, each for its own objectives and each a necessity for the other."[7]

We can now see, in retrospect, that proposals developed by the Committee on the Costs of Medical Care in its Final Report constituted, in effect, the first truly comprehensive design of a social policy for health in the United States, and that its specific recommendations could have provided the framework for a sound program of action.

Sydenstricker was one of the members who dissented from the Committee's Majority Report—but not because it proposed going too far or too fast toward effecting reforms and improvements in the health and medical care system but because it proposed too little and relied too much on voluntarism and private action.[8]

IV. Health Measures in the Social Security Act

I referred earlier to the national events that led to the design of a program for social security in the United States that would deal with illness as one of the major common threats to security. Being

in charge of the studies and formulations concerned with illness
and disability, Sydenstricker wrote for various audiences, first on
what was being developed and later on what had been achieved.
The two papers concerned with that period and reprinted here
have to be read with regard for their dates and their relation to the
stage of program development in Washington.

When the first of these papers—"Health Insurance and the
Public Health"—was presented on April 16, 1935, before the
Academy of Political Science, President Roosevelt had already
transmitted his Message on Economic Security to the Congress
(January 17, 1935), the Economic Security Bill had been introduced the same day, and the legislation which was to become the
Social Security Act of 1935 was being considered in the committees of the Congress. The message had endorsed and the bill had
included our recommendations for development of broad public
health measures. But other major elements of the national health
program we had recommended in our Final Report of March,
1935, were still being considered by the (Cabinet) Committee on
Economic Security. Consequently, in this paper Sydenstricker
could present the concepts being pursued and the guidelines that
we thought should be followed, and he could refer specifically to
the elements already presented to the Congress. He was not free,
however, to reveal more of what was in the as-yet unreleased
Final Report he and I, and our adjunctive staff colleagues, had
prepared. That Report was not actually transmitted by the Cabinet
Committee to the President until June 15, 1935.

Accordingly, Sydenstricker's paper was devoted to needs and
to opportunities for the development of a broadened concept of
public health. This, he proposed, should embrace not only the
traditional fields of public health but also medical care and protections against costs as essential components in a national program
of health conservation and of national well-being. He discussed at
some length the guidelines for health insurance which had been
included in the Cabinet Committee's report of January 15, 1935,
and which had been given to the Congress along with the President's message.

The second of these papers—"Health under the Social Security Act"—appearing in March, 1936, could at that point in time refer to what had been incorporated in the Social Security Act, passed by the Congress and signed into law by the President on August 14, 1935. He could refer specifically to the enactment of the newer supports for public health (Title VI of the Act) and for maternal and child health and welfare and for crippled children's services (Title V), and he could appraise them as "the greatest single step forward in the development of a national public health program that has ever been taken" (p. 152). But, with our staff report to the Cabinet Committee and the Committee's recommendations to the President still not yet made public, he could only proceed to a further reasoned discussion about needs still unmet toward policies for national health and for economic security against the risks arising out of ill health.

Had our Final Report been released and transmitted to the Congress, it would have presented:

1) A comprehensive assessment of the nature and the magnitude of the risks to security which arise out of ill health;
2) Further explanation and support for the strengthening of the public health services for the prevention of illness;
3) Development of the public (tax-supported) medical facilities and services;
4) The specifications for a Federal-state system of temporary disability insurance (covering wage-loss only); and
5) The specifications for a Federal agency to administer Federal grants-in-aid to states which elect to establish health insurance programs that meet at least minimum standards suggested for prescription in federal law, accompanied by suggestions for state legislation.

As noted earlier, much of this became available in 1938 through the agenda of the National Health Conference of that year. But the failure to submit the whole program, including health insurance, to the Congress in 1935 is what various students of the health and medical scene have named "the missed opportunity" and "the lost reform." Many years were to elapse before the mistakes of that time would be repaired.

It was a great disappointment to Sydenstricker, as it was to me, that so little of what we and our staff associates had developed for the Cabinet Committee came to fruition in the Social Security Act. Nevertheless, I remember well that he found great satisfaction in having had the opportunity to contribute to the national scene the framework for a national health policy, and of seeing at least some major elements of an implementing national health program enacted into law.

Many in the health field who reflect on the early social security period tend to emphasize what was needed but not done and would remain to be done in the years ahead. However, the health enactments that were incorporated in the Social Security Act of 1935 were no slight achievements. They laid foundations for much of great value that was built upon them in subsequent years. And these are monuments to Edgar Sydenstricker and to his vision for advancement of the public health.

Notes and References

1. Warren, B. S. and Sydenstricker, E., "Health Insurance, Its Relation to the Public Health." Public Health Bulletin No. 76. Washington: Government Printing Office, 1916.
2. *Ibid.*
3. Sydenstricker, E., Health and Environment. New York: McGraw-Hill Book Company, Inc., 1933.
4. Medical Care for the American People, The Final Report of the Committee on the Costs of Medical Care. Chicago: The University of Chicago Press, 1932. Reprinted by the Public Health Service, Department of Health, Education and Welfare. Washington: Government Printing Office, 1970.
5. Falk, I. S., "The Present and Future Organization of Medicine," Milbank Memorial Fund Quarterly 12: 115–125, April, 1934.
6. Sydenstricker, E., A Study of Standards for Health Insurance, in Social Security in the United States. New York: American Association for Social Security, Inc., 79–88, 1934.
7. Falk, I. S., Financing for the Reorganization of Medical Care Services and Their Delivery, Milbank Memorial Fund Quarterly 50: 205–206. Part 2. October, 1972.

8. Sydenstricker's views, not explained in his dissenting statement, were closely similar to those spelled out in the statement submitted by Walton H. Hamilton, pages 189–200 of the Final Report, *op cit.*

I. S. Falk, Ph.D.
Professor Emeritus of Public Health
  (Medical Care)
Yale University School of Medicine
  also
Executive Director
Community Health Center Plan
New Haven, Conn.

1

Health Insurance, the Medical Profession, and the Public Health

Including the Results of a Study of Sickness Expectancy[1]

B. S. WARREN AND EDGAR SYDENSTRICKER

The interest manifested by the medical profession and by health officials in the proposals for governmental health insurance in this country is as commendable as it is necessary. Any measure that may effect the quality and extent of medical service or that possesses possibilities in the prevention of disease is, it will be generally conceded, a proper subject of personal and professional concern to the physician, and a matter of vital consequence to public health administration. Health insurance—at least in some of the forms in which it has been suggested—without doubt is such a measure. In fundamental ways it proposes to modify some of the existing conditions of the practice of medicne. In a quite definite manner it promises to involve the social efficiency of all who are engaged in the work of conserving the health of individuals and of communities.

The physician and the health official, furthermore, perform a distinct service if they judge the various plans for health insurance by the criterion which these considerations suggest. It is proper, it is necessary, that certain questions be asked the proponents of any proposed form of governmental health insurance:

[1]Read at the annual meeting of the Medical and Chirurgical Faculty of Maryland at Baltimore, Apr. 25, 1917.

108

What effect will it have upon the professional work of the practicing physician and upon the quality of medical service?

In what ways does it afford the promise of more effective and extensive activities in disease prevention on the part of existing public health agencies?

Will the physician be enabled to do his work more efficiently, or will he have even greater handicaps than he already has?

Will public health administration be helped or hindered?

Sickness Insurance

For purposes of clearness it may be well first to state in a few words what health insurance, or, as it was formerly termed, "sickness insurance," means. Sickness insurance is a method by which the economic loss caused by sickness is distributed among a group of persons. The distribution is effected by the payment of periodic premiums on the part of the members of the group. In this way the cost of sickness arising from the stoppage of income, from fees of doctors, nurses, and hospitals, from expenditures for medicines, and the like, does not come as a sudden financial burden to the insured individual. This kind of insurance is now provided in the United States by many commercial companies and by thousands of fraternal orders and benefit associations of a wide variety of types, and is taken advantage of by a large proportion of those who are thrifty enough and financially able to pay the premiums. In the principal European countries sickness insurance of wage earners has been made a governmental function, but with certain fundamental differences from that form of sickness insurance which exists in this country. Among these differences are its extension to all wage earners upon a compulsory basis, the addition of medical and hospital service and certain other benefits to the cash payments to the sick, and the distribution of the cost of insurance not only among the insured, but also among the two other groups —employers and the public—who are considered responsible, in some degree, for the conditions which affect the health of the insured.

Health Insurance

The proposals for governmental "health insurance" in the United States not only adopt the principles just mentioned, but include additional features. Among these are an adequate medical service for the insured, and definite provisions for rendering the health-insurance system an aid to disease prevention. It has been proposed that the preventive force of governmental health insurance should not be limited to the financial relief during sickness, to the medical service afforded, and to the possible economic incentive to reduce sickness, but that it should be greatly increased by linking the health-insurance system to the existing public health agencies. In this sense, "sickness insurance," it is believed, would become a real health measure. It would not be merely a variety of commercial or mutual insurance or another type of public relief, but a practicable method of improving and extending the present facilities for the prevention of disease.

From the viewpoint of the physician and of the public health official, the principal points which suggest themselves for the consideration of "health insurance" are as follows:

1. The sickness expectancy, i.e., the amount of sickness for which medical and surgical service must be provided.

2. Methods of providing adequate medical and surgical relief.

3. Methods of adequate prevention of sickness.

1. Sickness Expectancy

Although in the absence of accurate statistics of morbidity in the United States it is impossible to arrive at accurate estimates of the amount of sickness occurring among wage earners, nevertheless considerable information concerning sickness expectancy may be obtained by a study of the experience of establishment sick benefit funds. Several estimates have been ventured, some of which have been based on extremely scanty material and some on more reliable data from surveys of actual sickness in industrial communities and from records of disability among employees of establishments. The wide difference in these estimates, from 6 to 9 days of sickness a year per wage earner, has served to call attention to the urgent need for accurate statistics.[1]

a) *Investigations concerning sickness expectancy.*—In the last two years the results of several "sickness surveys" or censuses have been published and have added materially to the very scanty American morbidity experience previously existing.

By the survey or census method the number of persons found sick on a given day in an enumerated population and recorded, affords the basis for computing the sick rate per 1,000 of the censused population as a whole or in sex, age, and other groups. In 1915–1917, 579,197 persons were censused in various localities by agents of the Metropolitan Life Insurance Co.; two censuses were made of certain districts in New York City by the department of health of that city; a survey was made of Dutchess County, N.Y., by the State Charities Aid Association; and several surveys have been made in a number of textile villages in South Carolina by the United States Public Health Service. Without attempting to present and discuss in detail the variations in rates among persons of different sex, ages, occupations, localities, income, or other conditions, reference may be made to indicate morbidity rates and annual days of sickness per person among populations 15 years of age and over.

In the following table the experience from the above-mentioned sickness censuses is summarized. The results of the Dutchess County survey are not in a form that is comparable with the results of other surveys, and are omitted from the table.

[1]The American Association for Labor Legislation in 1911 estimated that the American wage earner loses on an average 8.5 days per year on account of sickness. The Federal Commission on Industrial Relations, in its staff report estimated from such records as were then available that the average loss of time from disabling sickness and nonindustrial accidents was about 9 days per year per wage earner. The Social Insurance Commission of California in 1917 from a study of the records of American Benefit Association that were collected by the Federal Bureau of Labor a number of years previous and of such data as were available from similar records in California, estimated that the average loss of time per year per person was 6.5 days.

TABLE I Cases of disabling sickness and rate per 1,000 of various
populations 15 years of age and over, and indicated average annual number
of days of disabling sickness per person

Source of data	POPULA-TION CEN-SUSED	CASES OF SICKNESS		INDICATED NUMBER OF DAYS OF SICK-NESS PER PERSON PER YEAR OF—	
		Number	Rate per 1,000	300 days	365 days
Records of sick leave of Government clerks in Washington, 1914[1]	16,000	256	16.0	4.8	5.8
Sickness surveys in various localities by the Metropolitan Life Insurance Co., 1915–1917[2]	376,573	8,636	22.9	6.9	8.4
New York City Health Department "illness census" of health district No. 1, 1916[3]	20,169	552	27.4	8.2	10.0
U.S. Public Health Service sickness census of 7 textile villages in South Carolina, 1916[4]	2,367	114	48.2	14.5	17.6

[1]Warren, B. S. Sydenstrucker, Edgar. Statistics of Disability—A compilation of some of the data available in the United States Public Health Reports, Apr. 21, 1916.
[2]See appendix B: Combined Sickness Experience of the Company's Surveys, 1915 to 1917, of the Metropolitan Life Insurance Co.'s publication, "Sickness Survey of Principal Cities in Pennsylvania, and West Virginia," by Lee K. Frankel, Ph.D., third vice president, and Louis I. Dublin, Ph.D., statistician. The "combined sickness experience" referred to included the results of sickness surveys made in localities in Pennsylvania, West Vir-

ginia, and North Carolina, Kansas City (Mo.), Boston, Rochester, Trenton, and Chelsea (New York City).
[3]Wynne, Shirley Wilmott. Second Illness Census in the Experimental Health District. Monthly Bulletin of the Department of Health of the city of New York, November, 1916.
[4]Sydenstricker, Edgar, Wheeler, G.A., and Goldberger, Josehp. Disabling Sickness Among the Population of Seven Cotton Mill Villages of South Carolina, in Relation to Income. Public Health Reports, Nov. 22, 1918.

With reference to the rates in Table 1 it should be noted that the rate for Government clerks is probably for a preferred occupation. The rate approximates quite closely that for office employees afforded in the experience of the Leipzig local sickness fund during 1887–1905.[1]

The extremely high rate among the population of South Carolina textile villages, on the other hand, is probably due to a relatively low economic status.[2]

b) The authors' investigation concerning sickness expectancy.—In the investigation here described, data were collected from over 400 sick-benefit associations, covering, in the majority of instances, an experience of three years, have been collected. These data consist of records of disability due to sickness and nonindustrial accidents for which cash benefits have been paid under the various regulations of the associations, and afford this kind of sickness experience among over three-quarters of a million wage earners engaged in many different industries and occupations. The collection and tabulation of the information

[1]See Twenty-fourth Annual Report of the United States Commissioner of Labor, vol. 1, pp. 1281–1341.

[2]For a discussion of the sickness rate among persons of different family income in the population censused see Public Health Reports for Nov. 22, 1918. *Sup. cit.*

have not been completed, but it is possible, for purposes of illustration, to present some preliminary figures for groups of wage earners who are members of one or two types of sick-benefit funds. It should be kept in mind that any conclusions suggested by these statistics ought to be regarded as tentative for the reason that more complete data covering a larger sickness experience are yet to be compiled.

More trustworthy information, it is believed, will be afforded when certain inquiries now under way are completed and when the systematic reporting of morbidity among wage earners is begun. An effort is now being made by the United States Public Health Service to collect such statistics of disability as are at present available in the experience among employees of industrial establishments.*

For presentation here the disability records of those sick-benefit associations which pay no benefits for the first three days of sickness, or for illnesses of less than four days' duration, have been selected because a similar provision has been included in the health insurance bills that have been introduced in various State legislatures. Data for 23 of these associations have so far been collected. They include approximately 150,000 members,[1]

---

*[See: Industrial Establishment Disability Records as a Source of Morbidity Statistics. p. 186. ED.]

[1] It may be noted that the members of the 23 associations were nearly all males, the females constituting a negligible proportion, and, so far as could be ascertained, were adults of the usual wage-earning age period. They were employed in a variety of industrial plants and in various occupations; their sickness experience, however, is not large enough to permit of accurate indications of the influence of occupation. Since industrial accidents are not included, and since the members are fairly well distributed among different occupations in the groups presented in the table which follows, the occupational factor may be disregarded for the purposes of this illustration. To a considerable extent the members are a selected group; some of the associations require applicants for membership to pass a physical examination and to be under 45 years of age, and nearly all had provisions which operated to exclude casual laborers from their membership. The possible influence of administrative methods and practices upon the sick rate is more difficult to determine; the possible effect of the amount of the cash benefit, however, may be disregarded for purposes of approximation, since, for the most part, the cash benefits provided ranged between one-third and one-half of the wages.

for the great majority of whom a three years' (1914, 1915, and 1916) experience is available, which makes possible a consideration of 463,714 years of exposure of membership.[1] The regulations of the associations, however, are not uniform with respect to the maximum length of the period for which benefits can be paid; for this reason the statistics are presented according to groups of associations having the same or nearly the same maximum benefit period. The statistics follow:

TABLE II   Sickness and nonindustrial accident statistics of 22 establishment sick-benefit funds having a three days' waiting period, for 1914, 1915, and 1916: Classified according to length of benefit period

Maximum period for which benefits can be paid (weeks)	Number of funds	Years of exposure of membership[1]	CASES OF SICKNESS		DAYS OF SICKNESS		
			Total number	Rate per 1,000 per year	Total number	Per case	Per member per year
16 and under	13	18,335	6,130	334	81,382	13.3	4.4
23 to 26	4	4,688	1,840	392	28,100	15.3	6.0
52 and over	6	440,691	213,312	484	3,898,576	18.3	8.8
Total	**23**	**463,714**	**221,282**	**477**	**4,008,058**	**18.1**	**8.6**

[1]By "years of exposure of membership" is meant the number of members for whom a 1 year's sickness and nonindustrial accident record was obtained. The ap- . proximate number of persons who were members of the funds can be obtained by dividing the years of exposure of members by 3.

It will be noted that, as may be expected, the waiting period being the same for all associations considered, the average days of compensated sickness per case tends to increase according to the maximum length of the benefit period, and determines the trend of the average days of sickness per member. The importance of the length of the benefit period in determining the amount of sickness for which benefits are to be paid under a system of health insurance is thus suggested. The sickness experience covered in the foregoing statistics is too small to afford definite indications of the experience under any given benefit period except, probably, for those associations having benefit periods of 52 weeks or more. For those six associations, with 440,691 years of exposure, we have a rate of 8.8 days of sickness per year per member.

[1]Years of exposure of membership were ascertained from the records of the associations by securing the average memberships for each month in each year and computing the average yearly membership by dividing the total of the monthly membership by 12.

The sickness expectancy for associations having a maximum benefit period of 26 weeks is, however, of especial interest because some of the health insurance bills introduced in State legislatures contain a similar provision. Unfortunately, until the data obtained are more completely tabulated and adjustments made for varying waiting and benefit periods, our statistics are rather meager. The rate of 6 days of sickness per member per year and of 392 cases of sickness per 1,000 members per year for the group of associations having benefit periods of 23 to 26 weeks appears to be conservatively low,[1] especially when it is compared with the indicated experience obtained in several recent "sickness censuses" in the United States, to which reference has been made, and with the experience of the German sickness insurance system during the five years prior to the war. With similar waiting and benefit periods, the German experience for the years 1909–1913 showed an average of 8.4 days of compensated sickness per member per year. This was a considerable increase over the rate in 1900 and in years prior, which was about 6 or 7 days.[2]

While the increase was in some measure undoubtedly due to changes in the provisions of the sickness insurance law, it can be interpreted at least partly as an indication of improvements in the

[1]If the average annual case rate of 477 per 1,000 for the entire group of 23 associations included in the foregoing table be used as possibly a more accurate base, the days of sickness per member per year for the 4 associations with a benefit period of 23 to 26 weeks would be 7.3.

[2]The following table presents the German sickness insurance experience for the years 1885, 1890, 1895, 1900, and 1905–1913 (compiled for the years indicated from Statistik des Deutschen Reichs: Die Krankenversicherung):

Year	Average yearly number of members	Cases of sickness and confinement	Days of sickness and confinement	AVERAGE NUMBER OF DAYS OF SICKNESS—		Average number sick during the year per 1,000 members
				Per sick member	Per insured member	
1885	4,290,000	1,804,829	25,301,178	14.1	5.89	420
1890	6,579,539	2,422,350	39,176,689	16.2	5.95	368
1895	7,525,524	2,703,632	46,470,023	17.2	6.17	359
1900	9,520,763	3,679,285	64,916,827	17.6	6.82	386
1905	11,184,476	4,451,448	88,082,296	19.8	7.87	398
1906	11,689,388	4,423,756	87,444,605	19.8	7.48	378
1907	12,138,966	4,956,388	97,148,780	19.6	8.00	408
1908	12,324,094	5,206,148	103,894,299	20.0	8.43	422
1909	12,519,785	5,045,793	103,368,412	20.5	8.25	403
1910	13,069,375	5,197,080	104,708,104	20.1	8.01	398
1911	13,619,048	5,772,388	115,128,905	19.9	8.45	424
1912	13,217,705	5,633,956	112,249,064	19.9	8.49	426
1913	13,566,473	5,710,251	117,436,644	20.6	8.65	421

medical care of the sick, of the placing of a greater emphasis upon "medical inadvisability to work" rather than on actual "inability to work" as a principle in determining the return of disabled workers to employment, and of a clearer realization of insured persons as to their rights under the insurance system. It would therefore appear that all of the increase can not be attributed to malingering. Without venturing to assume that conditions affecting the health of German wage earners before the war were comparable in all respects with conditions in this country or that the German sickness rate is any guide to the sickness expectancy here, it seems reasonable to have under consideration the probability that the expectancy of sickness which is to receive cash benefits under State or other health insurance laws in the United States will be larger than that indicated by the experience of existing sick-benefit funds, especially if an adequate medical service is afforded.

Probably a conservative estimate of the total amount of sickness which will require medical service under the proposed health-insurance measures would be something between 8 and 9 days per insured person. This includes, of course, the first 3 days of sickness and sicknesses lasting less than 4 days for which medical service must be provided. With a sickness expectancy of 9 days per insured person per year, the physician with 1,000 insured persons on his list might expect to have 20 to 40 of these constantly sick. That would mean making some 20 to 40 professional visits a day, though a certain proportion will be office visits. This estimate applies only to insured persons; if the families are to be included in the medical benefits and if the average family consists of wage earner, wife, and child, the amount of medical work would be increased at least 200 per cent, for it may be safely estimated that the sickness expectancy in the family is at least twice as great as for insured persons.

Methods of Providing Adequate Medical and Surgical Relief

The question of adequate medical relief has become a serious economic problem. The advances made in medical science, the new discoveries, the refinements in technique of diagnosis and treatment, have added to the seriousness of the problem, until now it is often stated that only the rich and some of the very poor are able to obtain the latest and most up-to-date medical and surgical treatment.

For the general practitioner the question of rendering his best service is becoming more onerous. The examination which he is now equipped for carrying out requires so much time and patience that it becomes a question of increasing his charges to where the cost is prohibitive for the man of ordinary income, or doing his increased service at the old rate of pay and finding that he is not able to earn a decent living for his family.

The physician, when he faces this situation, must decide to confine his practice to the well-to-do, to drop back into the old method of a hurried and inadequate service for a large clientele, or to render his best service to all and content himself in his poverty with the knowledge that his life is worth while.

In another sense an important underlying cause of the present medical and surgical service inadequacy is an economic one. The income of the physician is dependent upon the misfortune of his friends. When his friends are not sick the doctor's income stops. In other words, when his friends are without income they have the further burden of a doctor's bill. This is, to say the least, economically unsound. If the practice of medicine is to be on a sound economic basis the cost of sickness should be met during the period of employment, when there is an income. The problem, then, is to furnish an adequate medical and surgical service to the wage earner, the cost to be met during the period of employment. To guarantee that it be within the reach of all employed persons, provision must be made for the continuance of a substantial part of the income during sickness, else many will not be able to stop work even when sick. Under present practices of the medical profession there is a premium placed on sickness. That is to say, the patient who is sick often, or for long periods, is worth much more to his doctor than the patient who is seldom sick. This should be reversed; the premium should, in so far as practicable, be placed on health. With a premium on health payable to the doctor,

it goes without saying that it would be an added incentive to him
to keep his patients well, and to cure them as quickly as possible
when sick. The question, then, is as to the practicability of working out some plan by which all of the good features in present
practice may be retained and at the same time add an economic
incentive as a further inducement for the doctor to keep his patient well.

If health insurance is to come, and changes in methods of
medical practice are to be made, certainly the opportunity is an
extraordinary one for placing these practices on an economically
sound basis, and for making "sickness" insurance actually a
"health" insurance.

It should be thoroughly understood that adequate medical and
surgical relief is not possible without adequate pay. Any plan
which proposes to reduce the average net income of the physician
will surely fail to provide adequate relief. If, as is often stated, a
large proportion of the people are not receiving adequate medical
treatment, the readjustments made necessary in order to provide
proper treatment for all insured persons would very probably
mean an increase in the average net income of the physicians.
Surely no plan should be countenanced which will make matters
worse.

In this connection it is well for physicians to consider the
experience of foreign countries under sickness insurance, and the
experience of this country under workmen's compensation laws.
In Germany, the plan of administration of medical benefits which
led to the "doctors' strike,"* would hardly offer inducements to us
to copy the German plan. In Great Britain, the plan has been the
subject of much criticism, mainly because of the incentive to
malingering, and delays in payments, and methods of payments to
the physicians.

After the British law had been in operation for something more
than a year, Mr. Lloyd George made the statement that there had
been an average increase in the annual income of the physicians
of $750 occasioned by the act, and that 22,000 of the 25,000

---

*[Physicians in Cologne, in 1910, in a dispute with the sickness insurance
funds, withheld services from the funds' beneficiaries. ED.]

physicians in England had registered on the panels. The experience in this country under workmen's compensation laws is too well known to need discussion here. That this experience has not been satisfactory is mainly the fault of the physicians themselves. They sat quietly by while the laws were being enacted and made little effort to have the proper provisions incorporated into these acts. The question naturally arises, shall the physicians spend their time and money fighting these proposed measures, or shall they direct all their efforts toward working out satisfactory plans, and insist on their inclusion in all the bills proposed in any State legislature?

Turning now to the discussion of the plans for providing medical and surgical treatment, and the methods of payment, the following have been proposed:

1. The establishment of a panel upon which any licensed practitioner so desiring may register. From this panel insured persons are allowed to select their physician, subject to the right of the physician to refuse under certain regulations.
   Payments to be made on a capitation or fee basis, or a combination of both.
2. Contract physicians employed on an annual salary basis, or a capitation basis, from which number the insured persons are allowed to select.
3. District physicians, paid on part-time basis.
4. Combinations of numbers 1, 2, and 3.

The success or failure of any of these plans will, of course, depend largely upon their administration. Two plans for the organization of the administration have been proposed; one, with an administrative board composed entirely of employers and employees, with an advisory medical committee; the other, with an administrative board composed of a chairman, employer, and employee directors, together with a medical director and a health director, with an advisory medical committee. It would appear obvious that in the administration of medical and health matters, medical and health men should have an active part in the management instead of only an advisory authority. The State should have representation through the selection of the chairman and the health director, and physicians should insist on having proper representation on the local and district boards which are to administer the medical benefits, and not be satisfied with an advisory position.

As to the plans for providing medical benefits, it seems to be conceded that free choice of physicians must be provided wherever practicable. Whether this will always provide the best medical service is a question, but the demand of individual freedom in this matter is too strong to be limited, even though the individual may at times exercise this freedom of choice to his own detriment. Furthermore, the efficiency of a physician's treatment would be seriously affected when attending a patient who did not prefer his services. Much may be said in favor of freedom of choice. It would avoid a disturbance of the time-honored relation of the family physician to his patients. With the right to change doctors at will, physicians would still have operative all of the present incentive to please their patients.

It would be through the method of payment that an opportunity would be afforded to take the premium off of sickness and place it indirectly upon health. By fixing the payments on a capitation basis, the physician would receive the same amount per patient per year, whether his patients were sick or well. This would indirectly result in making the healthy patient the most desirable to the physician. Under this system there might be some patients left over who had been refused by all of the physicians as undesirable on account of the frequency of their demands on the medical attendant's time. This, however, is liable to occur under any system of free choice. If the number of these left-over patients is small, they may be allotted pro rata. If the number is large, a salaried physician may be employed to attend them. Surely when the patients have the power to change physicians at will, the physician will have the same incentive as he now has to please and render his best service. Furthermore, he will realize that by doing everything possible to keep his patients in health his work will be reduced. On a visitation basis of payment the physician who had sickly patients would have the better income, so that there would be no indirect financial incentive to keep his patients well; on the contrary, the more visits he made, the greater his income. This plan of so much per visit would probably be too expensive for the insurance system, unless in making up the annual budget a fixed amount were allotted for the payment of medical benefits. Such an allotment of a definite amount per insured person would really be equivalent to capitation payment, as it would limit the payment to a fixed amount per capita. It would, however, have the defect of putting a premium on the sick patient.

In this discussion of plans for providing adequate medical and surgical relief, the remuneration of physicians must be presumed to be adequate, else the conditions are liable to be worse under health insurance than they are now. For this reason it might be provided in the organic act that the rate of remuneration must be adequate, and provisions made for a commission to fix the rates. Furthermore, if members of the families of insured persons are to be included in provisions for medical benefits, the rates should be fixed according to the number entitled to medical benefits and not according to the number of insured persons. Obviously, the physician who is to furnish medical treatment to an insured person with wife and child is entitled to three times more than he would be if he is only to furnish it to a single insured person with no dependents, for, as stated above, the sickness expectancy of women and children is very probably as great as that of men in the wage-earning age group.

Before leaving this question of medical benefits it should be stated that it is not just to oppose a proper health insurance bill on the ground that it means cheap contract practice, with all of its known evil. Contract practice can not be objectionable if the physician is paid enough so that he will not have to slight his work in order to make a living.

Contract practice is in successful operation in this country in many government services, and in many large business establishments. Furthermore, based on a capitation payment, where there is competition for patients, the contract practice is likely to

prove satisfactory, provided always that there is no opportunity for
cutting the rates of payments.

Methods of Adequate Prevention of Sickness–Plan for Making Sickness Insurance Actually Health Insurance

The foregoing discussion has related to sickness insurance as a
relief measure. If it is to be enacted on the grounds of a health
measure and is really to be health insurance then ample provision
should be made for the prevention of disease. It is not sufficient to
create a financial incentive for the reduction of the sickness rate.
Definite provision should be made for preventive machinery.
Some of the existing State health departments are too inefficient
to be depended upon. They should be strengthened, to meet the
needs in this field. If millions of State funds are to be expended for
health work, surely these funds should be spent to prevent disease, and not simply for relief.

With the appropriations for "health insurance" running into
millions of dollars annually it goes without saying that legislative
bodies will not materially increase the appropriations for their
health departments. Owing to this fact there is a decided probability of sickness insurance acts endangering the very existence of
State health departments by absorbing all of the funds available
for health work. Our statesmen and lawmakers must therefore be
careful that proper and ample provisions are made for health
machinery in any sickness insurance act.

No provisions have been made in any of the insurance systems
of foreign countries for coordinating them with the health agencies; though to a limited extent provisions are made by some for
disease prevention and medical research. The English experience has been such that the ministry of health bill now pending
provides for the transfer of the national insurance system to the
health department.

We should profit by this experience and make ample provision
for disease prevention through existing State health agencies. All
proposals for health insurance in this country should therefore be
carefully scrutinized and all sections providing for disease pre-

vention amended so as to definitely place these functions under the jurisdiction of the health departments. Otherwise there will be duplication of work, confusion of administration and waste of funds. The weightiest of the arguments presented by the proponents of health insurance are based on the probable effect it will have in preventing disease. The question then would seem to be whether existing health agencies shall be utilized or new agencies created. Surely some plan can be worked out whereby existing health agencies can be coordinated with health insurance systems and obviate the necessity of creating new machinery. Even if new machinery were created it would be unwise to create it to work independently, so that, after all, existing health agencies would need to be coordinated with the new system.

The general outlines of a plan for coordination were approved by the Annual Conference of State and Territorial Health Officers with the Public Health Service, May, 1916. This plan proposes to utilize the medical referees in carrying it into effect. It is proposed to have these appointed by the State, and commissioned to act as referees for the health insurance system and as health officers for the health department, under the jurisdiction of both agencies.

Following out this general outline, a scheme of organization has been suggested which, it is believed, would work out satisfactorily to both. It is pretty well conceded that medical referees will be required in every locality to see and keep in touch with each sick person in order to certify to his disability prior to the payment of cash benefits. Experience has shown that it is not right to impose the duty of signing the disability certificate upon the physician treating the case. Since the medical referee is considered necessary in the scheme of sickness insurance, and since his duties as referee will require him to pass upon claims in which three parties are interested, viz., the insurer, the insured, and the treating physician, it would appear but proper that he be employed by the State. The additional duties required of him as health officer would not interfere with his usefulness as referee; in fact, they would add to his efficiency and clothe him with the authority of the health department. Such authority would make of him one unit in the health machinery for the health insurance system.

The organization proposed would be about as follows:

1. Make the State commissioner of health an ex officio member of the State health insurance commission.
2. Detail a medical director from the State health department to assist the commission in supervising the administration of the medical benefits and to act as health adviser and director.
3. Detail district medical directors from the State health department to aid in the administration of the medical benefits in their respective districts.
4. Detail from the State health department a sufficient number of local medical officers to act as medical referees and to sign all disability certificates, and to perform such other duties as may be authorized by law or regulation.

To give some idea of the size of such a corps, it may be tentatively estimated that it would require one medical referee to every 4,000 insured persons. In a State with 1,000,000 wage earners, this would mean 250 local medical officers giving their entire time to the study of the health of the insured persons. This, of course, would be in addition to the medical treatment furnished by the panel physicians.

The objection could not be offered that such a corps would be too expensive, for it must not be forgotten that all the measures now advocated provide for medical referees. The only additional expense incurred by this plan would be for the medical director and the district medical directors.

Even if the expense of the whole corps were an additional expense, the cost would not be prohibitive because the medical referees would more than save their salaries in the disallowances of unfair claims. Furthermore, while an estimate can not be made of the amount to be saved by the work of these health experts, it is safe to say it would be many times more than the sum of their salaries.

At first glance this plan has been considered by some to be impracticable because they thought it gave too much authority to the health departments. It, however, does not add to the authority of health departments, it only extends their field of usefulness.

The duties of the referee as related to the insurance system would be to see and keep in touch with the sick insured, to certify to their disability, to advise with the treating physician, to advise the insuring agency as to measures calculated to shorten disabilities, and to prevent disabilities among insured persons.

The duties of the referee as related to the health department would be almost identical with the above, with the additional duties of sending duplicates of morbidity and mortality reports to the department, and advising as to any assistance he may need for research into the causes of sickness in his jurisdiction.

For the proper performance of these two sets of duties he would be responsible to each department. But under the organization proposed, a referee would receive State appointment, subject to duty anywhere within the State, so that if for any reason his services were not locally satisfactory he might be shifted to another locality; in fact, there should be a limit to his tour of duty in any one locality to prevent him becoming too thoroughly identified with the local politics or other conditions which might give a bias to his decisions or actions.

The plan has been criticized owing to the fact that it does not place employment of the referee under the control of the local insuring agency, one of the parties interested in his decisions as referee. It would seem obvious that a referee should not be employed by one of the parties at interest. Further criticism has been made that the treating doctors would not submit to supervision by a representative of the State health department. It is hard to understand why they would object to the physician employed by the State but would have no objection to the same supervision by a physician employed by the local insuring agency.

In order to secure the best men for medical referees, it is proposed in the plan to require an examination, physical and mental, as to qualifications, and after a probationary period of satisfactory service to make the appointment permanent, subject to efficiency and good moral conduct. It is believed that the prestige of a State appointment, and the permanent tenure of office, will obtain better men at the same salary for these offices than employment by local insuring agencies on a contract basis, with the liability that the contract may not be renewed on its termination. Furthermore, organized into a State corps with central control and direction, with a strong *esprit de corps,* there would be developed a health machine protecting every home, consisting of men trained to see unhygienic conditions, with a vision for the total environment, and clothed with all the present powers of the health department to look into conditions that are liable to cause disease, and with such influence as the prestige of State appointment may give to their opinions and acts.

Public Health Reports
April 18, 1919

2

Group Medicine or Health Insurance: Which Comes First?[1]

EDGAR SYDENSTRICKER

There are about enough doctors, nurses, and others who render or assist in rendering medical services—about a million persons all told—to take care of all illness and to do nearly all the preventive work for individual patients that we now know how to do. There is being spent annually by the American people enough money —about three and a half billion dollars—for doctors, nurses, medicines, and all sorts of medical services, good and bad, to purchase reasonably adequate medical care at current average prices.

Yet in a year's time—even in a prosperous era—thousands upon thousands of families cannot afford to obtain any medical care; millions upon millions of cases of sickness which ought to have medical attention are unattended; less than 7 per cent of the population have even a partial physical examination and less than 5 per cent are immunized against some disease; much preventable sickness occurs; and the death rate among adults of middle age is increasing. Although medical science is still far from having solved all the mysteries of ill health, only a little of the knowledge already gained is applied to *all* the people needing it. A large proportion of doctors and others who apply this knowledge do not receive an adequate or even a decent living income and, with a

[1]Address at the Twenty-seventh Annual Meeting, American Association for Labor Legislation, at Philadelphia, December 27, 1933.

deep sense of social duty, render much medical service without any direct remuneration.

In so stating the problem of medical care, certain objectives are assumed to be socially sound. And if they are sound, they may be regarded as postulates for any satisfactory program of action. They are:

1) Medical care should be provided to all who need it. It is assumed that such medical care is necessary to the maintenance of the health of the people and, conversely, if it is not so provided, the health of the people is not being maintained to the extent that we now know how to maintain it.

2) It is assumed (a) that the medical care of indigent and dependent sick is an obligation of society to be discharged either through official or philanthropic agencies or both; (b) that the institutional care of the mentally diseased, the tuberculous, and possibly other diseased persons is a concern of society; and (c) that measures for the control of communicable diseases are public functions.

3) Those who render medical services should be adequately and promptly paid. It is assumed that medical care cannot be rendered efficiently without proper compensation, and it is clearly shown by the facts that much care is not paid for at all and a large proportion of those who render it are underpaid.

Since we are practical minded, two further postulates may be added, namely:

4) Any program of action to be given serious consideration at present should assume the continuance of the economic system under which we now live—a system that is characterized by a grossly unequal distribution of wealth and of ability to pay for the essentials or the luxuries of life. Obviously, such an assumption does not preclude a course of action that may be followed by some other nation existing under an entirely different economic system. We can have even a better socialization of water supply than the U.S.S.R. or a more commonsense individualism in hygiene than China without being either communistic or ancient.

5) Any arrangement for medical services which may seem advisable for the attainment of the objectives implied in the

foregoing statements should interfere as little as possible with the conditions of private practice as they actually exist in the United States, whether they be economic or professional.

These, then, are some of the conditions under which the problem must be met. Many proposals have been made, but the principal suggested approaches to a solution may be summarized as follows:

1) The further commercial organization of medicine and medical services along lines similar to those in which public utilities and railroads have been developed, namely, mass production and distribution at prices regulated by the public.

2) Conversion of all medical services into a governmental function, either by the gradual development of public medical services along lines already fairly well established, or by some rather revolutionary action. In either case, it would mean that all those who render these services would be employed by the public and that all institutions and facilities for such services would be owned and operated by the public.

3) The gradual organization of medical practice along the lines of "group medicine" that already have been somewhat clearly developed in our urban centers, in order to lower costs and render medical care more easily available.

4) Application of the well-tried principle of compulsory insurance on a state-wide or on a nation-wide basis. This would involve governmental control and operation of health insurance, contracts with physicians and allied medical institutions, contributions from all insured persons and from employers, and a close coordination of the provisions for medical care with public health functions.

There seems to be a general unanimity against any approach to the solution in the first direction mentioned above, namely, the mass organization of medicine. It is safe to say that any solution of this nature would be unsatisfactory and repugnant to the medical profession in spite of the fact that the profession itself is composed of individual entrepreneurs who render services for profit. A more cogent objection is that the real economic problem would not be met for the simple reason that a large majority of the population are unable to pay for adequate services at any reasonable cost unless they have accumulated sufficient reserve funds. Furthermore, business methods have so far failed signally in solving other problems of rendering services on a universal scale.

The solution proposed in the second direction, public medicine, is regarded as repugnant by many and as impractical by others. It is, in effect, being tried in Russia, and although some think that ultimately it may be the wisest solution, it is obvious that it would not be possible for a long time in the United States. The fact that certain types of medical services are being slowly assumed by the public in this country because they are too expensive or because they have for their primary purpose the control of infectious diseases, does not, I think, give us any warrant for concluding that "state medicine" or complete public medical service, is a feasible solution.

However that may be, our discussion is concerned with the two last proposals which we may now examine in more detail.

The concept of group medicine as placed before the public has been defined briefly in the recommendation of the Committee on the Costs of Medical Care which reads as follows:

> "The Committee recommends that medical service, both preventive and therapeutic, should be furnished largely by organized groups of physicians, dentists, nurses, pharmacists, and other associated personnel. Such groups should be organized, preferably around a hospital, for rendering complete home, office, and hospital care. The form of organization should encourage the maintenance of high standards and the development or preservation of a personal relationship between patient and physician."

The Committee understood that by an "organized group," it meant a "group which is so organized that each professional person in it is responsible to the group for the quality of his work rather than solely to himself." A number of suggestions were made but the principal one was that of community medical centers. "The keystone of the concept of a satisfactory medical service for the nation," said the Committee, "is the development of one or more non-profit 'community medical centers' in nearly every city of approximately 15,000 population or more."[1]

This concept of group medicine was based upon careful studies of medical practice in different parts of the United States, of the trend toward specialism, and of specific developments of group medicine in many localities. The principal objections to the idea of group medicine as thus visualized was that a "medical hierarchy" would be established in every community; that the "continuance of the personal relationship of the physician and patient would not be possible"; and that the proposal was not only "far-fetched and visionary" but had "no practical relationship to the question the Committee set itself to solve." The report submitted by a minority of the Committee somewhat contemptuously said that "it seems to [them] an illustration of what is almost an obsession with many people, namely that 'organization' can cure most if not all human ills."

It is only fair to point out that the first two of these objections are against details of the specified type of organization proposed rather than against the essential principle of group medicine. In fact, "group medicine" is a term often misinterpreted by some to involve the doing away with the responsibility of the individual physician for the welfare of the patient, and that it sets up a group responsibility instead. This, as I understand it, was not in the minds of any member of the Committee. On the contrary, it was definitely proposed that in every medical center, a physician, preferably a general practitioner, would be responsible for the

[1]The Committee's report described such a center in the following words: "This center would include a well-equipped general hospital, an out-patient department, and pharmacy. It would provide offices for physicians, dentists, technicians, and subsidiary personnel, and headquarters for nurses. All facilities necessary for the practice of modern scientific medicine would be available, such as X-ray, laboratory, and physiotherapy equipment, and a well-stocked library. In large communities there would doubtless be several medical centers. The number of persons served by each center might vary widely and each might have branches at various convenient places. In communities with only one center, the headquarters of the voluntary health agencies of the medical, dental and nursing societies, and perhaps of the public health department might be located there."

care and treatment of each of its patients. The grouping of physicians, spatially and professionally, was intended to cut down
overhead costs, to increase physical and mechanical facilities for
diagnosis and treatment, and make more easily available the services of the best qualified specialists in each community as well as
improve medical practice in other ways. Experience with organized medical service shows that there is no necessary incom-
patibility between integration of services and retention of desirable, non-financial personal relations between doctor and patient.

The third objection appears to be cogent, namely, that group
medicine *per se* does not solve the practical question at issue. It is
a method of providing better medical care at lower cost to be
attained gradually and by voluntary means. Group medicine does
not meet the "heart of the problem" which, as the Committee
itself defined it, "is the equalizing of the financial impact of
sickness."

What the majority of the Committee on the Costs of Medical
Care had in mind was a sort of ideal procedure. They did recommend voluntary systems of group payment; but they emphasized
as the *first step*, the use of organized, efficient group practice.
Then, when the organization of medical service would have progressed to the point where it would be possible to guarantee the
quality and sufficiency of service, the voluntary system should be
made compulsory. But this is clearly a counsel of perfection.

One may pertinently ask: What is to encourage the rapid and
effective organization of medical facilities? Certainly there is no
ground in recent experience to warrant the view that the desired
objective will be reached by waiting upon the experiments now in
progress. There is at least as much likelihood that the current of
events will lead to the predominance of exploited contract practice as that it will entrench desirable forms of voluntary insurance.
Commitment to voluntary schemes holds no promise that it will
bring us to that threshold which would warrant the establishment
of a compulsory scheme. The reorganization of medical practice
which is badly needed will not come of itself, the product of
laissez faire. It will come — if at all — only as the fruit of strong and
directed labors, the product of compelling forces.

Now, of all the forces which society can muster in a program of medical reformation, the strongest is "the power of the purse." Thus, the case is inverted. Instead of organizing for the payment of medical costs *after* we have effected organization of service, it seems commonsense to say that we must *first* provide for payment *in order to effect organization of service.*

The type of health insurance that is adopted in the United States is, however, of utmost importance. The misuse of a device for distributing costs may defeat the very purposes for which it is designed. It is essential, therefore, that certain considerations be kept in mind. I should like to present briefly, for discussion, some of these considerations of health insurance in addition to those already presented:

1) Quality of medical care should not be sacrificed to economy in costs. Free choice of physician and other means to this end are assumed to be essential.

2) Group payment should be planned for a large population and preferably on a state-wide basis because of the need for actuarial stability and for administrative coordination with existing public health and public welfare facilities.

3) The plan should be compulsory.

4) The insurance for, and the provision of, medical care should be divorced from cash benefits for wage loss or other purposes (except perhaps to remunerate employed women for wage loss preceding and following confinement and except for low income families when the lack of even small cash resources interferes with the effectiveness of medical care).

5) The plan should not include proprietary or profit-making agencies.

6) There should be no independent intermediary between the potential patient and the medical agencies.

7) Administrative procedures should be determined by the joint action of professional and lay groups, and the plan should provide for the professional administration of professional personnel and activities.

8) The plan should provide opportunity for diverse arrangements in the provision of medical care, depending upon local

conditions in respect to availability of facilities and ability to pay
for medical care, except (a) that the care provided should, so far as
possible, cover complete home, office, and hospital service including necessary health examinations; (b) that economy should
be assured by proper organization of the practitioners and agencies furnishing service; and (c) that the quality of service rendered
should be insured, so far as it can be insured, by the joint professional responsibility of the groups of practitioners rendering the
service.

9) The plan should provide for maximum integration of the
medical provisions with public health and other governmental
authorities engaged in medical activities.

Of even greater importance than any of the foregoing, however, is the scope of health insurance. Shall it be restricted—as in
most foreign countries—to those who earn small wages? Or shall
it be extended to a larger portion of the population? The first
objective, it must be remembered, is to provide a system of distributing costs so that those who are ordinarily self-sustaining in
other matters are enabled, by fixed periodic payments, to assure
themselves of reasonably adequate medical care and to protect
themselves against the financial burdens of unusual medical
needs.

An analysis of this point, taking into account the size of medical costs, the normal variations in these costs, and the relation of
these costs to the budgets of families with various incomes, com-
pels the conclusion that the *family* rather than the individual or
the wage-earner should be taken as the primary unit. Furthermore, if the quality of care is to be high and practitioners are to be
adequately remunerated, and if health insurance is to be really a
health measure, it becomes necessary to embrace more than the
lowest income classes and it is highly desirable to include the
self-employed as well. We ought not to seek—and the professions
should not tolerate—in the United States the "poor-man's" health
insurance common in foreign countries.

In this discussion we are concerned with the advantages and
disadvantages of two apparently contrasting courses of social ac-

tion. We have, in effect, been asked to choose between an evolutionary policy and a program of definite action; between voluntary efforts to develop facilities for medical care through group practice and a business-like application of a well-tried method of distributing costs over that part of the population which is now unable to budget medical costs; between a plan which essentially is aimed at the *improvement* of medical care, and a program which has for its aim the *provision* of medical care.

Now the opposition between these two proposals really lies *in the choice of which to do first*. For obviously they are not antithetical; on the contrary, they are and should be complementary. A system of health insurance, if efficiently and effectively established with the cooperation of the public and the professions, should bring an increased total expenditure for medical care with a simultaneous elimination of the burdens of variable costs; provide an increased and more stable financial support of practitioners and institutions; contribute to improvements in the quality of medical practice; result in a vast increase in the public receipt of medical service and a concurrent reduction in the use of cultists and quacks and in the consumption of nostrums; extend the practice of preventive mddicine; and aid the development of group medicine, if that be found efficient.

The American Labor Legislation Review
June, 1934

3

Health Insurance and the Public Health

EDGAR SYDENSTRICKER

Health insurance, although an accepted governmental procedure in most modern nations, is now so controversial a subject in this country that I may be pardoned, perhaps, for confessing to a certain degree of wariness since I have found that the subject has not been discussed without some degree of heat and unreason. In this audience of academicians, however, I am less uneasy on this score, although I am not learned in the field of political science. Furthermore, I shall be obliged to impose upon myself the limitation that I am not at liberty to discuss at this time the results of the studies of health insurance which I was requested by the Committee on Economic Security to conduct in connection with the President's program for economic security. These results as well as proposals from other sources are now before the committee for consideration. Whatever views I express are, of course, upon my own responsibility and must not be interpreted as reflecting the attitude of any organization with which I happen to be connected.

I

I would like to approach the subject of health insurance primarily from the viewpoint of its possible use as a means of health conservation rather than that of economic security, although the two are necessarily interrelated. Health insurance, as the term is commonly used, is a method of distributing among population groups and over periods of time two kinds of financial burdens resulting from illness: 1) loss of wages due to temporary disability; and 2) the costs of medical care. One enables the insured person to prevent the standard of living of himself and his family from being too seriously lowered or from reaching zero during his illness; the other enables him to have medical care when he or a member of his family is ill and, incidentally, enables those who render care to be paid and to be paid promptly. In so far as the method of insurance actually will assure medical care of good quality to persons with modest and low incomes who cannot now receive it without sacrificing other necessities of life or without begging for it, it properly can be regarded as a direct public health measure.

The concept of public health which we are gradually coming to accept is much broader than what is now usually connoted by the term. Whether the general welfare clause of the Federal Constitution be interpreted strictly as the power to levy taxes for the welfare of the people or more loosely as the power to promote the welfare of the people in any way possible, it has always been and still is generally held that society is responsible for the health of all its members. At first this responsibility was limited to community conditions such as sanitation, pure water and food, and the control of infectious diseases. In recent years this responsibility has been gradually broadened to include the early diagnosis of certain diseases and impairments, the prevention of infant and maternal mortality, the promotion of child health, the education of individuals in the principles of personal hygiene and the medical care of persons afflicted with mental disorders, cancer, orthopedic defects and certain other diseases. The general medical care of the indigent has long been assumed to be a public responsibility, although only poorly discharged. In New York State, for example, the Welfare Law definitely says that, "the public welfare district shall be responsible for providing necessary medical care for persons under its care and for such other persons otherwise able to maintain themselves who are unable to secure medical care." The newer concept is much broader. Society has a basic responsibility (in addition to functions already being exercised) for assuring, so far as it can, to all of its members, healthful conditions of housing and living, a reasonable degree of economic security, proper facilities for curative and preventive medicine and adequate medical care—in fact the control (so far as means are known to science) of all of the environmental factors that affect physical and mental well-being. Such a concept in no way postulates any particular form of government nor does it prescribe any specific method. There is no reason why society cannot discharge this responsibility under any form of government in which it can express its will. Although the older public health functions have been and are exercised, more or less, under the police power of the community, many of the newer measures for the maintenance of health are, to a certain extent, carried on by voluntary organizations, by private practitioners of medicine, and by various combinations of public functions with the activities of private organizations and individuals.

Quite aside from these rather theoretical considerations, however, is a very practical reason for regarding medical care as an essential part or complement of society's efforts to conserve health. Experience has shown that the effectiveness of a specific public health procedure is in direct ratio to the amount of efficient medical or other service actually rendered. Sanitation for an entire community is not possible until the community itself provides facilities for sewage disposal. A safe water supply is generally impossible for a community until community water-purification plants are provided. The control of smallpox and diphtheria, for example, has been found to be impractical unless vaccination or immunization actually is accomplished. Public health agencies are beginning to realize that it is uneconomical for a public health nurse, for example, to educate an expectant mother in a family with low income in the principles and practice of maternal hygiene unless medical and nursing facilities are provided for her during prenatal, delivery and post-partum periods. To put it bluntly, society's responsibility for the health of its members cannot be discharged until and unless medical services and facilities are made available to the entire population. This does not mean "socialized", "sovietized", or "state" medicine. It does mean that medical care is a necessity of life to the individual and care is essential to national well-being.

II

I do not suppose that it is necessary for me to discuss before such an audience as this the present situation as regards health and medical care. I think we all realize that notwithstanding great advances in medicine and public health protection, the American people are not so healthy as they have a right to be. Millions of persons are suffering from diseases and annually thousands upon thousands die from causes that are preventable through the use of existing scientific knowledge. Numerous inquiries have shown that there is a direct correlation between low income and high mortality and high morbidity. Carefully conducted studies of considerable samples of our population have proved beyond doubt that a large porportion of families cannot afford to obtain medical care and that hundreds of thousands of cases of sickness needing medical attention are unattended. These are sweeping statements. They have been challenged by some who are under the impression that because individual physicians render medical care to the poor who call upon them, it is therefore to be had. Many physicians, social workers and nurses are daily aware of the actual situation and competent students have established the accuracy of the statements regarding it.

Now, if we grant that medical care is a necessity of life and of national well-being, and if we are aware of the fact that a large proportion of the population is deprived of this necessity, we are confronted with the serious question of how those who need medical care can be assured of it. It is not an easy question to answer. It involves the choice of the methods that are or will be most effective under the existing economic system, the existing organization of medicine, without forcing radical changes in our habits or violating too seriously our traditions. This is, I admit, a pragmatic approach and assumes the superiority of evolution over revolution; it is much easier to plan revolutions than to appraise correctly the conditions under which social evolution is proceeding and to benefit from the process. Medical care is an economic as well as a social service. Most of it is on sale. A minority of the public can purchase it without financial difficulty. Another minority must beg for it. The majority can purchase it only when it is urgently needed. Four-fifths or more of the producers of this service are professionally and expensively trained persons who, within certain legal restrictions and self-imposed limitations, are engaged as entrepreneurs for profit and in rendering a social service as well. We must assume that for a while, at least, some of the population will be poorer than their neighbors. We assume also that any arrangement for medical services which may seem advisable should interfere as little as possible with the conditions of medical practice as they have been developed in the United States.

III

The choice of the method or methods best suited to a solution of the problem may be approached in several ways.

One way, of course, is by definition not even an approach since it proposes no definite or planned action but trusts to a process of trial and error or, at most, to more or less casual experimentation. Another approach might be through the commercial organization of medicine and medical services on a large scale. I think it is safe to say that any solution of this nature would be unsatisfactory and repugnant to the medical profession. It would be ineffective because the real economic problem would not be met; for even if medical care could be sold according to department store methods, a large proportion of the moderate- and low-income families could not afford to buy it. A third approach is to make all medical services governmental functions either by the gradual development of public medical services along lines already fairly well established, or by some revolutionary action. This approach is through the method of "state medicine" in its complete form and would result in the socialized practice of medicine in the same way that the postal service or public education is socialized. It is regarded by many as unwise, impracticable and destructive of quality of service. I hold no brief for it.

The fourth approach is through the application of the principle of insurance. It is significant, I think, that all efforts to find a solution are actually based upon the principle of distributing the costs of medical care, as well as loss of wages due to sickness, among members of a group or over a period of time, or both. For example, many physicians employ a sliding scale of charges in order that the rich may aid in paying for charity practice. Some commercial organizations for the sale of medical services are being tried in some sections of the United States. Various voluntary schemes of health insurance have long been in operation among various groups in this country. Agencies are being formed for the payment of medical bills on the installment plan; group hospitalization for the insurance of hospital costs is finding favor in many communities; industrial establishments are providing medical care to the workers and in some instances to their families as well, either on a compulsory or on a voluntary basis; more commercial insurance companies are already considering the provision of medical care as one of the benefits of group sickness insurance. In a few places, county medical societies have organized service bureaus to adjust the medical fees charged to the worthy poor. In the Pacific Northwest there has been an important development of medical service bureaus which apply the principle of insurance to medical care provided under the auspices of the medical society. And, as you all know, health or sickness insurance has been in vogue in Europe, in Great Britain and in Japan for varying periods of time. Whether a solution based on the insurance principle is fully adequate or not, it is a significant fact that not a single country which has adopted health insurance has ever thrown it aside—though each country which has practised health insurance has from time to time made changes in the plan, its coverage and its operation.

In this country, the question of health insurance has again come to the fore after a lapse of nearly twenty years. Bills have been introduced in a number of states. The President's Economic Security Committee was charged with the study of health insurance as a measure of meeting the risks to economic security arising out of ill health. Since health insurance must involve the physician, the medical press has given much attention to the discussion of health insurance. The non-medical press and periodicals have discussed the pros and cons of various proposals.

IV

As I have said, I cannot, of course, discuss at this time the results of the studies made under the auspices of the President's Committee. Perhaps I may suggest for your consideration, however, some general conclusions to which I have been led by my own studies. I am not, on this occasion, presenting any argument for health insurance, but *if* insurance against the costs of medical care and insurance against loss of wages resulting from illness are to be adopted in this country, I suggest that at least the following propositions should be given serious attention:

1. The two types of insurance—insurance against loss of wages resulting from illness and insurance against the costs of medical care—should be regarded as separate and distinct. One is a form of unemployment insurance although it differs from insurance against unemployment from other causes in that its actuarial basis is easily established and no large reserves are necessary. It may be pointed out, however, that the principal reason for the separation of the two forms of insurance is an administrative one, namely, that the physician who certifies the disability of the insured person in order to draw cash benefits should not be the attending physician nor a physician who competes with private practitioners.

2. If a national system of insurance against the costs of medical care is the ultimate goal, it should be of the federal-state permissive type and should be so designed as to allow each state the greatest possible latitude in shaping the pattern of its system in order to draw a modest federal subsidy. The federal subsidy should be sufficiently large to encourage sound standards of administration and of protection for the medical profession. The states should, as far as possible, decide the populations to be covered and the kinds of medical services to be included. These proposals seem to me to be wise because existing facilities for medical care, the size of the easily insurable population groups,

medical traditions and practices, and economic and social conditions differ widely in various sections. They are wise, also, because as states come into a federal-state system, if they do, they will come slowly and thus provide a period of greatly needed experimentation.

3. *For the groups to be covered,* insurance against the costs of medical care should be compulsory. All European experience points to this conclusion. As an individualist, I bow to the necessity of compulsion only when it is the last resort in efforts for social betterment. I shall await with interest, therefore, the results of the many experiments now going on in this country. If voluntary insurance can be proved successful, I shall be among the first to rejoice.

4. As to the scope of insurance against the costs of medical care, it has been proposed that the family rather than the employed individual should be the unit. This proposal is obviously in the interest of making medical care available to a larger proportion of the population. Furthermore, it has been proposed that the insured families should not be restricted to the lowest income classes. Most of the European systems are inadequate in this respect. Granting that the indigent and dependent fractions of the population must be furnished medical care by the public in any case, most of the European systems make no provision for the great bulk of the population which is otherwise self-supporting but which cannot purchase adequate medical care on a fee-for-service basis. Medical benefits furnished under such "poor man's" systems, limited as they are by inadequate financial resources, obviously cannot be adequate in quality or sufficient in volume or variety and cannot furnish a decent income to the practitioner or the institution. It has been estimated that if the coverage is sufficiently broad to include income groups which, taken as a whole, can afford the costs of good medical care, the average costs will not greatly exceed, under insurance, what is now being spent by the average family within this group.

5. Proper provision should be made to safeguard the quality of medical service and to maintain the advantages of private medical practice. We must, I believe, postulate responsibility to the medi-

cal profession in respect to the control of professional personnel and practices and the supervision of professional service. Complete exclusion of proprietary and profit-making agencies and of intermediaries between the practitioner and the potential patient should be a basic principle. Physicians should be free to engage in insurance practice or not, as they please. Insured persons should be free to choose their physician from among all practitioners who engage in insurance practice, and the insurance practitioner should be free to accept or reject insured persons as potential patients. Furthermore, the physician who chooses to engage in insurance practice should be free to engage in private or non-insurance practice. The system of payment for professional services should be sufficiently flexible to provide for payment on a fee, salary or capitation basis, in accordance with the conditions of a given locality or the type of medical service, and the form of payment should be chosen by the practitioners of a given locality or district. The scope of medical services should include at least home and domiciliary care from the general practitioner, specialized services when needed in the home, office, clinic or hospital, and hospital, clinic and laboratory services. In addition, wherever possible, the services should include essential dental services, nursing service in the home when such service is necessary, and possibly expensive medicines and appliances when prescribed by the physician.

V

It should be kept in mind, however, that even if insurance against loss of wages resulting from illness and insurance against the costs of medical care are developed, either through the adoption of a federal-state permissive system, or by a state compulsory system, or by voluntary systems, these measures alone cannot discharge the full responsibility of society for the maintenance of public health. Insurance will be no panacea. At best it can be only a part of society's efforts to conserve health if integrated into a statesmanlike program. Other parts of such a program are important. The further extension of public health services, through larger appropriations, is absolutely necessary in order that every locality be provided with community facilities. I am happy to say that this recommendation of the Committee on Economic Security was approved by the President and placed before Congress in the pending economic security bill. In addition, adequate hospitals, laboratories and clinic facilities should be provided to the many localities, for the most part rural, now lacking them. Furthermore, the medical care of the dependent sick, although thoroughly established as a governmental procedure in communities before the present depression, and greatly developed by the use of federal relief funds for medical care, is a component part of an adequate plan for conserving health. The provision of medical care from public funds for persons afflicted with tuberculosis, mental diseases and other diseases which have a community interest is essential. All these are matters of not only professional interest to those who render medical and health services but are the concern of the public. For, as Disraeli said some generations ago: "The Public Health is the foundation upon which rests the happiness of the people and the welfare of the nation. The care of the public health is the first duty of the Statesman."

4

Health Under the Social Security Act

EDGAR SYDENSTRICKER

I

The scope of the inquiries conducted by the Committee on Economic Security in the field of health was undoubtedly broader than any study of the subject ever before made by a national body which had for its primary purpose the formulation of a social security program. Although the Committee undoubtedly recognized that any measure which renders the wage-earning family more stable would indirectly contribute to lessening sickness as well as aid in meeting the costs of sickness, it also considered more direct measures. Among these were methods of distributing loss of wages due to temporary disability and invalidism and of distributing costs of medical services, provision of more adequate tax-supported medical services and facilities, and the extension of public health measures. There were sound reasons for the broad scope of the Committee's interest in this field. When the Committee first began its work, health insurance was designated as the principal topic for inquiry on the general ground that health insurance is almost universally included in other modern countries as a form of social insurance. But soon after the technical staff, to which the subject of health was specifically assigned, got to work, it was realized that health insurance was only one method by which certain risks to economic security might be lessened. It was

146

pointed out that ill health itself is a risk to economic security. It soon became obvious, therefore, that risks to economic security arising out of ill health could not be dealt with adequately unless problems of the national health and of the health of under-privileged individuals and their families were considered in as comprehensive way as the time allotted for the study would permit.

In thus surveying the entire problem of health in relation to economic security, the Committee on Economic Security, in a sense, followed the example of the National Conservation Commission under President Theodore Roosevelt. This Commission, it will be recalled, surveyed the problem of health protection as an integral part of the larger question of the conservation of national resources, and produced a memorable report entitled *Report on National Vitality: Its Wastes and Conservation*.[1] This document undoubtedly served to call attention to the need for national action in health conservation, as did the White House Conferences on Child Health in later years under President Hoover. But none of these efforts resulted in a definite national program backed by federal appropriations.

II

During the quarter of a century since the *Report on National Vitality* was published, extraordinary advances in medicine and in community health protection were made, although the national government continued to give niggardly support to medical science and public health measures. In pointing with just pride to the accomplishments of medicine and public health, physicians and sanitarians too frequently overlook failures in the wider application of scientific knowledge in all communities. The fact is, as all students of the subject know, that preventable sicknesses and premature deaths still impose a tremendous and unwarranted

[1]Professor Irving Fisher, *Report on National Vitality: Its Wastes and Conservation* (Bull. 30 of the Committee of One Hundred on National Health, prepared for the National Conservation Commission; Washington: Government Printing Office, 1909).

burden upon industry, still needlessly mar the happiness of hundreds of thousands of homes, still handicap millions of children, and still cause a frightful waste of human vitality.

The Committee on Economic Security[2] properly gave emphasis to the gigantic annual money loss in wages caused by sickness in families with small and modest incomes in the United States, which is estimated to be not less than nine hundred million dollars, and to the still larger expenses of medical care, which probably are not less than one and a half billion dollars. These are only the direct costs. The much larger costs of depreciation in capital values of human life are incalculable. Even the direct costs could be borne if they were distributed equally, but they are not. It was pointed out, also, that among an average 1,000,000 persons in the United States, there will occur annually between 800,000 and 900,000 cases of illness. It may be predicted for this average 1,000,000 persons that, though 470,000 will not be sick during a normal year, 460,000 will be sick once or twice, and 70,000 will suffer three or more illnesses. Of those who become ill, one-fourth will be disabled for periods varying from one week to an entire year.

Science has not yet given us the means with which to prevent all of this sickness or to enable everyone to live healthfully until the end of the natural span is reached. But, as I have tried to emphasize in an earlier paper,[3] the plain fact must be faced that, notwithstanding great advances in medicine and public health protection, the American people are not so healthy as they have a right to be. Millions of them are suffering from diseases, and over a hundred thousand die annually from causes that are preventable through the use of existing scientific knowledge and the application of common social sense. Ample evidence exists to support this sweeping statement.

The ravages of typhoid fever, diphtheria, and smallpox have been enormously lessened; they ought to be and can be eradi-

[2]*Report to the President of the Committee on Economic Security, January 15, 1935* (Washington: Government Printing Office).

[3]"Health in the New Deal," *Annals of the American Academy of Political and Social Science*, November, 1934.

cated. The infant death-rate has been cut in half in the last quarter-century, but it can again be cut in half. Mortality from tuberculosis has been reduced by 60 per cent since 1900, and could be halved again. Two-thirds of the annual thirteen thousand maternal deaths are unnecessary. At least three-fourths of a million cases of syphilis are clinically recognized annually; but more than half of these do not obtain treatment at that stage of the disease when the possibility of cure is greatest. We have been rather vociferous in recent years over the health and welfare of children; yet it is estimated that three hundred thousand are crippled, a million or more are tuberculous, and nearly half a million have heart damages or defects.

The mortality of adults of middle or older ages has not appreciably diminished. The expectation of length of life at forty is about the same now as it was in 1850, 1890, or 1900. The mortality of adults who should be in their physical prime—twenty to forty-four years of age—is almost as great as that of the younger group, which includes babies and children. The mortality of persons who ought to be in full mental vigor and still capable of many kinds of physical work is over three times that of the younger adults. In the young adult ages, twenty to thirty-four years, tuberculosis still tops the list as a disease; accidents and homicides snuff out about one life in a thousand annually; organic heart disease appears in even this young age period as the third most important cause of death. All careful studies of illness and physical impairments corroborate these ghastly records; in fact, they reveal even more impressively than mortality statistics the extent to which the vitality of the population is damaged in the most efficient period of life. This disconcerting evidence of impaired efficiency among our adult population takes on a graver significance in view of the changing age of our adult population.

Such facts as the foregoing cannot easily be overlooked in the formulation of any sensible program for economic security. If a simple analysis is made of the problem for practical purposes, the principal risks to economic security arising out of ill health may be classified as follows: 1) loss of efficiency and health itself, and, thus, loss or impairment of the capacity to be employed; 2) loss of

earnings resulting from disabling illness among gainfully employed persons; 3) cost of medical care to gainfully employed
persons and their families.

No single method of attacking all these risks has as yet been
devised. It has been argued by some that greater economic security for families with modest and low incomes, through unemployment compensation, old-age annuities, wage increases,
stabilization of employment, or other means, will solve the question. We know, however, that even if everyone had what Dr.
Townsend* proposes for persons over sixty years of age, many
could not bear the expenses of serious illness—if the physician is
to be adequately paid and the hospital kept out of debt. Slum
clearance and effective housing programs; the better distribution
of the so-called supplementary food supplies and the application
of the newer knowledge of nutrition through education; the extension of facilities for physical training, recreation, and education in hygiene; sound methods of "population control"—all
these are desirable ways in which to aid in health conservation
but, even taken all together, do not constitute a completely effective attack upon the problem. In addition to these indirect approaches, it was clear that the Committee on Economic Security
had in mind the formulation of a more direct program.

In the consideration of such a more direct program, however,
the student of the problem is faced with a legion of proposals, a
bewildering variety of methods that have been tried in our own
country as well as abroad, a conflict in opinions and a confusion in
thought among those who might be affected. Space does not
permit even a brief presentation of these differences. Broadly
speaking, the various measures which have actually been employed with some degree of success are generally recognized as
falling into three groups, namely:

1. The reduction of sickness and the promotion of mental and

*[Dr. Francis W. Townsend (1867–1960) proposed a pension plan by which
every person over age 60 would receive $200 per month from Federal funds with
the requirement that it be spent within the month. The Townsend Plan received
wide attention and extensive popular support, but a bill for its enactment was
defeated in the House of Representatives. ED.]

bodily vigor through community or organized preventive methods of proven effectiveness. These are essentially public health services.

2. The provision through government funds of certain kinds of public medical services to the entire population, and of general medical services to indigent and dependent individuals and families.

3. The distribution of income loss due to illness and of the costs of medical care over periods of time and among groups of individuals of that fraction of the population which is financially unable to budget individually against such costs. This procedure is ordinarily termed "health" or "sickness" insurance.

It was along these general lines that the Committee's staff proceded and, aided by several technical groups of advisers, made a series of recommendations for the Committee's consideration.

III

Of the Committee's recommendations, only those in the field of public health and a few specific ones in the extension of medical services and facilities aided by public relief and works funds have been carried into effect.

As regards public health, the Committee's report to the President said:

It has long been recognized that the Federal, State, and local Governments all have responsibilities for the protection of all of the population against disease. The Federal Government has recognized its responsibility in this respect in the public-health activities of several of its departments. There are also well-established precedents for Federal aid for State health administration and for local public facilities, and for the loan of technical personnel to States and localities. What we recommend involves no departure from previous practices, but an extension of policies that have long been followed and are of proven worth. What is contemplated is a Nation-wide public-health program, financially and technically aided by

the Federal Government, but supported and administered by
the State and local health departments.

Under this general recommendation the Committee proposed
that the appropriations to the Federal Public Health Service and
the Federal Children's Bureau be increased for federal public
health work and that federal grants-in-aid to states be made for the
extension of health protection in localities unable to finance public health programs, the grants to be allocated by the two federal
services. These proposals were embodied in President
Roosevelt's message to Congress in which he transmitted the
report of the Committee on Economic Security, and appropriations totaling $13,800,000[4] were later authorized under the Social
Security Act of August 14, 1935. These provisions constitute probably the greatest single step forward in the development of a
national public health program that has ever been taken. As Dr.
E. L. Bishop, in his presidential address at the 1935 meeting of the
American Public Health Association, said, "Passage of the Social
Security Act by the last Congress presents the public health profession of this country with the greatest opportunity to establish
constructive programs of health service that has been given to any
group in our history."

IV

The provision of medical care of certain kinds to the community, as well as to those groups of individuals who, for one reason or
another, are unable to obtain medical care except as charity patients of generous physicians, has long been established in tax-
supported medical services. It has been estimated that these services amounted to something like $600,000,000 annually before
the depression. The services have included more or less general
medical care for persons who are without incomes and for whom
some government unit has assumed economic responsibility. It
included, also, some medical care, particularly hospital services,

[4]In addition, $4,350,000 was authorized for crippled children and child wel-
fare.

for individuals ordinarily self-sustaining who could not, because of insufficient income, meet the so-called catastrophic medical expenses at the time of illness. In addition, institutional care for certain conditions, especially mental disease and tuberculosis, for practically the entire population is a long-recognized practice in this country. The care for certain diseases of public health interest, for example, syphilis and certain other communicable diseases, and diseases of crippled children, is thoroughly recognized. It is a well-known fact, however, that these services are extremely uneven in their distribution. Many communities do not possess facilities for the diagnosis and treatment of diseases which have a definite public health interest. Recent surveys have shown that some rural areas are without any physicians. Other studies have brought to light the fact that in many communities a large proportion of persons with little or no incomes are unable to receive any medical care whatsoever.

Such problems as these obviously could not be met by any scheme of contributory health insurance. They are too large to be adequately dealt with through private philanthropy. Whether they should be regarded as purely local problems is a debated question; the fact is that they have not been solved satisfactorily in a very large number of local communities. Upon the broad assumption that national health is of national concern, the federal government has a definite responsibility for aiding in the solution of these local problems as well as in the task of disease prevention.

Under existing legislation, both of an emergency and of a more permanent character, it would seem that many of these problems should be dealt with by the co-operation of federal, state, and local governments. In many communities there is a distinct lack of hospital beds for mental disease and tuberculosis; and several hundred rural areas are without any hospital facilities. Some localities have been aided by the federal public works program. In areas where there are no physicians, or an insufficient number of physicians and other medical facilities, it would appear that federal assistance is as necessary as in the provision of public health facilities. The provision of medical care for individuals on federal relief was definitely recognized by the relief administration; yet no provision has been made for medical care of persons on work relief, although such persons are obviously not in a position to pay for it and hospitals in many localities are overburdened with indigent persons or persons on relief and work relief.

All these needs constitute a problem of national magnitude, which is more serious in some sections of the country than in others. It has never been fully met by any well-conceived program of the federal government. The recommendations of the Committee on Economic Security as regards this problem have as yet not been made public.

V

There is a wide divergence of opinion as to the best methods of obtaining a better distribution of medical care among those who are not economically dependent but who are unable to provide against risks to security arising out of sickness. There are still a few who are satisfied with the *status quo*. Others take the view that before any state-wide and national plan is considered, local experimentation with various ways of paying for medical care should be carried on. Some of these experiments have been in operation for some time, and new ones are being started. This is an encouraging sign of a growing consciousness of the situation on the part of the medical profession and of the public. Other proposals involve programs on a larger scale. One recently made is that all persons participating in the old-age annuity plan and unemployment compensation under the Economic Security Act and all others having annual incomes of less than $2,500 should be given "public care for costly illness," including facilities for accurate diagnosis, obstetrical care, hospital care, home nursing, and the treatment of chronic diseases. Various forms of health insurance frequently have been proposed; and, as pointed out in the report to the President by the Committee on Economic Security, the subject of health insurance was under consideration by its staff as well as by the Committee itself. The Committee said:

> We are not prepared at this time to make recommendations for a system of health insurance. We have enlisted the cooperation of advisory groups representing the medical and

dental professions and hospital management in the development of a plan for health insurance which will be beneficial
alike to the public and the professions concerned. We have
asked these groups to complete their work by March 1, 1935,
and to make a further report on this subject by that time or
shortly thereafter.

So far, no report on health insurance has been made public, and no
announcement has been made as regards the plans of the Social
Security Board in dealing with the question of the better distribution of medical care and of wages losses caused by sickness. As is
well known, these questions were considered by the Committee's
staff at length, in collaboration with technical experts of the American Medical Association, as well as with the medical and other
advisory committees already referred to. The only statement so
far authorized which reveals what the Committee had in mind is
that contained in its report of January 15, 1935. This statement
says:

   It seems desirable, however, to advise the professions concerned, and the general public, of the main lines along which
   the studies [health insurance] are proceeding. These may be
   indicated by the following broad principles and general observations which appear to be fundamental to the design of a
   sound plan of health insurance.

The report then goes on to outline these broad principles and
general observations as follows:

1. The fundamental goals of health insurance are: (a) The provision of adequate health and medical services to the insured
   population and their families; (b) the development of a system
   whereby people are enabled to budget the costs of wage loss
   and of medical costs; (c) the assurance of reasonably adequate
   remuneration to medical practitioners and institutions; (d) the
   development under professional auspices of new incentives
   for improvement in the quality of medical services.
2. In the administration of the services the medical professions
   should be accorded responsibility for the control of professional personnel and procedures and for the maintenance and

improvement of the quality of service; practitioners should have broad freedom to engage in insurance practice, to accept or reject patients, and to choose the procedure of remuneration for their services; insured persons should have the freedom to choose their physicians and institutions; and the insurance plan shall recognize the continuance of the private practice of medicine and of the allied professions.

3. Health insurance should exclude commercial or other intermediary agents between the insured population and the professional agencies which serve them.

4. The insurance benefits must be considered in two broad classes: (a) cash payments in partial replacement of wage-loss due to sickness and for maternity cases, and (b) health and medical services.

5. The administration of cash payments should be designed along the same general lines as for unemployment insurance and, so far as may be practical, should be linked with the administration of unemployment benefits.

6. The administration of health and medical services should be designed on a State-wide basis, under a Federal law of permissive character. The administrative provisions should be adapted to agricultural and sparsely settled areas as well as to industrial sections, through the use of alternative procedures in raising the funds and furnishing the services.

7. The costs of cash payments to serve in partial replacement of wage loss are estimated as from 1 to 1¼ per cent of pay-roll.

8. The costs of health and medical services, under health insurance, for the employed population with family earnings up to $3,000 a year, is not primarily a problem of finding new funds, but of budgeting present expenditures so that each family or worker carries an average risk rather than an uncertain risk. The population to be covered is accustomed to expend, on the average, about 4½ per cent of its income for medical care.

9. Existing health and medical services provided by public funds for certain diseases or for entire populations should be correlated with the services required under the contributory plan of health insurance.

10. Health and medical services for persons without income, now mainly provided by public funds, could be absorbed into a contributory insurance system through the payment by relief or other public agency of adjusted contributions for these classes.

11. The rôle of the Federal Government is conceived to be principally (a) to establish minimum standards for health insurance practice, and (b) to provide subsidies, grants, or other financial aids or incentives to States which undertake the development of health insurance systems which meet the Federal standards.

VI

What I have said in the foregoing pages and what I shall say by way of a concluding comment should not be interpreted in any way as reflecting the views of the Committee on Economic Security except in so far as its report to the President has been directly quoted. No one who has studied, with a fair degree of sincerity and earnestness, the practical possibilities of mitigating the risks to the economic security of the moderate- or low-income family which arise out of sickness and ill health, can escape the conclusion that public health, in its broad sense, is a national as well as a local responsibility. The prevailing concept of public health responsibilities has been and is too narrow. It is restricted to a few activities such as community sanitation, water supplies and food inspection, control of infectious diseases, education in hygiene, the medical care of the tuberculous and mentally diseased, and the medical care of the indigent. A newer concept which many sanitarians are coming to accept is much broader and far more sound. The public health of the future demands some sensible co-ordination of public health functions with private medical practice, some solution of the economic problems that are involved in obtaining preventive and curative medicine, some set of procedures by which the physician, sanitarian, and social worker can do their best work in preventing disease, in the care of the sick, and in the rehabilitation of the unfortunate. Such a concept in no way postulates any particular form of government. There is no reason why society cannot discharge this responsibility under any form of government through which it can express its will. Nor does this concept postulate "state medicine," "regimentation of physicians," or "Sovietized" control of those who render health services. A comprehensive program based upon such a concept is an integral part of any effective effort to enhance the economic security of all of the population.

The Social Service Review
March, 1936

4

ILLNESS AND
ILLNESS SURVEYS

COMMENTARY

GEORGE W. COMSTOCK

Modern epidemiology has many faces. So differently do some of its disciples view it that it is tempting to accept the apocryphal saying that epidemiology is what an epidemiologist does. Some of the variety in definitions may arise from the fact that "epidemiology can be thought of either as a body of knowledge, and the inferences derived from this knowledge, or as a method or discipline".[1] These two aspects and the relationships between them were recognized by Frost when he wrote, "Epidemiology at any given time is something more than the total of its established facts. It includes their orderly arrangement into chains of inference which extend more or less beyond the bounds of direct observation . . ."[2]

Epidemiology as a discipline can be subdivided by type of activity as descriptive, experimental, and theoretical.[3] Descriptive epidemiology not only deals with more or less routine observations of diseases in population groups but also with "natural experiments" which occasionally reward those who are both fortunate and attentive. Experimental epidemiology is exemplified both by controlled epidemics in laboratory animals and more recently by controlled clinical trials in man. Theoretical epidemiology deals with mathematical models of disease in populations, aided tremendously by simulations on modern computers. Epidemiology can be further classified by the techniques employed to collect data, such as clinical or serological epidemiology, or by its uses, as Morris has done in his stimulating book.[4]

Each of the preceding activities can also be categorized by their scope in time and place. On the one hand, there are one-time studies in small geographic areas, usually for highly specific purposes. At the other extreme, there are broad and continuing studies aimed at delineating the health of nations.

Several of these facets of epidemiology were included in Sydenstricker's wide range of public health activities. Some, exemplified by the selections in Section 5, were epidemiological studies in the classical sense, aimed at elucidating specific conditions. But Sydenstricker also looked at epidemiology in its broadest aspect. In the opening paragraph of the second paper in this section, he states, "Epidemiology is yet an undeveloped science largely because it lacks the basic data which it must draw from the field of vital statistics. Clinical medicine and bacteriology have made available a large body of material for its use, but since the epidemiological method is essentially the statistical method and epidemiological data are chiefly statistical data, the growth of this new branch of knowledge has so far been one-sided. We cannot hope for its uniform development until accurate and complete statistics of disease incidence in different population groups and under varying conditions of environment are collected currently and in considerable detail" (p. 186). He did not stop at a diagnosis; he and his colleagues, notably Dean K. Brundage and Selwyn D. Collins, did much to overcome this deficiency of epidemiology by initiating a variety of studies of morbidity and demonstrating their usefulness.

It is now difficult to realize how little was known about the health of the nation or about the health of any of its political subdivisions as recently as 50 years ago. At that time, there were only four general sources of information: death statistics, reports of notifiable diseases, prevalence of illness from two U.S. Censuses, and a few scattered surveys of illness prevalence and incidence.[5] Each of these sources provided data that was unsatisfactory on several counts.

Death statistics had the longest history. In this country, they are said to have been fairly complete for Massachusetts as far back as 1857, but it was not until 1933, when the last state qualified for the Death Registration Area, that national mortality data could be examined. But even with complete coverage, it is obvious that deaths give a very narrow view of a community's health. This limitation of mortality statistics must have been impressed upon Sydenstricker during his work in South Carolina. Pellagra, the principal focus of those studies with Joseph Goldberger, rarely killed its victims; mortality statistics gave only a feeble reflection of the burden pellagra imposed upon a community. Sydenstricker's subsequent illness surveys drove home the point more forcibly. In each of the last three papers in this section, he comments cogently on the inadequacies of mortality as an indicator of community health.

In 1880 and again in 1890, the U.S. Census collected information on persons who were ill on the day of the census.[5] However, this information was gathered only for certain parts of the country and only limited tabulations were published. State censuses in Michigan in 1884 and in Massachusetts in 1905 gave age-specific rates for certain illnesses present at the time of enumeration. Although these data added considerably to the picture of illness and health, their value was limited by the fact that the counts reflected prevalence only, thereby giving undue weight to chronic conditions.

A methodological advance came with studies of living conditions of several disadvantaged groups. Conducted by the U.S. Bureau of Labor in 1893 and 1896 primarily for economic information, these surveys included a history of illnesses occurring during the preceding 12 months, thereby giving acute and chronic conditions nearly equal opportunity to be counted. The illness rates were surprisingly low, probably because of poor recall for any but the most recent or the most severe illnesses.[6]

Sydenstricker's initial venture into the field of illness surveys came in 1916. This was a study of disabling illness in seven cotton-mill villages in South Carolina, the communities where he worked with Goldberger and Wheeler on their studies of pellagra. Although the principal measure was prevalence of disability on the day of interview, the addition of information on duration of disability allowed them to look at acute and chronic conditions separately. It was thus possible to see if disability, measured either as frequency or duration, was related to socio-economic status.

In these villages, socio-economic status was largely influenced by family income. Sydenstricker was careful to obtain accurate estimates of family income, to validate them by comparisons with mill payrolls, and to relate them to family needs. The latter refinement is all too often neglected, in spite of the obvious inference that living standards for families on similar incomes can vary markedly according to their basic requirements. Other things being equal, large families will have a lower standard of living than small families, and families composed of adults of working age will need more than similar-sized families with small children. This kind of careful workmanship made it unlikely that his findings would be in error; their concordance with those in other diverse populations suggested that economic status was truly related to morbidity in some way.

Such short-term studies in specific population groups might be useful for establishing relationships of various factors with morbidity, but they could afford only tantalizing glimpses of the total illness pattern that Sydenstricker felt was needed to complete the epidemiological picture. The second paper in this section illustrates a practical approach toward this broader perspective. A number of industries—or rather sick-benefit associations among their employees—were already collecting information on disabling conditions lasting for more than a specified period of time, usually 3 to 7 days. If some of these associations could be persuaded to keep their statistics in a standard fashion and submit reports to a central office, the occurrence of illnesses in a large segment of the general public could be recorded and analyzed. This was undertaken in cooperation with a committee of the American Public Health Association.

Several useful observations were apparent from even a preliminary analysis. Disability was much more common in the winter than in the summer, largely because of the winter excess of respiratory illnesses and diseases of the pharynx. Women not only became sick oftener but were disabled longer than men. Marked variations were found between industries. Even with the virtual absence of "occupational poisonings" from the reported illnesses, this finding suggested that differences in morbidity between industrial establishments might be useful for identifying occupational risks, the alleviation of which could improve the health of workers. A sidelight of considerable interest for modern epidemiologists was the finding that males had only a slight excess in morbidity attributed to diseases of the circulatory system, an excess which was more than accounted for by the much higher illness rate from hemorrhoids among men than among women. The case rate for "endocarditis and other organic heart diseases" was almost 40 per cent higher among females than among males.

Although records from industrial groups afforded a practical way to obtain estimates of the occurrence of illnesses in the population, they still left much to be desired. The major deficiency was that no information was obtainable about groups most likely to suffer illness—the very young, the old, and persons whose disabilities prevented them from working. To remedy this deficiency, the Hagerstown Morbidity Studies were initiated by the U.S. Public Health Service in 1921. As Sydenstricker put it, "The chief aim of the study was a record of illnesses, as ordinarily understood, that were experienced by a population group composed of persons of all ages and both sexes, and in no remarkable way unusual" (p. 212). Hagerstown was chosen as the site because it seemed reasonably typical of much of the country at that time, it could be easily reached from Washington, D.C., where Sydenstricker and his colleagues were stationed, and local contacts had already been made as the result of a health demonstration project. Its selection for the morbidity studies and for later studies on child growth and dental caries caused the name of Hagerstown to become known in public health circles throughout the world.

To achieve its principal goal, the morbidity study had to be conducted over a sufficient period of time to keep seasonal influences from distorting the estimates of annual incidence rates and to allow reasonable numbers of the less frequent diseases to develop. Resources for the project were inadequate to allow the entire city to participate. Consequently, a sample was selected with the purpose of obtaining fair representation of the various economic strata and at the same time of facilitating repeated home visiting. Typical of Sydenstricker's thoroughness was his demonstration that certain characteristics of the interviewed sample closely resembled those of persons in the 1920 Census of Hagerstown and the United States.

Sydenstricker also recognized and dealt with many of the fundamental problems of health surveys. He had to arrive at a working definition of "illness" and to decide, whenever more than one illness or cause was mentioned, which should be tabulated. He showed that informants reported a higher frequency of illnesses for themselves than they did for other household members. And he knew that recollection of minor illnesses could be fleeting and that even major events were often forgotten after a few months. Modern surveyors of the public health will find Sydenstricker's work of more than historical interest.

To account for the fact that information could not be gathered from everyone in the sample areas for the full study period of 28 months, the illness incidence rates were expressed as numbers of illnesses per 1000 person-years of observation. The tabulations show a number of items of current interest. Vaccination against smallpox carried a distinct penalty, 2.3 illnesses per 1000 persons per year being attributed to this cause. The rate per 1000 vaccinations must have been very much greater. The sex ratios for three major rubrics, tuberculosis, diseases of the heart, and cerebral hemorrhage and apoplexy, have reversed since the 1920's. In striking contrast to the present situation, all three conditions were then more than twice as common among females as among males.

In conducting the Hagerstown studies, Sydenstricker still had his eye on a broader goal, namely "to develop an epidemiological method whereby human populations could be observed for as complete an incidence as possible of various diseases, so far as they are manifested in illness, under actual conditions of community life" (p. 233). There can be no question but that he succeeded in this endeavor by laying a major part of the foundations for the current National Health Interview Surveys. In addition, he recognized the need for supplementing interview data with physical and laboratory examinations of the general population in order to account for both recognized illnesses and unrecognized abnormalities, as has been done in the National Health Examination Surveys. These two sample surveys have finally yielded the first reasonably complete picture of the nation's health. Together they have begun to provide the kind of data that Sydenstricker called for in order to achieve a more uniform development of epidemiology. Both can be traced back through a chain of studies, the most prominent of which were the National Health Survey of 1935–1936 and the canvass conducted by the Committee on the Costs of Medical Care in 1928–1931, to Sydenstricker's work in Hagerstown, industry, and the cotton-mill villages of South Carolina. His illness surveys, by stimulating and starting the collection of national morbidity statistics, may well prove to have been Edgar Sydenstricker's most enduring and influential contribution to epidemiology and public health.

References

1. Sartwell, P. E., Preventive Medicine and Public Health, 9th Edition. New York: Appleton-Century-Crofts, 1965, pp. 1–19.
2. Frost, W. H., In Snow on Cholera. New York: The Commonwealth Fund, 1936, p. ix–xxi (Introduction).
3. Lilienfeld, A. M., Epidemiology of infectious and non-infectious disease: some comparisons. The first Wade Hampton Frost lecture. American Journal of Epidemiology 97: 135–147. 1973.
4. Morris, J. N., Uses of epidemiology. Edinburgh and London: E & S Livingstone, Ltd., 1957.
5. Collins, S. D., Sickness surveys. In Administrative Medicine, ed. by Emerson, H. New York: Thomas Nelson & Sons, 1941, pp. 185–213.
6. Collinson, J., and Linder, F. E., Vital Statistics. In Administrative Medicine, ed. by Emerson, H. New York: Thomas Nelson & Sons, 1941, pp. 325–353.

George W. Comstock, M.D.
Professor of Epidemiology
School of Hygiene and Public Health
The Johns Hopkins University

1

Disabling Sickness Among the Population of Seven Cotton–Mill Villages of South Carolina in Relation to Family Income

EDGAR SYDENSTRICKER,

G. A. WHEELER AND

JOSEPH GOLDBERGER

I. Introduction

In connection with the study of the relation of dietary, economic, and other conditions to pellagra incidence in seven cotton-mill villages of South Carolina in 1916,[1] a census of disabling sickness among the population was made during May and June, 1916. Statements were also obtained by the enumerators as to the number of days lost from work by wage-earning persons on account of disability and from other causes during the period from January 1, 1916, to the date of inquiry.

These data have been correlated with certain facts concerning the economic status of mill workers' families as ascertained by the same study, and the results are presented in the following pages.

The study covered 747 households, which, at the date of the census, were composed of 4,161 individuals. Only households of white cotton-mill workers (operatives) were included. The vil-

---

[1]Goldberger, J., Wheeler, G. A., and Sydenstricker, E., A Study of the Diet of Nonpellagrous and of Pellagrous Households in Textile Mill Communities in 1916. Journal American Medical Association, Sept. 21, 1918 (71:944–949).

lages are situated in the northwestern part of South Carolina. Each had a population of between 500 and 800 persons, and each constituted a separate and distinct industrial community in which practically the only opportunity for employment was in the cotton mill. The villages may be regarded as generally typical of cotton-mill communities in that section of South Carolina, from the standpoints both of community conditions affecting health and of the economic status of the population. While the morbidity experience afforded by this study is not extensive and caution should be exercised in drawing broad conclusions, the data are presented for the reason that the results seem definite enough to be suggestive of the value of considering differences in family income along with other conditions, in analyzing differences in disability incidence.

The bases and method of the census and of the classification of the population according to family income are first briefly explained. The tabulations then follow.

II. Method of Census

Experienced enumerators visited each mill worker's household in the seven mill villages on a date between May 1 and June 30, 1916, and secured, among other data, facts as to the sex, age, occupation, earnings, and regularity of employment of each individual member of the household and as to the income of the family as a whole. Such individuals as were found to be unable to work on account of sickness or accident at the time of the visit were noted and the length of such disability up to the date of inquiry was ascertained.

The definition of disability used in certain recent "sickness surveys" was adopted in order to render the results of this study as comparable as possible to the results of other censuses. According to this definition persons classified as "sick" were those who were "unable to work" on account of sickness or accident, including persons "up and about but unable to work," as well as persons confined to bed at home or in hospitals on account of disease and accident.[1] A distinction was made, however, between accidents suffered while actually engaged in millwork (i.e., those which were plainly industrial accidents) and accidents suffered under other circumstances; industrial accidents were not included as causes of disabling sickness. The number of such accidents was extremely small and, if included, would not modify appreciably the rate per 1,000 for any group of persons considered. Statements as to the duration of each illness to date of inquiry were also secured.

The terms of the definition, "unable to work," obviously had to be interpreted in such a manner as to obtain data for persons at home (i.e., not employed for wages) that would be as comparable as possible with the data obtained for persons employed for wages. For such persons as were confined to bed the definition was easily interpreted in nearly all instances, but it was more difficult to draw the line between disabling and nondisabling sickness for sick persons who were "up and about." The difficulty was experienced principally in the cases of children under the age of employability in the mills (12 years at the time the census was made) and of nonwage-earning women. The enumerators were instructed to note all doubtful cases in detail, and the evidence in each case was considered at the time the schedules received their preliminary editing in the field. Since the enumerators spent from a half hour to an hour or more in each household, it was believed

---

[1]Cf. Instructions to Agents, Community Sickness Survey, Rochester, N.Y., September, 1915, by Leo K. Frankel, sixth vice president and Louis I. Dublin, statistician, Metropolitan Life Insurance Co., U.S. Public Health Reports, p. 3, Feb. 25, 1916 (Reprint No. 326). The instructions to agents defining sickness and duration of sickness were as follows:

"The sick should include:

"a) Those persons who are up and about, but are unable to work because of sickness or accident.

"b) Those persons who are confined to bed at home because of disease or accident.

"c) Those persons who are receiving treatment in hospitals or other institutions for the sick.

"The question 'how long sick to date' should be answered definitely in days, weeks, or months."

that sufficient opportunity was afforded to "size up" the situation with a fair degree of accuracy in all such cases. Finally, in order to have a conservative basis for analysis of the data, all cases of sickness and accident which, after final editing of the schedules, appeared doubtful as to actual disability, were not classified as disabling. These classifications were completed before computations of family income were begun. The resulting tabulations may be described as statements of the minimum rather than the maximum amount of disability as found by the census.

III. Classification of the Population According to Income

In classifying the population of the seven cotton-mill villages according to their economic status, family income was used as the basis. Practically all (89 per cent) of the individuals composing the population were members of families who subsisted from family income. The small proportion not subsisting from family income were boarders in the families studied, and may be regarded as living under almost the same conditions as the members of the families with which they boarded. The total population considered thus has been classified according to the income of the families of which they were members or with which they boarded.

1. *Data.*—The data relating to family income were secured at the time of the census by inquiries made of the housewife or of some other responsible member or members of each family, and were supplemented by data from the mill pay rolls. The information obtained from the families covered (*a*) the rate of daily earnings for each member earning wages during the preceding half month and the rates of daily earnings of all members who had been employed during the 12 preceding months; (*b*) days not at work for all members who had worked for wages during the 12 preceding months; (*c*) income from all other sources during the preceding half month, as well as during the preceding 12 months, this information being secured in detail for each source of income. On the basis of this information from the family it was possible to

approximate the total income of each family for the half month preceding the visit of the enumerator and, roughly, for any period in the preceding year or for the entire preceding year. It was believed, however, after trial tabulations of the results, that family income during the half month preceding the week in which the enumerator's visit was made would be a fairly accurate and representative indication of family income during the general period under special consideration (the late spring of 1916). Since it was found that approximately 90 per cent of the total incomes of the families studied came from the earnings of wage-earning members, the family statements of earnings during this half-month period were compared with the records on the mill pay rolls. In the great majority of instances the family statements were found to be substantially correct; but, in order to reduce the error from even slightly inaccurate statements, the mill companies' pay-roll records were used instead of the family statements to supply the earning data. Thus the total income of each family for the half-month period[1] was (a) the amounts earned by wage-earning members employed in the cotton mills as shown by the mill pay rolls, (b) the amounts earned by wage-earning members employed elsewhere, and (c) the amounts received from all other sources, as indicated by statements of responsible informants, during the half-month preceding the week of the enumerator's visit. The basis for classifying families with respect to income, therefore, strictly was the total money income of each family during a 15-day period in May or June, 1916, thus affording a cross-section view of the economic status of the population.

2. *Method.*—For the purpose of classifying cotton-mill families according to income, the conventional method of using total family income for a given period was found to be so inaccurate in many instances as to be misleading. The average total cash income of all of the families for which income data were secured was about $700, and relatively few had annual incomes of over $1,000; the range of total income thus was relatively small and the

[1]A half-month period was used, because a majority of the mills in the villages paid at semimonthly intervals. The pay-roll data from the other mills were adjusted to a half-month basis.

families were, from this point of view, fairly homogeneous. They differed, however, very markedly in size and with respect to the age and sex of their members. Manifestly it was improper to classify, for example, a family whose half-month's income was $40, and which was composed of only a man and his wife, in the same income class as a family whose half-month's income was also $40, but which was composed of a man and his wife and several dependent children. Since family income, for the purpose of this study, was used as an index of the economic status of the individuals who composed the family group, it was necessary to take into consideration the number of such individuals in comparing one family with another. A per capita statement of income, however, while more accurate than the statement of total income, was subject to the inaccuracy arising from differences in the age and sex of the members of the families to be compared. It appeared advisable, therefore, to employ a common denominator to which could be reduced the individuals of both sexes and of all ages in order to afford a more nearly representative method of expression of the relative size of the families to be compared. In the absence of a better common denominator for this purpose, the Atwater scale of basal food requirements was employed, and the size of each family was computed according to this scale and expressed in terms of "adult male units."[1] The assumption in the use of this scale was that the expenditures for individuals varied according to sex and age in the same proportion as their basal food requirements. The assumption is by no means as accurate as could be desired; in its favor, however, it may be said that since family

[1]Principles of Nutrition and Nutritive Value of Food, by W. O. Atwater, U.S. Department of Agriculture, Farmers' Bulletin No. 142 (1915 ed.), p. 33. The scale used was as follows:

Age	EQUIVALENT ADULT MALE UNIT	
	Male	Female
Adult (over 16)	1.0	0.8
15 to 16	.9	.8
13 to 14	.8	.7
12	.7	.6
10 to 11	.6	.6
6 to 9	.5	.5
2 to 5	.4	.4
Under 2	.3	.3

expenditures in the great majority of cases equaled total family income, and since food expenditures were nearly half (among poorer families considerably more than half) of total expenditures, a scale based even on food requirements alone is obviously very much more accurate than one omitting any consideration whatsoever of the number, sex, and age of the individuals to be compared with respect to income.[1]

[1] In order to establish a more accurate basis for computing the size of families in comparing their incomes, a detailed study of expenditures for individuals in a number of representative families in cotton-mill villages was undertaken during 1917. While the tabulations of these data have not yet been completed, it is indicated that the Atwater scale is roughly indicative of the variations, according to sex and age, in the consumption of all articles for which there are individual expenditures. It should be noted that before using the Atwater scale in the preliminary computations of family income, several published estimates of the cost of maintenance for individuals of various ages were examined. These estimates were based, in several instances, upon the results of investigations of actual expenditures of individual members of families. Using the estimated expenditures for an adult male as 100, the estimates for individuals of other ages of either sex were expressed relatively and compared with the Atwater scale. It appeared that, in most instances, the scales were fairly similar. The following table, computed from probably the most pertinent data available, indicates the relative cost of maintenance (at "a fair standard of living") for a year of individuals of various ages as estimated for Southern cotton-mill workers by the United States Bureau of Labor in 1911, in comparison with the Atwater scale for basal food requirements:

Age	MALES		FEMALES	
	Individual expenses (Bureau of Labor)	Food requirements (Atwater)	Individual expenses (Bureau of Labor)	Food requirements (Atwater)
Adult (over 16)	100	100	89	80
15 to 16	85	90	79	80
13 to 14	72	80	67	70
12	61	70	57	60
10 to 11	56	60	59	60
6 to 9	45	50	46	50
2 to 5	34	40	35	40
Under 2	26	30	26	30

The individual expenses estimated were for food (estimated by the Bureau of Labor, according to the Atwater scale), clothing, medical attendance and medicines, insurance, amusement, tobacco and school books. See Report on Condition of Women and Child Wage-Earners in the United States: Vol. XVI, Family Budgets of Typical Cotton-Mill Workers by Wood F. Worchester and Daisy Worthington Worchester (Sen. Doc. 645, 61 Cong. 2d. Sess.) 1911, p. 150.

For preliminary purposes, therefore, the total income of each family, as defined above, has been divided by the number of "adult male units" subsisting on the family income, and the resulting figure has been termed the "family income per adult male unit."

3. *Classification.*—The 747 families for which income data were sufficiently accurate and complete for consideration have been classified by this method and grouped into four convenient classes, each containing a fair proportion of the total number and affording, at the same time, opportunity for contrasting families with the lowest incomes with those having the highest incomes. Table I presents this classification as well as the resulting classification of individuals and their equivalent "adult male units."

TABLE I   Number of families and members of families and their equivalents in adult male units in seven cotton-mill villages of South Carolina, classified according to family income during a 15-day period between Apr. 15 and June 16, 1916

Half-month family income per adult male unit	Families	Persons[1]	Equivalent adult male units[2]
	Number	Number	Number
Less than $6	217	1,289	866.2
$6 to $7.99	183	972	675.9
$8 to $9.99	139	704	529.2
$10 and over	208	800	607.1
All incomes	**747**	**3,765**	**2,678.4**
	Per cent	Per cent	Per cent
All incomes	**100.0**	**100.0**	**100.0**
Less than $6	29.1	34.2	32.4
$6 to $7.99	24.5	25.8	25.2
$8 to $9.99	18.6	18.7	19.8
$10 and over	27.9	21.3	22.6

[1]Exclusive of persons paying board and including only those dependent upon family income.   [2]According to the Atwater scale for basal food requirements.

The differences in income are also indicated in Table II, which shows the average income during the half-month period per family, per person, and per "adult male unit."

It will be noted that Table II is clearly suggestive of the fact that the same *general* differences in *average* incomes for the four groups are indicated by any of the three methods of classification according to income to which reference has already been

TABLE II   Average half-month family income, computed in terms of "per family," "per person," and "per adult male unit,"[1] for various income classes of the population in seven cotton-mill villages in South Carolina

Half-month family income per adult male unit	All family income during a half month	AVERAGE INCOME DURING A HALF MONTH		
		Per family	Per person[2]	Per adult male unit[2]
Less than $6	$3,990.45	$18.38	$3.09	$4.61
$6 to $7.99	4,780.85	26.12	4.92	7.07
$8 to $9.99	4,642.29	33.40	6.55	8.77
$10 and over	7,777.99	37.39	9.72	12.81
All incomes	21,191.58	28.36	5.63	7.92

[1]According to the Atwater scale for basal food requirements.   [2]Exclusive of persons paying board, and including only those dependent upon family income.

made—total family income, income per capita, and income per "adult male unit."[1] The "adult male unit" method, however, is believed to be more accurate than either of the two other methods, for reasons already stated, for the actual classification of individual families.

IV. Disability Incidence According to Income

Upon the foregoing basis of income classification the sickness rate among persons who were members of households with low incomes was found to be markedly higher than among persons with a more favorable economic status. This condition was found to prevail not only among wage-earning persons, but also among non-wage-earning persons. The data are given in Table III and the rates are plotted in Figure 1.

[1]The relative average income in the four classes according to each method has been computed in the following table, the average income of all families according to each method being used as the base:

Family income per adult male unit	RELATIVE AVERAGE INCOME DURING A HALF MONTH PER—		
	Family	Person	Adult male unit
All incomes	100	100	100
Less than $6	65	55	58
$6 to $7.99	92	87	89
$8 to $9.99	118	116	112
$10 and over	132	173	162

TABLE III Cases of disabling sickness and rate per 1,000 persons, as ascertained by a census of seven cotton-mill villages of South Carolina during May and June, 1916, classified according to family income

ALL PERSONS

Half-month family income per adult male unit[1]	Number of persons considered	SICK PERSONS[2]	
		Number	Per 1,000 persons considered
Less than $6	1,312	92	70.1
$6 to $7.99	1,038	50	48.2
$8 to $9.99	784	27	34.4
$10 and over	1,027	19	18.5
All incomes	**4,161**	**188**	**45.2**

WAGE-EARNING PERSONS

Less than $6	450	36	80.0
$6 to $7.99	426	22	51.6
$8 to $9.99	426	8	18.8
$10 and over	538	8	14.9
All incomes	**1,840**	**74**	**40.2**

NONWAGE-EARNING PERSONS

Less than $6	862	56	65.0
$6 to $7.99	612	28	45.8
$8 to $9.99	358	19	53.1
$10 and over	489	11	22.5
All incomes	**2,321**	**114**	**49.1**

[1]According to the Atwater scale of basal food requirements. [2]Exclusive of disability due to confinement.

The results of the sickness census are corroborated, as far as wage-earning persons are concerned, by the records of working days lost on account of disability during the period January to May, 1916. These records are presented in brief form in Table IV.[1]

[1]It will be noted that the percentages of working days lost on account of disability during the five-months' period (Table IV) appear to be lower in most instances than the percentages of wage earners actually found to be incapacitated on the date of inquiry (Table III). When the percentages of working days lost on account of disability were compared for months, it was also seen that the rate of disability was somewhat higher in May than in preceding months. This higher rate, as shown by the census in May–June and by percentages of working days lost, was probably due in part to the fact that instances of short illnesses prior to the date of inquiry were not recalled by the informants. In view of the relatively high rate of pellagra prevalence in May and June, however, it appears proper to suggest that a higher rate of disability in May and June probably actually occurred, partly, at least because of pellagra.

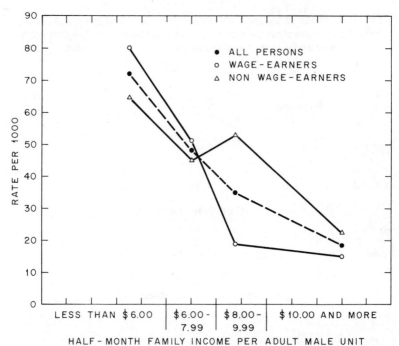

Figure 1   Disabling sickness in seven cotton-mill villages, as ascertained by a census in May and June, 1916, among all persons, and wage-earning and nonwage-earning persons, classified according to family income. (See Table III.)

It is of interest to compare the sick rate per 1,000 persons of different family incomes in these cotton mill villages with that found in other sickness censuses. The sick rate per 1,000 persons (only sickness involving inability to work being considered) as ascertained by a number of community-sickness surveys conducted in various localities in the United States by the Metropolitan Life Insurance Co. was found to be 18.8 for 579,197 persons of all ages.[1]

[1]See Appendix B. Combined Sickness Experience of the Company's Surveys, 1915 to 1917, of the Metropolitan Life Insurance Co.'s publication, "Sickness Survey of Principal Cities in Pennsylvania, and West Virginia," by Lee K. Frankel, Ph.D., third Vice President and Louis I. Dublin, Ph.D., statistician. The "combined sickness experience" referred to included the results of sickness surveys made in localities in Pennsylvania, West Virginia, and North Carolina, Kansas City, (Mo.), Boston, Rochester, Trenton, and Chelsea (New York City).

TABLE IV Number and per cent of total possible working days lost from all causes and from disability by wage-earning members of families in seven cotton-mill villages of South Carolina during January–May, 1916, the wage earners being classified according to family income

			Days not at work				
	Average number of wage-earning persons per month	Total number of possible working days	FROM ALL CAUSES		FROM DISABILITY		Per cent of total days not at work, lost on account of dis-ability
Half-month family income per adult male unit			Number of days	Per cent of total possible working days	Number of days	Per cent of total possible working days	
Less than $6	395	49,753	7,736	15.5	2,938	5.9	38.0
$6 to $7.99	349	44,948	4,631	10.3	1,611	3.6	34.7
$8 to $9.99	306	39,191	3,114	7.9	1,005	2.6	32.3
$10 and over	491	50,026	5,326	10.6	1,153	2.3	21.6
All incomes	**1,541**	**183,918**	**20,807**	**11.3**	**6,707**	**3.6**	**32.2**

If this rate of 18.8 may be considered as a normal one, the suggestion is afforded that in these South Carolina mill villages the normal sick rate was approximated only among those persons who were members of families with half-month income per adult male unit of $10[1] and over, and that in families with incomes lower than this level the sickness rate was markedly higher.

That possible differences in sex and age of the persons comprising the various income classes do not account for differences in the sickness rate among persons of different incomes is indicated in Table V, in which are shown the rates among males and females of different ages in families with incomes above and below the average.[2]

In practically every age period for either sex the sick rate was distinctly greater in families of low incomes than in families with

[1]Expressed in terms of gross annual family income this would be approximately $800, for a "normal" family of 3.3 adult male units (man, wife, and three children under 14 years of age). To render this figure comparable to family income statistics for typical communities elsewhere in the United States, an addition should be made for higher rent expenditures since the rent cost for cotton mill families in the villages studied was relatively low. Allowing for an expenditure for rent similar to that for families of this income in other localities, as shown by various studies of workingmen's family budgets, the equivalent annual income would be approximately $900 or over.

[2]The average half-month income per adult male unit for all families in the villages studied was approximately $8 ($7.92).

TABLE V   Cases of disabling sickness and rates per 1,000 persons as ascertained by a census of seven cotton-mill villages of South Carolina in May and June, 1916, the persons being classified according to income, sex, and age

ALL INCOMES

Age	Total			Males			Females ALL CASES			Females EXCLUSIVE OF CONFINEMENT CASES	
	Number of persons	Number sick¹	Rate per 1,000	Number of persons	Number sick	Rate per 1,000	Number of persons	Number sick	Rate per 1,000	Number sick	Rate per 1,000
Under 5 years	648	43	66.3	339	24	70.8	309	19	61.5	19	61.5
5 to 9 years	609	12	19.7	313	6	19.2	296	6	20.3	6	20.3
10 to 14 years	537	20	37.3	279	6	21.5	258	14	54.3	14	54.3
15 to 24 years	977	37	37.9	463	12	25.9	514	32	62.2	25	48.7
25 to 34 years	606	27	44.6	287	8	27.9	319	23	72.1	19	59.6
35 to 44 years	392	21	53.6	200	10	50.0	192	15	78.1	11	57.4
45 to 54 years	213	12	56.4	109	5	45.9	104	7	67.3	7	67.3
55 to 64 years	107	9	84.1	48	6	125.0	59	3	50.8	3	50.3
65 years and over	72	8	111.2	33	3	90.9	39	5	128.2	5	128.2
Total	**4,161**	**189**	**45.4**	**2,071**	**80**	**38.6**	**2,090**	**124**	**59.3**	**109**	**52.2**

FAMILY INCOME OF LESS THAN $8 PER ADULT MALE UNIT

Age	Number of persons	Number sick	Rate per 1,000	Number of persons	Number sick	Rate per 1,000	Number of persons	Number sick	Rate per 1,000	Number sick	Rate per 1,000
Under 5 years	422	30	71.1	212	15	70.8	210	15	71.4	15	71.4
5 to 9 years	417	10	24.0	215	4	18.6	202	6	29.7	6	29.7
10 to 14 years	344	18	52.3	187	5	26.7	157	13	82.8	13	82.8
15 to 24 years	427	27	63.2	200	11	55.0	227	22	96.9	16	70.5
25 to 34 years	310	17	54.8	135	5	37.0	175	15	85.8	12	68.6
35 to 44 years	224	20	89.3	115	10	87.0	109	13	119.3	10	91.8
45 to 54 years	109	7	64.2	61	5	82.0	48	2	41.7	2	41.7
55 to 64 years	45	5	111.2	22	4	181.8	23	1	43.5	1	43.5
65 years and over	52	8	153.8	24	3	125.0	28	5	178.6	5	178.6
Total	**2,350**	**142**	**60.4**	**1,171**	**62**	**53.0**	**1,179**	**92**	**78.1**	**80**	**67.8**

FAMILY INCOME OF $8 OR MORE PER ADULT MALE UNIT

Age	Number of persons	Number sick	Rate per 1,000	Number of persons	Number sick	Rate per 1,000	Number of persons	Number sick	Rate per 1,000	Number sick	Rate per 1,000
Under 5 years	226	13	57.5	127	9	70.8	99	4	40.4	4	40.4
5 to 9 years	192	2	10.4	98	2	20.4	84				
10 to 14 years	193	2	10.4	92	1	10.9	101	1	9.9	1	9.9
15 to 24 years	550	10	18.2	263	1	3.8	287	10	34.8	9	31.4
25 to 34 years	296	10	33.8	152	3	19.7	144	8	55.6	7	48.6
35 to 44 years	168	1	5.9	85			83	2	24.1	1	12.1
45 to 54 years	104	5	48.1	48			56	5	89.3	5	89.3
55 to 64 years	62	2	32.3	26	2	76.9	36	2	55.6	2	55.6
65 years and over	20			9			11				
Total	**1,811**	**47**	**26.0**	**900**	**18**	**20.0**	**911**	**32**	**35.1**	**29**	**31.9**

¹Exclusive of disability due to confinement.

incomes above the average. The same condition is indicated when only wage-earning persons are considered, as shown in Table VI.

A comparison of the sickness rates among mill-working and nonmill working persons is possible only for females since practically all males of wage-earning age were employed in the mills. Females, however, were almost evenly divided among mill work-

TABLE VI   Cases of disabling sickness per 1,000 wage earners, as ascertained by a census of seven cotton-mill villages of South Carolina in May and June, 1916, the wage earners being classified according to income, sex, and age

ALL INCOMES

Age	TOTAL			MALES			FEMALES		
	Number of persons	Number sick[1]	Rate per 1,000	Number of persons	Number sick	Rate per 1,000	Number of persons	Number sick[1]	Rate per 1,000
10 to 14 years	235	9	38.3	137	5	36.5	98	4	40.8
15 to 24 years	799	27	33.8	449	11	24.5	350	16	45.7
25 to 34 years	406	14	34.5	279	8	28.7	127	6	47.2
35 to 44 years	238	13	54.6	194	9	46.4	44	4	90.9
45 to 54 years	107	5	46.7	98	4	40.8	9	1	111.1
55 years and over	55	6	109.2	50	5	100.0	5	1	200.0
Total	**1,840**	**74**	**40.2**	**1,207**	**42**	**34.8**	**633**	**32**	**50.6**

FAMILY INCOME OF LESS THAN $8 PER ADULT MALE UNIT

Age	Number of persons	Number sick	Rate per 1,000	Number of persons	Number sick	Rate per 1,000	Number of persons	Number sick	Rate per 1,000
10 to 14 years	145	3	55.2	87	5	57.5	58	3	51.7
15 to 24 years	325	20	61.5	194	10	51.5	131	10	76.3
25 to 34 years	191	9	47.1	135	5	37.0	56	4	71.4
35 to 44 years	130	12	92.3	110	9	81.8	20	3	150.0
45 to 54 years	58	4	69.0	54	4	74.1	4		
55 years and over	27	5	185.2	23	4	173.9	4	1	250.0
Total	**876**	**58**	**66.2**	**603**	**37**	**61.3**	**273**	**21**	**76.9**

FAMILY INCOME OF $8 OR MORE PER ADULT MALE UNIT

Age	Number of persons	Number sick	Rate per 1,000	Number of persons	Number sick	Rate per 1,000	Number of persons	Number sick	Rate per 1,000
10 to 14 years	90	1	10.9	50			40	1	25.0
15 to 24 years	474	7	14.8	255	1	3.9	219	6	27.4
25 to 34 years	215	5	23.3	144	3	20.8	71	2	28.2
35 to 44 years	108	1	9.3	84			24	1	41.7
45 to 54 years	49	1	20.4	44			5	1	200.0
55 years and over	28	1	35.7	27	1	37.0	1		
Total	**964**	**16**	**16.6**	**604**	**5**	**8.3**	**360**	**11**	**30.6**

[1]Exclusive of disability due to confinement.

ing and nonmill-working occupations. In Table VII is shown a comparison of the sick rate for nonmill-working and mill-working females in families of different incomes.

In order to put nonmill-working and mill-working females on as comparable a basis as possible—1) disability due to confinement was excluded, 2) only those females of the ages at which they were found to work in the mills were considered (i.e., roughly between the ages of 10 and 45), and 3) cases of invalidism were excluded from consideration as far as practicable by considering only those persons whose disability was less than three months up to the date of the inquiry.

The resulting sickness rates suggest that, without respect to the question of family economic status, mill-working females probably were more subject to disabling sickness than nonmill-working females. The suggestion is strengthened by the presumption that in enumerating cases of disability the tendency might have been to include some sickness among women not employed for wages which would not have been disabling had these women been employed.

The experience is too small to warrant the attaching of much significance to the relatively slight difference for mill-working and nonmill-working women without regard to economic status. When the females are classified according to family income, however, the indication is afforded that higher family income is a more striking concomitant of low sickness incidence than millwork. In fact, the suggestion is afforded by this study that the higher incidence among mill-working females was more pronounced among those whose family incomes were under the average than among those whose family incomes were on a higher level.

In this connection it is of interest to note that among the same persons (as classified in Table VII) the pellagra rate was the reverse of the sickness rate.[1] Among nonmill-working females the 1916 pellagra rate was approximately four times as high as that among mill-working females. Pellagra, therefore, appeared to be relatively an unimportant cause of the higher sickness rate among

[1]Cases of disabling sickness of less than three months' duration (exclusive of confinements), as ascertained by a census in May and June, 1916, and of pellagra during 1916, among non-mill-working and mill-working females between the ages of 10 and 45, in seven cotton-mill villages of South Carolina.

	NONMILL WORKING			MILL WORKING		
		CASES			CASES	
	Number of persons	Number	Rate per 1,000	Number of persons	Number	Rate per 1,000
Disabling sickness at date of census	664	26	39.2	619	28	45.2
Pellagra during 1916	657	33	50.2	625	8	12.8

The actual rate of pellagra prevalence during 1916 can not, of course, be compared with the rate of disabling illness as found for one day. The relative differences in rates according to occupation, however, are comparable, especially when the fact is taken into consideration that the majority of the pellagra cases had

TABLE VII Cases of disabling sickness of less than three months' duration (exclusive of confinement cases) among females between the ages of 10 and 45 years, as ascertained by a census of households during May and June, 1916, in seven cotton-mill villages of South Carolina, females being classified according to family income and employment in millwork

Half-month family income per adult male unit	NONMILL WORKING			MILL WORKING		
	Number of fe-males	Number sick	Rate per 1,000	Number of fe-males	Number sick	Rate per 1,000
Less than $8	403	20	49.6	265	18	67.9
$8 and over	261	6	23.0	354	10	28.2
All incomes	**664**	**26**	**39.2**	**619**	**28**	**45.2**

TABLE VIII The relation of family income to the duration of disabling sickness in families of mill workers, as ascertained by a census in May and June, 1916, of seven cotton-mill villages in South Carolina

BOTH SEXES

Nature of sickness	Half-month family income per adult male unit	NUMBER OF CASES				PERCENT OF CASES OF EACH DURATION			
		DURATION OF ILLNESS				DURATION OF ILLNESS			
		Any length	Less than two weeks	Two weeks but less than two months	Two months or longer	Any length	Less than two weeks	Two weeks but less than two months	Two months or longer
All cases	Less than $8	153	57	48	48	100.0	37.2	31.4	31.4
	$8 or more	49	23	17	9	100.0	46.9	34.7	18.4
Exclusive of con-finement	Less than $8	141	53	42	46	100.0	37.6	29.8	32.6
	$8 or more	46	22	15	9	100.0	47.9	32.6	19.6

MALE

| All cases | Less than $8 | 62 | 27 | 16 | 19 | 100.0 | 43.6 | 25.8 | 30.6 |
| | $8 or more | 17 | 8 | 7 | 2 | 100.0 | 47.0 | 41.2 | 11.8 |

FEMALES

Exclusive of con-finement	Less than $8	79	26	26	27	100.0	32.9	32.9	34.2
	$8 or more	29	14	8	7	100.0	48.3	27.6	24.1
Cases of confinement	Less than $8	12	4	6	2	100.0	33.3	50.0	16.7
	$8 or more	3	1	2		100.0	33.3	66.7	
All cases	Less than $8	91	30	32	29	100.0	33.0	35.2	31.9
	$8 or more	32	15	10	7	100.0	46.9	31.3	21.9

their onsets in May and June, the same months in which the census of disabling sickness was made.

It may be mentioned that the cases of pellagra occurred almost entirely among individuals whose family incomes were below the average. The data relating to pellagra incidence according to sex, age, occupation, economic status, etc., which were collected in the study of cotton-mill villages, will be presented in later publications.

mill-working females, and, conversely, the disability indicated by
the higher sickness rate in mill-working females appeared not to
influence appreciably the pellagra rate in this group. This does
not afford any support to the view entertained in many directions
that general debility is necessarily a contributing factor in the
production of pellagra.

A classification of disabling sickness according to duration to
date of inquiry among persons of different family economic status
has been attempted in Table VIII.

The condition is suggested that, for both males and females, a
greater proportion of disabling sicknesses were of long duration
(two months or longer) in families with incomes below the average than in families of higher incomes.

Conclusions

While extreme caution should be exercised in drawing broad
conclusions from so small an amount of data, the experience
derived from the census of sickness and from the records of working days lost on account of sickness in the seven cotton-mill
villages studied appears to suggest the following:

1. A higher sickness (involving inability to work) rate and a
greater amount of working time lost on account of such sickness
were found among members of families whose incomes were low
than among members of families with a more favorable economic
status. This condition appeared for persons of either sex and of
similar ages. Only when a family income approximated $10 per
half month per adult male unit (or about $900 a year for a family of
"normal" size in 1916) did the sickness rate appear to be as low as
that suggested by similar censuses in a number of localities in the
United States as the normal rate.

2. Low economic status appeared to be a more striking concomitant of high sickness rate among females than employment in
millwork.

3. A greater proportion of disabling illness, of relatively long
duration, appeared among persons whose family income was

below the average than among persons with a more favorable economic status.

To what extent low family income was a cause of higher sickness rate and to what extent it was an effect of disability (and thus of inability to increase income) can not, of course, be determined from these data. The condition, however, is manifest that a greater amount of disabling sickness existed among persons who were living under less favorable economic conditions than among persons whose economic status was more favorable—a condition which has been pointed out by previous observations in the literature on the social aspects of ill health and indicated by several recent studies.[1] The data here presented afford additional ground for the suggestion that in the analysis of morbidity facts the factor of economic status should be given proper emphasis.

Public Health Reports
November 22, 1918

[1]For example, physical examinations of garment workers in the cloak, suit, and skirt industry in New York City in 1914 showed that while "no vocational diseases peculiar to garment workers" were found, the condition was "clearly suggested * * * that the greatest number of poorly nourished, anemic tuberculous workers in an extremely seasonal industry were in that group composed of the lowest paid and the least regularly employed." (Health of Garment Workers—The Relation of Economic Status to Health, by B. S. Warren, surgeon, and Edgar Sydenstricker, public health statistician, with an introduction by J. W. Schereschewsky, surgeon, U.S. Public Health Reports, May 26, 1916, pp. 1298–1305, Reprint No. 341). Reference may also be made to the recent reports of infant mortality studies conducted in various communities by the Children's Bureau of the U.S. Department of Labor; to the studies of John Robertson, M.D., in Birmingham, England; and to others.

2

Industrial Establishment
Disability Records as a Source
of Morbidity Statistics*

EDGAR SYDENSTRICKER AND
DEAN K. BRUNDAGE

Epidemiology is yet an undeveloped science largely because it lacks the basic data which it must draw from the field of vital statistics. Clinical medicine and bacteriology have made available a large body of material for its use, but since the epidemiological method is essentially the statistical method and epidemiological data are chiefly statistical data, the growth of this new branch of knowledge has so far been one-sided. We cannot hope for its uniform development until accurate and complete statistics of disease incidence in different population groups and under varying conditions of environment are collected currently and in considerable detail.

The statistics of disease incidence which are now available are confined almost entirely to deaths. The grave shortcomings of mortality data as the basic data for statistical research in disease incidence have not, perhaps, been sufficiently realized. In fact, the statement may be ventured that we have been too satisfied with and have attached too much importance to epidemiological conclusions based upon data which relate to only one phase of disease incidence. We are yet greatly in the dark with regard to even the most important facts concerning predisposition to disease, the conditions under which disease begins, and the circum-

*Read at the Eighty-second Annual Meeting of the American Statistical Association, Atlantic City, New Jersey, December, 1920.

stances which affect or control its course in a population. What we need, what we must have, before satisfactory progress can be made, are morbidity data.

This has been said so often that it has become trite. May it not be said that we have fallen more or less into the habit of regarding complete and accurate morbidity statistics as an impracticable ideal, as a goal impossible of attainment? Is there not in such an attitude this element of danger—a tendency to relax in the endeavor to obtain the desired data simply because they cannot be obtained at once and with the methods which we are accustomed to use in recording mortality?

Before bringing to your attention a possible field for morbidity research, a brief consideration of the situation with regard to morbidity statistics seems pertinent.

The data upon which morbidity statistics are now based necessarily are less uniform, less complete, and less accurate than those which are the foundation of mortality statistics. A death is an event of which the local public, in the performance of certain governmental functions and in the observance of certain social conventions, must take cognizance. The fact that a citizen has ceased to live is usually recorded: at least, some statement of the cause of his demise is placed upon the public books, and certain facts as to his nativity, sex, age, marital condition, residence, occupation, and the like are ascertained. His remains cannot be disposed of until these things are done. We have, therefore, a set of mortality records which are gradually becoming more uniform, more complete, and more accurate. An illness, on the other hand, is a commonplace happening unless the affected individual is regarded as a menace to the community. A case of leprosy, of typhus fever, of bubonic plague, or even of smallpox or scarlet fever, is important enough in the public mind as a source of danger to be reported and isolated. But a disability resulting from tuberculosis or from a non-communicable disease equally as serious to the individual and, indirectly, to the community is such an every-day affair that only by the most searching inquiry can its occurrence be ascertained and recorded.

The obstacles actually encountered in obtaining morbidity

reports for a given population or population groups are well known to vital statisticians. The chief difficulties may be expressed in three statements:

1) Only such diseases can be reported as come to the attention of physicians and other diagnosticians. These diseases ordinarily are brought to their attention only at a stage when discomfort, pain, or disability is experienced; in their incipient and latent stages, when they are not noticed even by the individual affected or do not interfere with his normal activities, but when their importance is equally as great or even greater, they are not reported.

2) Only such cases are reported as are (a) notifiable under the law, and of these (b) only the ones that the physician or other reporting agency is willing to report.

3) Even when the occurrence of an illness is reported, the diagnosis is frequently less accurate than a statement of cause of death. This is inevitably so for the reasons that the illness itself may be merely a symptom of one or several diseases, that it is not always practicable to apply established tests, and that the individual affected cannot be under sufficiently close observation to obtain the necessary clinical evidence.

How, then, are we ever to obtain the necessary material for statistical analysis or epidemiological research?

Let us examine, for a moment, the possible sources of morbidity data. Keeping in mind the fact that the occurrence of disease in a population for which certain facts as to race, sex, age, and various environmental conditions can be known, is the goal, we may classify the various sources into three general groups, as follows:

1. Reports of diseases that are "notifiable" under the law, which are made by physicians and other diagnosticians to health authorities.

2. Disability or sickness records for persons associated into insured groups, or persons employed in certain industrial establishments maintaining fairly detailed supervision of the health of their employees, for persons living in various institutions, and in the armed forces of the United States.

3. Special surveys of observed groups of persons that are

made with the specific purpose of obtaining accurate records of the incidence of a given disease. These studies are, of course, researches in their purpose and character.

It will be seen at once that the first source of material mentioned—the reports of certain notifiable diseases which have accumulated in every health department—does not begin to satisfy the elementary requirements for statistics of disease incidence. The reports are by no means complete for any disease, even assuming the diagnosis to be trustworthy. They do not contain accurate or sufficient data regarding conditions under which the disease occurs. The decennial enumeration of the population as to specific occupation, for example, cannot be utilized, and the cases are not reported for any definitely enumerated population from any point of view. The third source of material obviously is of a special kind, and its scope and its usefulness are limited only by the amount of money and time spent and by the ability of those who are making the research. The second group of sources of data, on the other hand, afford at the present time more encouragement of a practical sort for obtaining *current* facts as to disease incidence for a definitely known exposure under a limited number of important conditions than either health department records or the results of special surveys.

In this belief, the attempt is being made by the statistical office of the Public Health Service to collect current records of disability (exclusive of those due to industrial accidents) occurring among employees of industrial establishments. The project was planned with the assistance of a committee of the American Public Health Association.* Since very few plants maintain records of specific causes of disability among their employees, it was necessary to utilize records of such sick-benefit associations of employees as

*The plan for standardized sickness records and reports is contained in the following Public Health Reports:

1. *Report of Committee on Industrial Morbidity Statistics,* Reprint No. 484.

2. *Continuation Report of the Committee on Industrial Morbidity Statistics,* Reprint No. 564.

3. *Sickness Records for Industrial Establishments,* Reprint No. 573.

4. *Diseases Prevalent among Steel Workers in a Pennsylvania City,* Issue of December 31, 1920.

were willing to conform to a standard system of records and reports. These records show for each case of disability the date on which cash "benefits" commenced (usually the third, fifth or seventh day of disability), the number of days for which benefits were paid, and the cause of disability as stated on a physician's certificate. At the present time, about sixty such associations are coöperating with the Public Health Service, although not all of them have made the changes in their method of recording and reporting disabilities that are necessary to conform to either of the "standard" methods suggested by the committee and the Public Health Service. The total membership of these associations at last report was approximately 250,000; because of reductions in force, this "exposure" will probably be considerably decreased. Two standard methods of recording and reporting disabilities were proposed to industrial establishments and sick-benefit associations in order to secure their sickness experience as well as to assist them in utilizing and analyzing their own records as a basis for preventive work. 1) One method requires a record of the number of persons considered by sex and occupation (or department within the plant), and a record of every case of disability for which sick benefits are paid, showing the date of onset, (*i.e.*, the date on which the disability commenced), duration (*i.e.*, the number of days for which sick benefits were paid), diagnosis, and occupation (or department) in which the disabled person is employed. 2) The other plan includes not only the data required in 1) but also contemplates a greater amount of detailed information, such as the age, race, length of time in occupation, etc., for both the persons considered and the cases of disability among such persons. The latter plan requires a rather detailed system of individual cards and only a few plants are at present in a position to put it into effect.

Although the work of utilizing these records after placing them on either of the so-called standard plans, is still in an experimental stage and the policy of retrenching as much as possible on all expenditures for records is being practiced in industrial plants generally at the present time, it is believed that the use of such records can be developed to serve two important purposes: 1) to furnish fairly current information regarding the incidence of disease among a representative group of wage-earners in different industries, and 2) to accumulate a mass of data relating to the causes of disability among a large number of adult persons of different race, sex, age, and occupation and industry.

Since the plan has been inaugurated only a few months, the material so far collected is not sufficient to warrant definite conclusions on any of the essential points. The data cannot be presented here in detail, but for purposes of illustration we will call attention to two tabulations. One shows the monthly variation in diseases which caused disabilities of seven days or longer in a group of plants during the first eight months of 1920; the other shows the incidence of various diseases causing a disability of more than one day during a 12-month period in a large industrial plant.

Taking up first the monthly variations in disease incidence among the members of certain sick-benefit associations of employees in a group of industrial establishments: The number of persons considered varied from 14,208 in January to 62,757 in July, and the number of industrial establishments from 8 in January to 25 in July. The annual incidence rates per 1,000 persons for sicknesses causing inability to work for seven days or longer by months were as follows: January 275, February 327, March 126, April 103, May 77, June 67, July 67, August 54. An extremely wide seasonal variation thus is manifested, the rate for February being approximately six times the rate for August. It will be recalled that the recrudescence of epidemic influenza occurred in the first three months of 1920, particularly in February, and in order to find out to what extent the epidemic influenced the seasonal variation in disease incidence, the following table and graph were prepared [Table I and Figure 1] showing the monthly incidence rates of influenza and grippe in comparison with the rates for the principal disease groups. Cases diagnosed either as influenza or as grippe were combined, because the terms were often used interchangeably in reporting the epidemic.

In the first two months of the year the frequency rate for influenza and grippe, it is seen, was larger than the frequency rate for all other diseases combined; in March, however, the number of new cases of influenza and grippe dropped perceptibly below the rate for all other diseases, and gradually diminished to the negligible incidence of 0.8 cases per 1,000 in July. The occurrence of the epidemic in the months in which sickness ordinarily is heavy accentuated markedly the usual seasonal variation. Even with influenza and grippe eliminated from the sickness rates, disease occurrence was about twice as frequent in winter as in summer.*

When influenza and grippe are subtracted, there still remains a surprisingly high frequency rate of sickness causing disabilities of seven days or longer. In January this rate was 132 new cases per 1,000 persons on an annual basis, and even in August, the month of lowest incidence in the 8-month period, the annual rate was over 50 per 1,000. This is true in spite of the fact that the members of a large proportion of the associations are a selected group.**

In lieu of a more satisfactory basis for classifying the diseases, and in accordance with the recommendations of the American Public Health Association's committee, the groupings appearing

*In regard to the more important diseases and groups of diseases occurring each month, it should be stated that the monthly fluctuations in their incidence, presently to be discussed, were indicated in a general way for each reporting association.

**Twelve of the 27 associations specify definite age limits for eligibility to membership, the average limits being from 17 to 55 years of age. In some other respects, too, industrial employees are a distinctly selected group. Temporary or casual laborers are seldom admitted to membership, and some may be too poor to afford the cost of insurance. Women have not the privilege of belonging to some of the reporting associations, and in those reporting associations which do have female members their number is relatively small, so that the sickness rates presented could not be affected to any appreciable extent by the greater frequency of illness among women. Furthermore, not all diseases are included in the tabulations, as sick benefits are denied for venereal diseases, and six of the 27 reporting associations in this group refuse to pay benefits for chronic diseases contracted prior to the date of joining the association. Sixteen of the associations do not pay for disabilities brought on by the use of intoxicating liquors; eleven decline to pay for disabilities resulting from the violation of any civil law; and eight for the results of wilful or gross negligence. Just how rigidly these rules are enforced is not known, but, considering these restrictions, the statistics should be regarded as a *minimum* statement of the disabilities actually occurring and lasting seven days or longer.

TABLE I
Frequency of influenza and grippe
compared with the frequency of the principal disease groups,
by month of onset, January to August, 1920*

Number of cases per 1,000 persons per year

Month of onset	Number of associations reporting	Membership	All diseases and conditions	Influenza and grippe	OTHER DISEASES AND CONDITIONS					
					Total	Diseases of respiratory system	Diseases of digestive system	General diseases†	Diseases of the nervous system	All other diseases
January	8	14,208	275.0	142.9	132.1	49.9	24.1	20.8	7.5	29.8
February	13	22,249	326.7	201.4	125.3	40.8	22.7	17.5	8.5	35.8
March	14	23,527	126.0	37.1	88.9	21.1	24.1	17.1	8.0	18.6
April	18	30,075	103.4	13.2	90.2	19.4	15.6	16.6	8.0	30.6
May	22	58,302	76.1	4.6	72.1	16.8	15.3	12.2	5.9	21.9
June	25	62,344	67.1	2.3	64.8	9.2	14.1	15.8	5.0	20.7
July	25	62,757	67.3	.8	66.5	8.1	15.2	8.7	3.8	30.7
August	24	60,304	54.4	1.1	53.3	9.1	13.9	9.4	3.8	17.1

*Annual number of cases per 1,000 members of certain sick benefit associations reporting to the Public Health Service. Only cases lasting 7 days or longer are included.
†Except influenza and grippe.

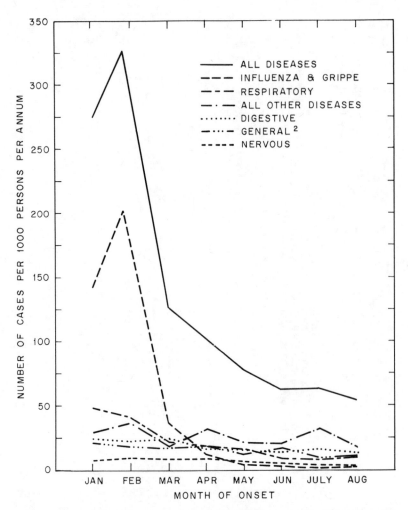

Figure 1 Frequency of influenza and grippe compared with the frequency of the principal disease groups, by month of onset, January to August 1920.
Annual number of cases per 1,000 members of certain sick-benefit associations reporting to the Public Health Service[1]
1) Includes only those sickness and non-industrial accident cases which caused absence from work for one week or more.
2) Except influenza and grippe.

TABLE II   Annual number of cases of sickness causing disability for one week or longer per 1,000 members of sick-benefit associations in certain industrial establishments reporting to the Public Health Service: by month of onset, January to August, 1920, and by disease causing disability

Disease or condition causing disability (with corresponding title numbers in parentheses from the International List of the Causes of Death)	Jan.	Feb.	Mar.	Apr.	May	June	July	Aug.
All Diseases and Conditions (a)	275.0	326.7	126.0	103.4	76.7	67.1	67.3	54.4
General Diseases	163.7	218.9	54.2	29.8	16.8	18.1	9.5	10.5
Typhoid fever (1)	1.7		.5	.5	.4		.4	.6
Influenza and grippe (10)	142.9	201.4	37.1	13.2	4.6	2.3	.8	1.1
Tuberculosis of the lungs (28)	2.5	1.1	3.0	.9	.9	2.3	1.2	1.3
Cancer—all forms (39–46)		1.1	.5	.9	.7		.6	.8
Rheumatism (47, 48)	6.6	6.8	5.5	7.6	5.0	6.7	3.0	3.6
Occupational poisonings (57, 58)						.2		
Others (2–9, 11–27, 29–38, 49–56, 59)	10.0	8.5	7.5	6.6	5.2	6.5	3.4	3.2
Diseases of the Nervous System	7.5	8.5	8.0	8.0	5.9	5.0	3.8	3.8
Neuralgia and neuritis (73)	4.2	2.8	2.0	.5	1.7	.8	1.4	1.3
Cerebral hemorrhage, apoplexy and paralysis (64–66)	.8		.5	.5	.2	.2	.2	
Insanity (67, 68)	.8	1.1	1.5	.5	.2	.2		.6
Others (60–63, 69–72, 74)	1.7	2.3	3.0	4.3	1.5	2.3	1.6	1.5
Diseases of the eyes (75)		.6		1.9	1.5	1.1	.4	.4
Diseases of the ears (76)		1.7	1.0	.5	.7	.4	.2	
Diseases of the Circulatory System	2.5	5.1	4.5	3.3	4.8	2.9	4.0	2.1
Diseases of the heart (77–80)	1.7	2.3	1.0	1.4	1.7	1.1	2.2	1.1
Diseases of the veins (83)	.8	2.3	2.5	1.4	1.7	1.5	1.4	.6
Others (81–82, 84–85)		.6	1.0	.5	1.3	.4	.4	.4
Diseases of the Respiratory System	49.9	40.8	21.1	19.4	16.8	9.2	8.1	9.1
Bronchitis (89, 90)	21.6	19.3	12.0	8.5	6.3	3.2	3.8	3.4
Pneumonia (91, 92)	15.8	12.5	2.5	4.7	5.0	1.9	1.6	1.9
Others (86–88, 93–98)	12.5	9.1	6.5	6.1	5.5	4.2	2.6	3.8
Diseases of the Digestive System	24.1	22.7	24.1	15.6	15.3	14.1	15.2	13.9
Diseases of the pharynx (100)	15.0	12.5	10.0	7.1	5.5	4.0	3.4	3.4
Diseases of the stomach (102, 103)	4.2	5.1	5.5	3.8	3.1	2.9	4.4	3.6
Diarrhea and enteritis (105)	1.7	1.1	2.0			1.3	1.0	1.9
Appendicitis (108)	3.3	2.3	2.5	1.9	2.8	2.5	3.4	3.0
Hernia (109)		1.1	1.0	2.4	2.4	2.1	.8	1.1
Others (99, 101, 106, 107, 110–118)		.6	3.0	.5	1.5	1.3	2.0	1.1
Diseases of the Genito-Urinary System	2.5	3.4	.5	1.4	1.7	1.1	1.4	.6
Acute nephritis and Bright's disease (119, 120)	2.5	.6				.6		
Others (121–133)		2.8	.5	1.4	1.7	.4	1.4	.6
The Puerperal State								
Diseases of the Skin and Cellular Tissue	5.8	7.4	2.5	5.2	2.2	2.7	4.9	2.5
Furuncle (143)	3.3	3.4	1.5	3.8	.7	1.3	2.6	.6
Others (142, 144, 145)	2.5	4.0	1.0	1.4	1.5	1.5	2.2	1.9
Diseases of the Bones and Organs of Locomotion	4.2	1.7	3.0	2.4	3.7	1.7	2.4	2.3
Diseases of the bones (146)	.8	.6		.5	.7		.2	.4
Diseases of the joints (147)			1.5	.5	1.1	.4	.8	.2
Others (148, 149)	3.3	1.1	1.5	1.4	2.0	1.3	1.4	1.7
Senility								
External Causes (155–186)	3.3	10.8	2.5	13.2	6.1	7.6	12.1	6.3
Ill-Defined Diseases and Conditions (187–189)	11.6	7.4	5.5	5.2	3.3	4.6	5.7	3.2

(a) Except those mentioned in the footnote on p. 192

in the International List of the Causes of Death have been utilized in our tabulations [Table II]. On this basis, the outstanding causes of disability are found in the "general" (from 10 to 219 per 1,000), the "respiratory" (from 8 to 50 per 1,000), and the "digestive" (from 14 to 24 per 1,000), these three groups accounting for from 49 to 86 per cent of all disabilities lasting seven days or longer. The wide fluctuation in the general diseases was caused almost entirely by influenza and grippe. Rheumatism does not show so great a seasonal fluctuation as might have been expected; the rate from this cause was high during the period January–June, showing a slight tendency to become less frequent in July and August. The tuberculosis rate varied between 1 and 3 per 1,000 persons per year which seems to indicate a relatively slight disability from tuberculosis lasting seven days or longer. It may be offered in explanation that many cases which actually began in the period under consideration probably had not yet reached a stage involving actual incapacity for work.

It is interesting to note that occupational poisonings are almost entirely absent in this list as a cause of disability. Two possible reasons for this fact may be advanced: (a) that poisonings do not ordinarily incapacitate for as long as seven days, and (b) that they are not accurately diagnosed. The group of respiratory diseases, as may be expected, exhibits a marked seasonal fluctuation. This variation is true of each and all of the diseases in this group, the disabilities caused by bronchitis and pneumonia being the outstanding features. The relatively high rate from the digestive diseases in the first three months of the year is accounted for chiefly by diseases of the pharynx, of which tonsillitis is the most important. Disability due to tonsillitis is shown to be astonishingly great. Eliminating pharyngeal affections, the digestive diseases exhibit a fairly constant rate throughout the 8-month period. Seasonal disabilities arising from these causes do not show the anticipated increase in the summer months.

When the frequency rates from all diseases are compared for establishments (see Table III), extraordinarily wide differences are shown in every month. In February, for instance, the frequency rate for association A was 118 per 1,000, while for associa-

TABLE III Annual number of cases of sickness per 1,000 for all reporting sick-benefit associations, and for each reporting association having more than 500 members, by months, January to August, 1920[a]

(Where blank spaces appear the statistics were not available)

Sick-benefit associations	Average member-ship	NUMBER OF CASES PER 1,000 PERSONS PER YEAR							
		Jan.	Feb.	Mar.	Apr.	May	June	July	Aug.
All reporting associations	41,721	275	327	126	118[b]	80[b]	71[b]	74[b]	59[b]
Group I[c]	34,936	266	283	118	109	71	67	67	55
A	8,528	170	118	60	45	26	38	36	38
B[d]	2,890	548	785	252	175	150	119	120	
C	6,813		272	133	102	77	61	75	53
D	4,125					108	101	98	72
E	18,671					61	52	46	59
F	3,169						64	48	40
G	5,286					59	65	62	17
H	4,301				204	125	130	170	112
Group II[c]	4,858	362	616	130	120	133	97	101	78
N	879	270	620	148	70	136	70	146	131
O	553		461	83	153	43	44	21	21
P	626	527	648	200	151	203	137	39	119
Q	697	328	700	152	157	135	122	101	118
R	1,134			85	55	94	76	101	51
S	1,193				175	190	97	191	30
T	922				113	111	133	133	95
Others[f]	1,927	132	338	212	208	145	115	154	92

[a]Includes only those sickness and non-industrial accident cases which caused absence from work for one week or longer.

[b]Rate for all reporting associations from April to August differs from the rate for all diseases shown in Table II, because association H, which does not report diagnosis, is included in this table.

[c]Associations which have more than 3,000 members.

[d]Included with the large associations because the membership is nearly 3,000.

[e]Associations which have less than 3,000 members.

[f]Associations which have less than 500 members.

tion B it was 785 per 1,000; and in July Association II had nearly five times as much sickness as Establishment A. It was observed that similar differences appeared in the rates among the smaller associations. These marked differences afford strong reasons for a careful study not only of the causes of illness in the different plants, but of the conditions which give rise to them. Although it is not the purpose to analyze these differences at this time, since the records for the different associations are not sufficiently comparable with respect to the period covered, the value of statistics of this nature will, it is believed, become more and more manifested as they accumulate.

As an example of the data afforded by records of sickness causing a disability of *one* day or longer, we present a tabulation of the experience of a rubber manufacturing company employing 18,000 persons during the year ending October 31, 1920 [Table IV]. Although this company endeavors to obtain the diagnosis of each case of illness by requiring employees resuming work after illness to check in through the medical department, there were a large number of unclassified cases. The illnesses for which no diagnoses were recorded, however, were of short duration, the average being less than 3 working days. It may be assumed, accordingly, that the more serious diseases have been properly classified, and that the unclassified cases probably are mostly colds, headache, constipation, dysmenorrhea, and other conditions that disable for only two or three days. The cases for which no diagnosis was recorded constituted 36 per cent of the male cases and 42 per cent of the female cases, and since the difference is slight, it is believed that comparisons of the recorded diseases according to sex are sufficiently accurate for all practical purposes.

This experience shows a frequency rate of sickness, based on reported cases which terminated within the year, of 1,933 per 1,000 among 16,400 male employees on the factory payroll (office workers not having been included in the record). This is virtually two cases of disabling sickness per man per year. The rate for the 1,625 female factory workers was considerably higher—i.e., 2,565 cases per 1,000.

In view of the estimate of 6.9 working days as the average loss of time per person per year, based on the sickness surveys of the Metropolitan Life Insurance Company in 1916 and 1917, it is interesting to find that the number of work days lost in the rubber manufactory during the year ending October 31, 1920, was 9.3 per male employee, and 13.8 per female employee. The average duration of disability was found to be 4.8 working days per male case, and 5.4 working days per female case. The women, therefore, not only were sick oftener, but failed to recover as rapidly as the men.

Considering first the incidence of the principal groups of diseases among persons of different sex, the statistics for this company show that the frequency of incapacitating illness was greater among the females for all disease groups except diseases of the circulatory system, diseases of the skin, and diseases of the bones, and in each of these three groups the number of female cases was not large enough to be conclusive, but only suggestive of the possibility that a larger number of cases might show the same results. The severity of disease as measured by the days lost per case was greater among the females for each principal disease group except diseases of the nervous system, non-industrial accidents, and diseases of the genito-urinary system. The comparatively short duration of disease of the genito-urinary system among the females is accounted for by the large number of cases and brief duration of dysmenorrhea.

But what specific diseases and conditions were most prevalent among the rubber workers under consideration? The most frequent cause of disability among the males was "excessive colds" for which the case rate was 196 per 1,000. Though severe colds were more frequent among the females than among the males, colds were not the first cause of disability among the women employees. Tonsillitis with a rate of 239 cases per 1,000 was the most frequent cause of female inability to work. There were 388 cases of tonsillitis among 1,625 women, causing an absence of 6.3 days per case, and a day and a half of lost time per woman per year. Severe colds among the men incapacitated on the average for 3.3 working days, causing a loss of 0.7 of a day per man per year. Among the women hard colds caused an average disability of 3.9 working days per case and 0.9 of a working day per person per year. Influenza and grippe ranked second in point of frequency among the males, and third among the females. Two thousand eight hundred and twenty-seven male cases averaged 7.2 working days lost, and 293 female cases, 8.2 working days lost. Dysmenorrhea was the fourth greatest cause of disability among the women, causing an absence of 2.6 working days per case.

Other interesting sex comparisons might be cited. Headache, for example, was only slightly more frequent among females than among males. The women were not attacked by bronchitis as frequently as were the men, and their rate for constipation was only one-third of the male rate. The female rate for rheumatism was less than the male rate, and the frequency of boils (furuncle) was only one-seventh of the male rate for this cause of incapacity for work. The women had neuralgia and neuritis more often than the men, and also diseases of the eyes; but men had more diseases of the circulatory system, possibly partly for the reason that a

TABLE IV Prevalence of disabling diseases among employees of a large rubber company during the year ending October 31, 1920

Based on reported cases which caused absence from work for one day or longer and which terminated within the year

Disease or condition causing disability (with corresponding title numbers in parentheses from the International List of the Causes of Death)		CASES PER 1,000		DAYS LOST PER CASE		DAYS LOST PER PERSON	
		Males	Females	Males	Females	Males	Females
All Diseases and Conditions		1933.0	2565.3	4.81	5.38	9.30	13.80
I General Diseases		275.1	297.2	9.79	12.16	2.69	3.61
Typhoid fever	(1)	.5		41.25		.02	
Malaria	(4)	1.5	4.3	5.04	4.57	.01	.02
Smallpox	(5)	3.0	3.7	13.61	12.00	.04	.04
Measles	(6)	9.9	14.7	11.81	16.29	.12	.24
Scarlet fever	(7)	7.8	16.0	18.47	28.77	.14	.46
Diphtheria and croup	(9)	1.0	5.5	7.94	6.33	.01	.04
Influenza and grippe	(10)	172.5	180.2	7.21	8.22	1.24	1.48
Dysentery	(14)	2.6	2.5	2.21	3.50		.01
Erysipelas	(18)	1.5	3.1	17.80	17.40	.03	.05
Mumps	(19)	18.5	14.8	10.06	11.96	.19	.18
Chicken pox	(19)	.6	.6	8.90	5.00		
Infections	(20)	9.6	15.4	7.73	5.60	.07	.09
Tuberculosis of the lungs	(28)	2.6	2.5	60.86	235.25	.16	.58
Acute miliary tuberculosis	(29)	2.0	2.5	47.94	36.00	.10	.09
Tuberculosis of other organs	(30-35)	.4		38.00		.01	
Syphilis	(37)	1.8	3.1	24.13	30.00	.05	.09
Gonococcus infection	(38)	6.1	3.1	9.72	14.60	.06	.04
Cancer—all forms	(39-46)	1.0		54.50		.05	
Rheumatism	(47, 48)	31.1	24.0	10.73	7.46	.33	.18
Diabetes	(50)	.2		59.25		.02	
Exophthalmic goiter	(51)	.2	.6	45.00	16.00	.01	.01
Anaemia	(54)	.5		70.13		.03	
Alcoholism	(56)	.2		3.33			
Chronic poisonings	(57-59)						
Other general diseases			.6		16.00		.01
II Diseases of the Nervous System		36.2	40.0	7.67	7.06	.28	.28
Cerebral hemorrhage, apoplexy, and paralysis	(64-66)						
Mental alienation	(67-68)	.4	.6	22.84	6.00	.01	
Epilepsy	(69)	.4		6.29			
Chorea	(72)		1.2		7.50		.01
Neuralgia and neuritis	(73)	6.8	12.3	5.71	5.65	.04	.07
Sciatica	(73)	1.8	1.2	22.24	30.50	.04	.04
Other diseases of the nervous system				29.00			
Diseases of the eyes	(75)	13.7	16.7	5.09	4.52	.07	.07
Diseases of the ears	(76)	13.1	8.0	8.94	10.92	.12	.09
III Diseases of the Circulatory System		12.2	9.1	9.05	26.47	.11	.24
Endocarditis and other organic heart diseases	(78, 79)	1.3	1.8	17.50	90.33	.02	.17
Hemorrhoids	(83)	5.2	1.2	7.92	11.50	.04	.01
Other diseases of the veins	(83)	.5	1.2	11.13	17.50	.01	.02
Other diseases of the circulatory system		5.2	4.9	7.82	8.50	.04	.04
IV Diseases of the Respiratory System		279.2	314.4	4.59	6.17	1.28	1.94
Excessive colds	(86)	195.8	219.0	3.31	3.91	.65	.80
Other diseases of the nasal fossae	(86)	20.7	26.5	3.73	4.35	.08	.12
Diseases of the larynx	(87)	5.2	6.8	3.41	6.45	.02	.04
Bronchitis	(89, 90)	43.1	37.5	7.95	16.18	.34	.61
Pneumonia	(91, 92)	6.2	11.7	14.98	20.79	.09	.24
Pleurisy	(93)	6.8	11.7	9.24	6.00	.06	.07
Asthma	(96)	1.2	.6	30.65	2.00	.04	
Other diseases of the respiratory system		.2	.6	12.00	3.00		
V Diseases of the Digestive System		394.3	422.2	4.51	5.68	1.78	2.40
Diseases of the mouth	(99)	12.9	23.4	3.63	5.95	.05	.14
Tonsillitis	(100)	171.7	238.8	4.99	6.29	.86	1.50
Other diseases of the pharynx	(100)	19.5	4.3	3.09	2.86	.06	.01
Ulcer of the stomach	(102)	.4	.6	31.43	6.00	.01	
Other diseases of the stomach	(103)	84.1	68.3	3.20	3.80	.27	.26
Diarrhoea and enteritis	(105)	26.7	25.2	3.03	3.07	.08	.08
Appendicitis and typhlitis	(108)	11.2	13.6	14.79	16.18	.16	.22
Hernia	(109)	4.1	1.8	21.93	12.33	.09	.02
Constipation	(110)	37.3	12.3	2.56	2.10	.10	.03
Other diseases of intestines	(110)	24.5	30.2	3.24	3.18	.08	.10
Biliary calculi	(114)	.2	.6	7.33	3.00		
Other diseases of the digestive system		1.7	3.1	10.57	13.00	.02	.04

TABLE IV—*Continued*

Disease or condition causing disability (with corresponding title numbers in parentheses from the International List of the Causes of Death)		CASE PER 1,000		DAYS LOST PER CASE		DAYS LOST PER PERSON	
		Males	Females	Males	Females	Males	Females
VI Diseases of Genito-Urinary System		5.4	190.1	14.35	5.71	.08	1.09
Nephritis and Bright's disease	(119, 120)	.8	5.5	28.21	56.56	.02	.31
Diseases of the bladder	(124)	1.2	7.4	5.68	4.08	.01	.03
Diseases of the testicles	(127)	2.7		7.38		.02	
Uterine hemorrhage	(128)		12.3		16.70		.21
Dysmenorrhea	(130)		151.4		2.58		.39
Other diseases of female genitals			13.5		10.82		.15
Other diseases of genito-urinary system		.7		40.18		.03	
VII The Puerperal State			16.6		24.93		.42
VIII Diseases of the Skin		51.5	25.8	5.62	6.38	.29	.16
Gangrene	(142)	.1	.6	4.00	4.00		
Furuncle	(143)	27.4	3.7	4.79	3.50	.13	.01
Acute abscess	(144)	5.2	9.9	8.93	6.94	.05	.07
Rash-benzine	(145)	5.1	2.5	7.48	4.00	.04	.01
Other diseases of the skin		13.7	9.1	5.34	7.73	.07	.07
IX Diseases of the Bones and Organs of Loco-motion		41.1	22.7	5.10	6.24	.21	.14
Diseases of the bones	(146)	1.2	.6	10.79	55.00	.01	.03
Diseases of the joints	(147)	.8	.6	7.15	7.00	.01	.01
Lumbago	(149)	13.2	3.7	5.43	8.00	.07	.03
Myalgia	(149)	20.5	14.8	4.12	4.08	.09	.06
Flat feet	(149)	4.6	1.8	7.08	6.00	.03	.01
Other diseases of the bones, and organs of locomotion		.8	1.2	3.14	2.50		
XII Senility				147.00		.01	
XIII External Causes		45.6	48.6	7.52	6.81	.34	.33
Poisoning by food or drugs	(164)	.4	3.7	5.20	6.83		.02
Fractures	(185)	.9	2.5	23.27	23.75	.02	.06
Other injuries	(186)	44.3	42.4	7.21	5.83	.32	.25
XIV Ill-Defined		792.4	1178.6	2.82	2.71	2.23	3.19
Headache	(2-189)	87.4	94.8	2.63	3.20	.23	.30
Others		705.0	1083.8	2.84	2.66	2.00	2.89

larger proportion were in the older ages. Other points will doubt-less suggest themselves to those who desire to examine the tables in greater detail.

Attention is called to Figure 2 which shows the duration of the most frequent causes of disability among both male and female employees of the company.

These two tabulations are presented merely as samples of the material which is afforded in the records of industrial establish-ments. It is obvious that they are not so complete or so accurate as may be desired, but it is believed that they constitute a definite advance over the fragmentary data available from health depart-ments. It is believed also that when the data are collected in a larger mass, for a longer period, and in greater detail for persons of different occupational status, race, sex, and age, they will afford

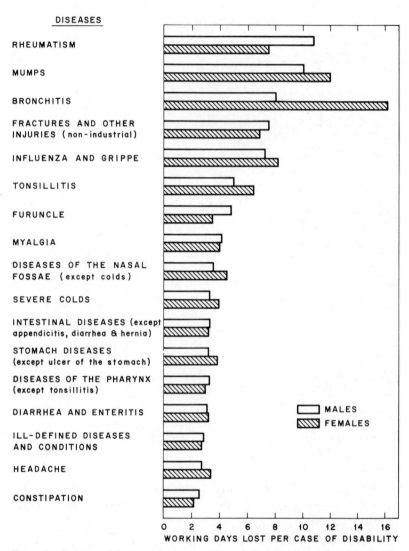

Figure 2   Duration of the most frequent causes of disability among employees of a rubber company in year ending Oct. 31, 1920.[1] Based on reported cases which caused absence from work for one day or longer and which terminated within the year.
1) Includes only those diseases having a frequency rate of more than 18 cases per 1,000 persons.

the first considerable body of dependable material for the use of
the statistician in the study of disease incidence as well as for the
student of industrial hygiene in its broader aspects. Certainly the
employer who desires to know definitely how he can improve
most effectively the health of his workers will be aided not only by
a more careful scrutiny of his own records when they are intelli-
gently tabulated and analyzed, but by the accumulated experience of other plants.

Journal of the American Statistical Association
March, 1921

3

A Study of Illness in a General Population Group

Hagerstown Morbidity Studies No. I:
The Method of Study and General Results

EDGAR SYDENSTRICKER

In a previous paper a report was given of the general results of a morbidity study in Hagerstown, Md.[1] These results were provisional, since they were based on a preliminary tabulation.

In the present communication a more precise and complete statement is made of—

1. The scope of the study and the method of observation;
2. The general character of the results obtained;
3. The procedure employed in classifying illnesses according to cause;

And some of the general results are given of a final tabulation of the data collected, including—

1. The incidence of illness and the causes thereof as observed over a period of 28 months;
2. The incidence of certain *acute diseases* in so far as they were observed, whether they were the sole cause or were complicating conditions or sequelae of a given illness;
3. The proportion of *persons* among whom certain diseases or conditions were incident or prevalent during the period.

In later papers it is planned to present other phases of the study.

[1]The Incidence of Illness in a General Population Group. Pub. Health Rep. Feb. 13, 1925, 40, 279–291. (Reprint No. 989.)

Scope of the Study and Method of Observation

A brief description of the scope and method of the study was given in the preliminary report, but for the sake of completeness and greater precision, as well as to afford the opportunity of making certain addenda, this description is somewhat revised and amplified here.

Location of study.—The city of Hagerstown was selected for this study partly because certain facilities were already afforded by the location there of a health demonstration and partly because it was a fairly typical small city in that part of the eastern section of the country which had not been influenced greatly by recent immigration. At the time when the study was made Hagerstown had a population of about 30,000 (29,878 estimated as of February 1, 1923, the mid-date of the period of observation). In 1920, 93 per cent of its population were native white and 88 per cent were native white of native parents. The foreign born comprised less than 2 per cent, and 5 per cent were colored. Of the total population 10 years of age and over, only 3 per cent were classed illiterate, and of the native white of the same ages only 2 per cent were classed as illiterate. No large or predominant industry is located in Hagerstown, the chief industries being those incident to the requirements of the surrounding area—retail and wholesale trade, a number of small factories, and transportation. Among the wage-earning group, railroad work probably predominates, the shops of the Western Maryland Railway being situated there.

Scope.—The study was planned to include between 1,500 and 2,000 families, and the sections of the city in which the observations were to be made were selected upon two grounds, namely, 1) representativeness of different economic classes, and 2) convenience for repeated visiting. The accompanying plat of the incorporated city shows the sections selected. Only white persons were included, since the number of negroes was too small to yield comparable results.

In the final tabulation of the results the observations made in 1,815 households were included. These households contained 8,587 persons for whom morbidity information at one or more

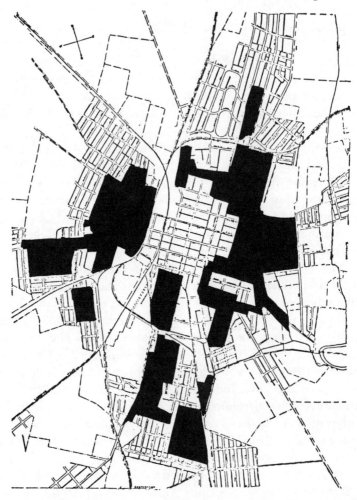

Plat of Hagerstown showing scattered areas in which the population was observed for incidence of illness from December 1, 1921 to March 31, 1924 by U.S. Public Health Service investigators.

canvasses was secured. The actual number of households visited was somewhat larger, the discarded households being of two kinds—those which moved away from the city or to some section of the city inconvenient for the field assistants to visit and those from which only unsatisfactory information could be secured. The proportion of the latter was small; in fact, the cooperation given by the families of all economic classes was very satisfactory and gratifying. As will be explained later, the data approximate a continuous record for 28 months. A certain amount of changes necessarily occurs in an ordinary population of this size, however. As stated above, 8,587 persons were included in the study, but the maximum population in any one month was 7,572. Obviously, births and deaths affected the population, and sons and daughters were married, sometimes living with a parent temporarily and later leaving the household for some part of the city not being canvassed. Occasionally no one could be found at home or the family was away on a vacation for a month or two in the summer. The following table shows, however, that 90 per cent of the persons were observed for one year and 50 per cent for 26 of the possible 28 months.

Per cent of persons observed for specified number of months in the Hagerstown morbidity study

Months under observation	PERSONS UNDER OB-SERVATION SPECIFIED NUMBER OF MONTHS	
	Number	Per cent of total
28 months	3,202	37.3
26 months or more	5,140	49.8
24 months or more	5,787	67.4
18 months or more	6,824	79.5
14 months or more	7,528	87.7
12 months or more	7,794	90.8
9 months or more	8,085	94.2
6 months or more	8,340	97.1
4 months or more	8,431	98.2

When the number of persons born or dying in the household which was observed 26 months or more is added we find that 63 per cent of the total persons of record were in the population classed as "Under observation 26 months or more."

If we express this total "exposure" in terms of persons for one year our population consists of 16,517 "years of exposure," of which 8,001 were for males and 8,516 for females. This is the *numerical* equivalent of a population of 7,079 persons observed continuously for 28 months, or an average monthly population of the same size.[2]

[2]This figure is somewhat smaller than that (7,200) used in the preliminary report because of the discarding of some families, as explained above.

Sex and age distribution of the population. —In selecting the population for study, some preference was given to those with children. As a result, the observed population has a greater percentage of children under 15 years of age and slightly fewer young adults from 20 to 35 years of age than the entire city. The percentage distribution of the observed population is compared with the total Hagerstown population in the table below:

**Percentage distribution of Hagerstown
population and of the observed population**

Age group	Hagers-town, census of 1920	Observed popula-tion 1921–1924	Differ-ence + or −
Total	**100.0**	**100.0**	
0–4	10.7	11.0	+0.3
5–9	10.2	13.0	+2.8
10–14	8.7	10.6	+2.1
15–19	8.4	8.6	+0.2
20–24	9.3	7.0	−2.3
25–34	17.9	15.3	−2.6
35–44	13.6	13.5	−0.1
45–64	16.3	16.0	−0.3
65 and over	4.8	5.0	+0.2

These differences are not great enough to prevent the observed population from being typical of the whole, an indication not without interest in itself since it suggests that in a city of this type there is a comparatively small number of unattached persons, and that family groups constitute almost the entire population. The differences shown in the table are so slight that if the total illness rate for persons of known age in the observed population is adjusted according to the Hagerstown population the rate is lowered less than 3 per cent. In fact, if we adjust the rate for sex and age to the population of the United States it becomes 1054 per 1,000 as against a crude rate of 1081, a difference of only 2 per cent.

Method. —The method of observation and recording the results may be described briefly as follows:

1) A preliminary house-to-house survey was made by members of the staff of the Office of Statistical Investigations in November, 1921, in the several sections selected, in the course of which the population of these sections was enumerated and records were made (*a*) for each individual, relating to color, sex, and

age, past occurrence of certain contagious diseases and present acute or chronic diseases or ailment, and (b) for each household relating to its general economic status, sanitary condition, method of excreta disposal, and water and milk supplies.

2) This survey was followed by a series of 16 canvasses, each household being visited by a trained field assistant at intervals of from six to eight weeks. At each visit a history of the incidence of sickness in the family since the preceding visit, with a statement of the date of onset, duration, extent of disabling effects, and attendance of physician, was obtained from a relatively responsible informant, usually the housewife.

3) In addition, other sources of information were regularly and systematically utilized in obtaining the record of disease prevalence, as follows: (a) weekly records of absence from school, specifying the nature of the illness whenever illness was the cause so far as the teacher could ascertain it; (b) reports of all cases treated in the various clinics maintained in conjunction with the Washington County Health Demonstration, all of the clinics being participated in by local physicians; (c) reports of notifiable diseases from practicing physicians; (d) reports of district nurses; (e) data collected in field investigations of child hygiene by the United States Public Health Service in cooperation with the Washington County Health Demonstration.

4) For all cases attended by physicians the statements made by the informant as to the nature or cause of illness were submitted to the physicians concerned for review and correction.

General Discussion of the Nature of the Results Obtained

As it was pointed out in the preliminary report, the result of these canvasses is not, of course, a complete record of all of the ill health prevalent in this population during the period of observation nor even an accurate statement of the causes of all the attacks of disease which were recorded. Such a record was impracticable for so large a population of this kind, and no false hopes of obtaining it were indulged in. Furthermore, it must be obvious from clinical experience as well as from considerations of a practical kind that the full extent of ill health and its specific nature can not be ascertained by any one method. Properly conducted physical examinations, supplemented by the necessary laboratory findings, will yield certain indispensable indications of the existence and the net results of various diseases and conditions, but they will not tell the whole story. A carefully obtained history, for each individual, of previous health, incidence of disease, occurrence of various symptoms, and exposure to certain possibly relevant conditions will add to the picture. Of undoubted importance is a period of observation during which the reactions of the individual under ordinary as well as specific circumstances are recorded; this record may be of the occurrence of various symptoms and of the extent to which the subject is affected—whether only slightly ill, or more or less continuously "below par," or unable to engage in his usual activities, or disabled for long periods, or dying. The detail and accuracy with which these observations are made depend, naturally, upon the means employed.

Our study was of the nature of the third method mentioned above, namely, *a series of observations which was directed as specifically as possible to the illnesses which occurred among a population during the period chosen.*

Now, it is evident that the length of interval between inquiries is one important determinant of *how much* sickness and what kinds of sickness will be recorded. A weekly inquiry will elicit information on more slight ailments than a monthly inquiry, and an inquiry made every six or eight weeks will fail to obtain information on many ailments of very short duration or of several days' duration but accompanied only by slight discomfort. From previous experience in sickness surveys and continuous morbidity records and disability records of industrial employees we were led to believe that the intervals between visits chosen for the present study would probably yield a fairly accurate record of *real illnesses.*

As a matter of fact, less than 5 per cent of the illnesses of exactly stated durations recorded in our study were one day or less in duration. Nearly 80 per cent were three days or longer, and 60 per cent were eight days or longer in duration.[3] Approximately 40 per cent were not only disabling but caused confinement to bed. It is evident, therefore, that in the main the illnesses recorded were more than trivial in their character, in spite of the fact that in some instances mere symptoms were given as diagnoses. The incidence of acute attacks of specific and generally recognizable diseases has been, we feel, recorded with a satisfactory degree of completeness. On the other hand, the incidence of mild attacks, as, for example, of coryza, and of slight disorders and even of serious conditions when such conditions were not accompanied by noticeable symptoms, is probably incomplete and in many instances inaccurate in spite of the fact that a record of 28 months was obtained for the same individuals. Cases attended by physicians may be said to be quite complete.[4]

The question properly may be asked: Exactly what is meant by "illness"? The question is hard to answer with a precise definition. In the first place, the records of "illness" obtained in this study were of illnesses as reported by the household informant (usually the wife) either as experienced by herself or as she observed them in her family; the definition of the term thus can not be refined any further than the common understanding of the word. In the second place, the records as obtained were of *attacks* rather than illness in the sense of ill health. As will appear later, of those persons affected with some chronic condition, only those who suffered ill effects of this condition *during the period* were

[3]The results of this study relating to duration of cases of illnesss will be presented and discussed in a later paper.

[4]During the same period in which this study was made every absence of school children in Hagerstown was recorded, with such information relating to cause of absence as could be secured from the children, parents, and teachers. The sickness rates for children in school based upon records obtained in house-to-house visits were compared with the rates based upon school records, with the result that the two rates for sickness lasting three days or longer were almost identical. About 50 per cent of sicknesses lasting one day or longer and about 75 per cent of those lasting two days or longer were recorded in the house-to-house canvasses, but a larger proportion of the short-time absences from school were ascribed to "headache" and other symptoms.

recorded as having this condition. It is undoubtedly true that had we employed this method of study over a period longer than 28 months more conditions of this nature would have been brought to light, since the factor of time is a fundamental one in recording and interpreting morbidity. At the same time it must be evident that there is a period beyond which additional observation of this kind will not yield much additional information, when, for practical purposes, the "law of diminishing returns" renders further expenditure of effort and patience unprofitable for the purpose in mind.

The reader is cautioned against putting too fine a point on the definition of illness as recorded in this series of observations. Perhaps it is sufficient simply to bear in mind that the chief aim of the study was a record of illnesses, as ordinarily understood, that were experienced by a population group composed of persons of all ages and both sexes, and in no remarkable respect unusual. This record, the first of its kind so far as we are aware, was regarded as desirable in order to give a picture of the sickness *incidence* in a general population group over a sufficiently long period of time to distinguish it from sickness prevalence as ascertained at a given instant in time by the cross-section method.

Classification of Illnesses According to Cause

When the stage of classifying the illnesses according to cause was reached in the course of this study, it was brought home to us that while a little knowledge is a dangerous thing, the task of dealing with a little more knowledge was a very puzzling and troublesome thing. The chief difficulty lay in the selection of the primary cause of illness when several possible causes were observed. This difficulty has been experienced, of course, in dealing with the so-called "joint" causes of death, and a more or less arbitrary statistical procedure has been developed. But in the case of our morbidity records it happened that for many individuals there was a series of observations covering some period of time, and this entire sickness history of an individual frequently had to be considered in determining the primary cause of a particular illness. In other words, we were in the position of knowing a good deal more about these individuals than we would learn from the entries ordinarily made on a death certificate. There were other difficulties, as well; but in dealing with them all it seemed to us that the primary purpose to be kept in mind was *the immediate cause of each specific illness*. The prevalence of any disease or the reason or reasons for the ill health of the individual concerned was regarded as another, although often related, matter, to be determined for another purpose. This we tried to do by adhering to the procedure outlined below.

1. The term "illness" was rigidly interpreted as "a continuous period of sickness"[5] regardless of complications, even though in some instances the coincident occurrence of two or more conditions seemed to be a matter of chance. Thus, a person who had grippe, measles, and chicken pox within one continuous period, i.e., without a definite statement from the family that some time intervened between the separate conditions, would be credited with only *one illness*. A person with several chronic conditions contributing to a more or less continuous condition of illness was counted as sick only once, and one condition was considered the primary cause and the others contributory causes. All respiratory illnesses were carefully edited to see that the same continuous sickness was not counted as two illnesses when due to what seemed to be *successive* or *progressive* conditions. Thus a person might report a cold followed by pneumonia; this would be counted only once as pneumonia. Similarly, many combinations of respiratory conditions were reported, such as cold and bronchitis, bronchitis and tonsillitis, tonsillitis and influenza. All were counted as *one illness*, and that condition which, from the obtainable information, was chiefly responsible for this particular illness was considered the sole cause.

2. In the many cases in which more than one cause of an illness or attending condition was recorded the following general

[5]The annual incidence rate determined by our final tabulation was 51 per 1,000 less than in the preliminary tabulation, a difference due primarily to a more rigid conformance to this interpretation.

rules were followed in selecting the primary cause under which the illness was classified:

(*a*) The *first* cause in order of occurrence, applied largely to acute conditions with common complications; such as influenza and pneumonia, measles and otitis media, scarlet fever and nephritis.

(*b*) *Acute* conditions ordinarily were given preference over an attack of some chronic condition. Thus, in case of grippe and chronic rheumatism, the grippe was considered primary.

(*c*) The condition or disease *most specifically associated with the period of sickness* was preferred over a minor condition which preceded or accompanied it. For example, tooth abscess and rheumatism; the latter was made primary. When it was difficult to determine the factual basis, the more serious condition was chosen.

(*d*) The *more specific* cause was given preference over a statement of a symptom.

(*e*) When none of the above rules could be applied, and the history of the individual gave no basis for decision, the condition mentioned first by the informant was made primary. The number of such cases was relatively small.

Rather frequently the informant mentioned more than one condition in telling about an illness, but when these conditions were in the nature of symptoms which simply amplified the information as regards a single cause of illness they were not tabulated as complications or contributory causes. For example, a person may have reported indigestion and a headache as the cause of illness, but only the indigestion was counted. In other words, *symptoms* were not made contributory causes unless it seemed quite certain they represented a condition *separate* and *distinct* from the primary diagnosis. On the other hand, all specific conditions were tabulated, even though they were very frequently complications of the primary disease. Thus, in the case of cold and indigestion, the cold was made primary, but the indigestion was tabulated as a complication.

The form of the classification used was the International List of Causes of Death, 1920 Revision. Some departures, dictated by considerations which we believe will be apparent to anyone more interested in the causes of illness than in a mere scheme of classification, were made from it; but in all the tables here presented the International List numbers are carried for definitive purposes.

The Incidence of Illnesses Classified by Cause

The basic data used in this report are presented in Table I. Here is shown the number of illnesses recorded during the 28 months, classified according to the sole or primary cause. The principal specific causes are shown separately and also the totals for groups of diseases according to the International List of 1920. In the last two columns of the table are shown the number of times each disease was reported as a complicating or contributory cause of an illness. Thus if it is desired to know the number of times otitis media was the primary cause of illness the first three columns in Table I show that there were 117 illnesses due to this cause, 57 males and 60 females; but the last two columns in the table show that otitis media was present in an additional 19 illnesses of males and 30 illnesses of females, and the sum of the two numbers for males and the two for females gives, therefore, the total number of times otitis media was either a primary cause or a contributory cause of illness.

From the point of view of the frequency of illness from various causes, the rate per 1,000 persons is a much more comprehensible term, although as a single expression it can not afford the detail given in Table I. In Table II, therefore, is shown the annual illness rate based upon our 28 months' experience. It should be observed that this rate is computed in all instances by dividing the number of cases recorded by the "years of exposure."

An illness rate of slightly more than one illness per person per year is indicated. This rate was somewhat higher than it would have been for two "normal" calendar years, for the reasons that the period of observation included nearly three winter seasons

TABLE I   Number of illnesses in which specified diseases or conditions were the sole or primary cause and the number in which each disease or condition was reported as a contributory cause in a canvassed population group of white persons in Hagerstown, Md., December 1, 1921–March 31, 1924

Diseases and conditions causing illness (numbers in parentheses refer to those given in the International List of the Causes of Death, 1920)	NUMBER OF ILLNESSES IN WHICH SPECIFIED DISEASE WAS THE SOLE OR PRIMARY CAUSE			NUMBER OF ILLNESSES IN WHICH SPECIFIED DISEASE WAS A CONTRIBUTORY CAUSE	
	Both sexes	Male	Female	Male	Female
Years of life exposed	**16,517**	**18,001**	**8,516**		
All diseases	17,847	7,541	10,306	216	444
Total respiratory (excluding operations) (11, 31, 97–107, 109)	10,844	4,746	6,098	55	77
Influenza and grippe (11)	2,366	1,009	1,357	5	11
Pneumonia (all forms) (100, 101)	111	57	54	18	15
Pleurisy (102)	33	13	20	3	2
Diseases of pharynx (109)	1,085	467	618	2	14
Tonsillitis	470	193	277	1	6
Sore throat	512	223	289		2
Quinsy	50	28	22	1	4
Other diseases of pharynx	53	23	30		2
Diseases of larynx (98)	188	80	108		
Laryngitis	95	25	70		
Croup	88	54	34		
Other diseases of the larynx	5	1	4		
Hay fever and asthma (105, part of 107)	95	33	..2	2	3
Tuberculosis, pulmonary (31)	52	16	36		3
Other diseases of respiratory system (including head colds, chest, and bronchial conditions) (97, 99, 103, 107)	6,914	3,071	3,843	25	29
Tonsillectomy, adenoidectomy, or both	120	63	57		
Other operations on throat and nasal fossae	8	6	2		
Epidemic, endemic, and infectious diseases (1–42, except 11 and 31)	1,448	731	717	9	8
Typhoid (1)	19	6	13		
Measles (7)	565	277	288	2	1
Scarlet fever (8)	34	18	16		
Whooping cough (9)	374	204	170		
Diphtheria (10)	45	21	24		
Chicken pox (25a)	229	138	91	1	2
German measles (25b)	18	7	11		
Tuberculosis, nonpulmonary (32–37)	14	5	9		
Venereal diseases (38–40)	27	6	21		5
Vaccinia (part of 42)	38	18	20		
Other diseases in this group (2–6, 12–24, 26–30, 41, and part of 42)	85	31	54	6	
General diseases (43–69)	359	113	246	6	16
Cancer (43–49)	22	3	19		
Rheumatism, acute and chronic (51, 52)	275	89	186	3	12
Diabetes (57)	15	2	13	1	
Exophthalmic goiter (60a)	9	1	8		
Other general diseases (50, 53–56, 58, 59, 60b,[1] 61–69)	38	18	20	2	4
Diseases of the nervous system (70–84, part of 205)	728	168	560	18	56
Cerebral hemorrhage and apoplexy (74)	11	2	9	3	1
Paralysis (75)	25	9	16		2
Epilepsy (78)	10	8	2	1	
Chorea (81)	20	4	16		
Neuralgia (part of 82)	101	20	81	5	15
Neuritis and sciatica (part of 82)	87	19	68	2	6
Headache (part of 82 and 205)	249	64	185		2
Neurasthenia (part of 84)	181	23	158	6	29
Other nervous diseases (71–73, 76, 77, 79–80, 83, part of 82, 84)	44	19	25	1	1
Diseases of the eyes and annexa (85)	123	71	52	2	14
Diseases of ears and mastoid process (86)	180	81	99	25	43
Otitis media	117	57	60	19	30
Mastoiditis	10	7	3		1
Other and unqualified diseases of the ear	53	17	36	6	12
Diseases of circulatory system (87–96)	303	113	190	34	60

[1]Includes simple goiter only when it caused some illness in the period.

TABLE I —*Continued*

Diseases and conditions causing illness (numbers in parentheses refer to those given in the International List of the Causes of Death, 1920)	NUMBER OF ILLNESSES IN WHICH SPECIFIED DISEASE WAS THE SOLE OR PRIMARY CAUSE			NUMBER OF ILLNESSES IN WHICH SPECIFIED DISEASE WAS A CONTRIBUTORY CAUSE	
	Both sexes	Male	Female	Male	Female
Years of life exposed	**16,517**	**8,001**	**8,516**		
Diseases of the heart (87–90)	166	51	115	17	39
Arteriosclerosis (part of 91)	20	11	9	6	6
Hemorrhoids (part of 93)	18	9	9		
High blood pressure (part of 96)	19	4	15	3	8
Adenitis (part of 94)	44	21	23	7	6
Other diseases of circulatory system (91, 95, part of 91, 93, 94, and 96)	36	17	19	1	1
Diseases and disorders of the digestive system (110–127, part of 108 and 205)	1,594	645	949	24	67
Ulcers of stomach and duodenum (111)	11	10	1		1
Indigestion and upset stomach (112)	716	313	403	8	15
Biliousness (part of 205)	156	54	102	4	12
Stomach trouble, unqualified (112)	125	56	69	3	9
Diarrhea −2 years (113)	75	36	39	2	2
Diarrhea +2 years (114)	136	58	78		4
Appendicitis (117)	85	26	59		14
Hernia (118a)	27	18	9		
Intestinal disorders, including constipation (118b, 119)	37	13	24	2	
Biliary calculi (123)	69	11	58		3
Cholecystitis (part of 124)	30	3	27		2
Jaundice (part of 124)	45	18	27		
Other diseases of liver (part of 124)	28	7	21	2	1
Other diseases of digestive system (110, 116, 126, and 108, excluding teeth and gums)	54	22	32	3	4
Diseases of teeth and gums (part of 108)	124	47	77	3	9
Diseases of kidney and annexa (128–134)	182	57	125	20	35
Acute nephritis (128)	9	3	6	3	2
Chronic nephritis (129)	43	16	27	9	17
Other and unqualified kidney trouble (131)	73	17	56	7	11
Cystitis and bladder trouble (unqualified) (133)	41	14	27	1	5
Other diseases in this group (132, 134)	16	7	9		
Nonvenereal diseases of genito-urinary system (135–142)	183	9	174	3	29
Diseases of male organs (125–136)	9	9		3	
Diseases of female genital organs (137–139, part of 141, 142)	99		99		11
Menstruation (part of 141)	48		48		4
Menopause (part of 141)	27		27		14
Puerperal state (143–150)	395		395		7
Abortion and stillbirth (part of 143)	33		33		
Confinements	324		324		
Other puerperal conditions (143–150)	38		38		7
Diseases of skin and cellular tissue (151–154, part of 205)[2]	291	165	126	14	16
Furuncle (152)	71	54	17	2	4
Abscess (153)	27	11	16	1	3
Impetigo contagiosa (part of 154)	24	12	12	1	
Scabies and itch (part of 154)	23	15	8	1	
Other and unqualified skin conditions (part of 154 and 205)[2]	146	73	73	9	9
Disease of bone and organs of locomotion (155–158, part of 205)	111	44	67	2	3
Lumbago, myalgia, and myositis (158)	49	26	23	2	1
Backache (part of 205)	37	7	30		1
Other diseases of bone or organs of locomotion (155, 156, part of 158)	25	11	14		1
Congenital malformations and infancy (159–163)	19	5	14		
Senility (164)	14	6	8		
External causes (165–203)	653	397	256	1	2
All poisonings (175, 176, 177)	46	28	18		
Burns (178–179)	35	19	16		
Fractures, wounds, injuries (ind.) (183–188, 201, 202)	116	113	3	1	
Fractures, wounds, injuries (nonind.) 183–188, 201, 202)	373	177	196		2
Fractures, wounds, injuries (not stated) (183–188, 201, 202)	51	43	8		
Other external causes (165–174, 181–182, 189, 190–196)	32	17	15		
Ill-defined and unknown	168	74	94		2

[2]Includes rash, hives, and sores on body

TABLE II   Morbidity from groups of causes and from certain specified diseases in canvassed population group of white persons of Hagerstown, Md., December 1, 1921–March 31, 1924

Diseases and conditions causing illness (numbers in parentheses refer to those given in the International List of Causes of Death, 1920)	ANNUAL RATE PER 1,000 PERSONS OBSERVED		
	Both sexes	Male	Female
All causes	1,080.5	942.5	1,210.2
Total respiratory (excluding operations) (11, 97–107, 109, 31)	656.5	593.2	716.1
Influenza and grippe (11)	143.2	126.1	159.3
Pneumonia (all forms) (100, 101)	6.7	7.1	6.3
Pleurisy (102)	2.0	1.6	2.3
Diseases of pharynx (109)	65.7	58.4	72.6
Tonsillitis	28.5	24.1	32.5
Sore throat	31.0	27.9	33.9
Quinsy	3.0	3.5	2.6
Other diseases of pharynx	3.2	2.9	3.5
Diseases of larynx (98)	11.4	10.0	12.7
Laryngitis	5.8	3.1	8.2
Croup	5.3	6.7	4.0
Other diseases of larynx	.3	.1	.5
Hay fever and asthma (105, part of 107)	5.8	4.1	7.3
Tuberculosis, pulmonary (31)	3.1	2.0	4.2
Other diseases of respiratory system (including head colds, chest and bronchial conditions) (97, 99, 103, 107)	418.6	383.8	451.3
Tonsillectomy, adenoidectomy, or both	7.3	7.9	6.7
Other operations on throat and nasal fossae	.5	.7	.2
Epidemic, endemic, and infectious diseases (1–42, except 11 and 31)	87.7	91.4	84.2
Typhoid (1)	1.2	.7	1.5
Measles (7)	34.2	34.6	33.8
Scarlet fever (8)	2.1	2.2	1.9
Whooping cough (9)	22.6	25.5	20.0
Diphtheria (10)	2.7	2.6	2.8
Chicken pox (25a)	13.9	17.2	10.7
German measles (25b)	1.1	.9	1.3
Tuberculosis, nonpulmonary (32–37)	.8	.6	1.1
Venereal diseases (38, 40)	1.6	.7	2.5
Vaccinia (part of 42)	2.3	2.2	2.3
Other diseases in this group (2–6, 12–24, 26–30, and part of 42)	5.1	3.9	6.3
General diseases (43–69)	21.7	14.1	28.9
Cancer, all forms (43–49)	1.3	.4	2.2
Rheumatism, acute and chronic (51, 52)	16.6	11.1	21.8
Diabetes (57)	.9	.2	1.5
Exophthalmic goiter (60a)	.5	.1	.9
Other general diseases (50, 53–56, 58, 59, 60b,[1] 61–65, 67–69)	2.3	2.2	2.3
Diseases of the nervous system (70–84, part of 205)	44.1	21.0	65.8
Cerebral hemorrhage and apoplexy (74)	.7	.2	1.1
Paralysis (75)	1.5	1.1	1.9
Epilepsy (78)	.6	1.0	.2
Chorea (81)	1.2	.5	1.9
Neuralgia (part of 82)	6.1	2.5	9.5
Neuritis and sciatica (part of 82)	5.3	2.4	8.0
Headache (part of 82, part of 205)	15.1	8.0	21.7
Neurasthenia (part of 84)	11.0	2.9	18.6
Other nervous diseases (71–73, 76–77, 79, 80, 83, part of 82, part of 84)	2.7	2.4	2.9
Diseases of eye and annexa (85)	7.4	8.9	6.1
Diseases of ear and mastoid process (86)	10.9	10.1	11.6
Otitis media	7.1	7.1	7.0
Mastoiditis	.6	.9	.4
Other and unqualified diseases of the ear	3.2	2.1	4.2
Diseases of circulatory system (87–96)	18.3	14.1	22.3
Diseases of the heart (87–90)	10.1	6.4	13.5
Arteriosclerosis (part of 91)	1.2	1.4	1.1
Hemorrhoids (part of 93)	1.1	1.1	1.1
Adenitis (part of 94)	2.7	2.6	2.7
High blood pressure (part of 96)	1.2	.5	1.8
Other diseases of the circulatory system (92, 95, part of 91, 93, 94, and 96)	2.2	2.1	2.2
Diseases and disorders of the digestive system (110–127, part of 108 and 205)	96.5	80.6	111.4
Ulcers of stomach and duodenum (111)	.7	1.2	.1
Indigestion and upset stomach (part of 112)	43.3	39.1	47.3
Biliousness (part of 205)	9.4	6.7	12.0

[1]Includes simple goiter only when it caused some illness in the period.

TABLE II—*Continued*

Diseases and conditions causing illness (numbers in parentheses refer to those given in the International List of Causes of Death, 1920)	ANNUAL RATE PER 1,000 PERSONS OBSERVED		
	Both sexes	Male	Female
Stomach trouble, unqualified (part of 112)	7.6	7.0	8.1
Diarrhea −2 years (113)	4.5	4.5	4.6
Diarrhea +2 years (114)	8.2	7.2	9.2
Appendicitis (117)	5.1	3.2	6.9
Hernia (118a)	1.6	2.2	1.1
Intestinal disorders, including constipation (118b, 119)	2.2	1.6	2.8
Biliary calculi (123)	4.2	1.4	6.8
Cholecystitis (part of 124)	1.8	.4	3.2
Jaundice (part of 124)	2.7	2.2	3.2
Other and unqualified diseases of liver (part of 124)	1.7	.9	2.5
Other diseases of digestive system (110, 116, 126, 108 excluding teeth and gums)	3.3	2.7	3.8
Diseases of teeth and gums (part of 108)	7.5	5.9	9.0
Diseases of kidney and annexa (128–134)	11.0	7.1	14.7
Acute nephritis (128)	.5	.4	.7
Chronic nephritis (129)	2.6	2.0	3.2
Other and unqualified diseases of the kidney (131)	4.4	2.1	6.6
Cystitis and bladder trouble, unqualified (133)	2.5	1.7	3.2
Other diseases in this group (132, 134)	1.0	.9	1.1
Nonvenereal genito-urinary system (135–142)	11.1	1.1	20.4
Diseases of male organs (135–136)	.5	1.1	
Diseases of female genital organs (137–142)	6.0		11.6
Menstruation (part of 141)	2.9		5.6
Menopause (part of 141)	1.6		3.2
Puerperal state (143–150)	23.9		46.4
Abortion and stillbirth (part of 143)	2.0		3.9
Confinements	19.6		38.0
Other puerperal conditions (143–150)	2.3		4.5
Diseases of skin and cellular tissue (part of 205,[2] 151–154)	17.6	20.6	14.8
Furuncle (152)	4.3	6.7	2.0
Abscess (153)	1.6	1.4	1.6
Impetigo contagiosa (part of 154)	1.5	1.5	1.4
Scabies and itch (part of 154)	1.4	1.9	.9
Other and unqualified skin conditions (part of 154 and 205)[2]	8.8	9.1	8.6
Diseases of bones and organs of locomotion (155–158, part of 205)	6.7	5.5	7.9
Lumbago, myalgia, myositis (part of 158)	3.0	3.2	2.7
Backache (part of 205)	2.2	.9	3.5
Other diseases of bones or locomotion (155, 156, part of 158)	1.5	1.4	1.6
Congenital malformations and infancy (159–163)	1.2	.6	1.6
Senility (164)	.8	.7	.9
External causes (165–203)	39.5	49.6	30.1
All poisonings (175, 176, 177)	2.8	3.5	2.1
Burns (178–179)	2.1	2.4	1.9
Fractures, wounds, injuries (ind.) (183–188, 201, 202)	7.0	14.1	.4
Fractures, wounds, injuries (nonind.) (183–188, 201, 202)	22.6	22.1	23.0
Fractures, wounds, injuries (not stated) (183–188, 201, 202)	3.1	5.4	.9
Other external causes (165–174, 181–182, 190–196)	1.9	2.1	1.8
Ill-defined and unknown	10.2	9.2	11.0
Years of life exposed	**16,517**	**8,001**	**8,516**

[2]Includes rash, hives, and sores on body.

and only two summers and that in 1923 an outbreak of influenza occurred. At the same time it is far below what a record of *all* respiratory attacks alone would show,[6] and very properly so, be-

[6]Unpublished records of respiratory attacks among members of families of medical officers of the Army, Navy, and Public Health Service showed a rate of about 2,000 attacks per 1,000 persons. The rate among college students as reported by themselves for a six months' period was even higher, but it included many cases which ordinarily would not be noticed.

cause the Hagerstown study was, as has been stated, a record of illnesses rather than of attacks that did not result in illness. The Hagerstown rate is about ten times the rate for illnesses causing absences from work among industrial workers (chiefly adult males)[7] for eight days or longer. The Hagerstown rate for males of all ages is more than twice the 1924 rate for illnesses causing absences of *two* days or longer among adult males employed in a group of establishments, while the Hagerstown rate for females of all ages is about 20 per cent higher than that for adult females employed in these establishments.[8] When the higher illness rate among children, old persons as well as other persons not employed, who are included in the Hagerstown study, are taken into account, it would appear that the Hagerstown rate compares very favorably from the point of view of completeness with the records of illness incapacitating for two days or longer. A more exact comparison, however, will be made in a later report when the records for persons of different ages are presented and discussed.[9]

The general picture of illness afforded by Table II is shown in graphic form in Figure 1. The relative importance from the point of *incidence*—not severity as measured by duration, incapacitation, fatality, or by other means—of the principal diseases and groups of diseases is indicated in such a way as to need no detailed comment, but a few general observations may be offered.

Doubtless it will be somewhat surprising that such diseases as tuberculosis, cancer, diseases of the heart, kidneys, etc., upon which so much emphasis is placed in public-health work, occupy

[7]Frequency of Disabling Illnesses Among Industrial Employees. Pub. Health Rep., Jan. 22, 1926, 41, 113–131. (Reprint No. 1060.)

[8]From unpublished data in the Offices of Statistical Investigations and Industrial Hygiene, United States Public Health Service, upon which a report will be presented shortly.

[9]In Tables I and II, under the heading of illnesses due to respiratory attacks, a large number (6,914 cases) are grouped under the subtitle "other diseases of respiratory system (including head colds, chest, and bronchial conditions)." During the second half of the period an effort was made to obtain more definite statements as to the nature of these attacks, the results of which will be presented in a later publication dealing with morbidity from respiratory diseases.

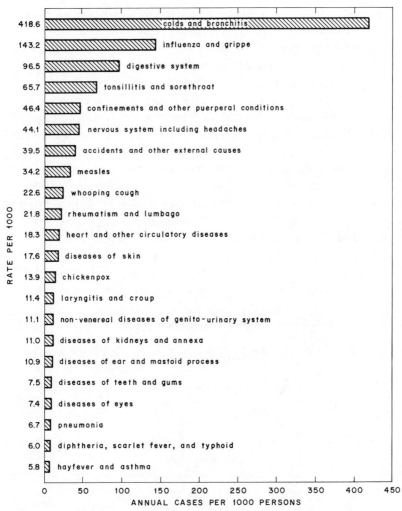

Figure 1   Principal causes of illness in Hagerstown—28 months.

such a low position in the list of diseases which cause illness.
Upon this indication two comments suggest themselves: 1) That
as *causes of illness* in a *general* population group, a group that has
not been considered heretofore to the same extent as special
groups of persons, these diseases are actually far less frequent
than the ailments which most of us, who are not suffering from

serious ill health, experience; 2) that the measure of the frequency
of these diseases was, in this study, the extent to which they
manifested themselves in illness; that is, our study was not an
intensive physical examination nor an exhaustive survey of ill
health. This observation is further supported by the evidence,
which will be elaborated in a later paper, afforded by records of
medical attendance which showed, for example, that all or practically all cases of tuberculosis, high-blood pressure, nephritis,
cancer, etc., recorded were those which were attended by physicians during the period of observation.

On the other hand, the general outline of the causes of illness
in a fairly representative population afforded by Tables I and II
seems to us to be extremely illuminating. It is shown that the
causes of illness present an aspect quite different from that presented by the causes of mortality as we now record and classify
mortality. Of the total illnesses observed, we find the proportionate distribution according to broad groups of causes as follows:

**Percentage distribution of illnesses
in each broad disease group**

General disease groups	Per cent of total illnesses
Respiratory	61.4
Epidemic, endemic, and infectious	8.1
General	2.0
Nervous system	4.1
Eye and annexa	.7
Ear and mastoid process	1.0
Heart and circulatory system	1.8
Digestive	8.9
Teeth and gums	.7
Kidneys and annexa	1.0
Genito-urinary (nonvenereal)	1.0
Puerperal	2.2
Skin	1.6
Bones and organs of locomotion	.6
External causes	3.7
Other	1.1

The fact that 61 per cent of the illnesses were due to respiratory diseases as against only 20 per cent of mortality in Hagerstown during the same period[10] is significant of the unsuitability of
mortality statistics as any indication of the causes of morbidity. On
the other hand, the fact that 35 per cent of the deaths as against 2.8
per cent of the illnesses were due to diseases of the circulatory

[10]Incidence of illness in a General Population Group. Pub. Health Rep., Feb.
13, 1926, 40, 279–291. (Reprint No. 989.)

system and kidneys and annexa is equally significant of the unsuitability of illness statistics (when cases of relatively short duration and slight severity are included) as indices of the causes of contemporaneous mortality. A relationship between morbidity and mortality exists, of course, but it is intricate and variable; the experience here presented confirms a wise dictum that no ratio between morbidity and mortality may be assumed for the great majority of diseases without a knowledge of their fatality.

Incidence of Certain Diseases as Revealed by Illness

Having clearly in mind the fact that the "statistical unit" in our study is an illness lasting approximately three days or longer, and having ascertained as best we could the causes of these illnesses and classified them accordingly, we may next consider the data as records of the incidence and prevalence of specific diseases.

It is obvious that the value of the observations in affording evidence on these important points must vary according to diseases in proportion to the extent to which an attack of a disease results in illness of that degree of severity which was recorded. Thus, many attacks of "colds" certainly were not recorded because only those resulting in "illnesses," according to the definition of the term, were observed. On the contrary, it is quite certain that a very much larger proportion of the cases of whooping cough were noticed. This suggests a point of refinement, however, that morbidity statistics are far from having attained, but which is well to keep in mind if one wishes to put data of the sort we are dealing with to uses involving rather fine shades of interpretation. It is reasonable to say, we believe, that the Hagerstown study affords a fairly complete indication of the incidence of most diseases occurring among a general population group the attacks or effects of which were severe enough to produce the condition of sickness.

With these limitations before us, two tables are presented for consideration.

One (Table III) shows the *annual* incidence rates for a number of acute diseases and diseases which manifested themselves in a more or less acute form, either as primary or as contributory causes of illness. It will be observed at once that some of the diseases are rather poorly defined, since they are grouped under general titles. This means that, while the information secured was sufficiently accurate to permit of a general classification as to their nature, it was not specific enough to warrant a very definite designation as to the exact disease or condition involved. For the great majority of diseases included in Table III, however, we feel that the specific classifications employed are justified by the information secured.

The rates in Table III require no particular comment. They are of unusual interest, it is believed, because they represent a rather extended and intensive series of observations upon a fairly typical population. For some diseases the rates will possess somewhat permanent value as a basis for comparison with other morbidity studies of a similar kind; for others, such as measles or whooping cough, the rates are characteristic only of the particular period in which they occurred.

In Table IV an entirely different phase of morbidity is presented. This table represents an attempt to answer the question, How many *persons* were affected by certain diseases and conditions of a more or less continuing or chronic nature? Here, again it must be kept in mind that only those chronic conditions were revealed which manifested themselves in illness or definitely morbid effects as a result of the disease or condition during the period of observation. It is evident, of course, that observations such as these can not yield the same kind of results as a physical examination of each individual. Latent or incipient diseases and conditions that did *not* manifest themselves in morbid effects obviously do not appear in the rates shown in Table IV. It is believed, however, that nearly all of the more serious of these diseases and conditions are portrayed. While the cases recorded of venereal diseases, for example, are probably too low—although we have no comparable data to judge by—the rate for active cases of tuberculosis, to cite another instance, is just about what we would expect in a population and under conditions of the kind observed. The facts that two-thirds of the persons were under.

TABLE III   Incidence of acute attacks of certain diseases resulting in illness during a 28 months' period in a general population group in Hagerstown, Md.

Diseases and conditions causing illness (numbers in parentheses refer to those given in the International List of Causes of Death, 1920)	NUMBER OF CASES			RATE PER 1,000 YEARS OF EXPOSURE		
	Both sexes	Males	Fe-males	Both sexes	Males	Fe-males
Acute respiratory:						
Influenza and grippe (11)	2,382	1,014	1,368	144.21	126.73	160.64
Pneumonia, all forms (100–101)	144	75	69	8.72	9.37	8.10
Pleurisy (102)	38	16	22	2.30	2.00	2.58
Diseases of pharynx (109)	1,089	466	623	65.93	58.24	73.16
Tonsillitis	476	194	282	28.82	24.25	33.11
Sore throat	514	223	291	31.12	27.87	34.17
Quinsy	55	29	26	3.33	3.62	3.05
Other diseases of pharynx	44	20	24	2.66	2.50	2.82
Diseases of larynx (98)	187	80	107	11.32	10.00	12.56
Laryngitis	94	25	69	5.69	3.12	8.10
Croup	88	54	34	5.33	6.75	3.99
Other diseases of larynx	5	1	4	.30	.12	.47
Colds and other respiratory diseases (including chest and bronchial conditions)	6,933	3,087	3,846	419.74	385.82	451.62
Epidemic, endemic, and infectious diseases:						
Typhoid fever (1)	19	6	13	1.15	.75	1.53
Measles (7)	568	279	289	34.39	34.87	33.94
Scarlet fever (8)	34	18	16	2.06	2.25	1.88
Whooping cough (9)	374	204	170	22.64	25.50	19.96
Diphtheria (10)	45	21	24	2.72	2.62	2.82
Mumps (13)	9	3	6	.54	.37	.70
Chicken pox (25a)	232	139	93	14.05	17.37	10.92
German measles (25b)	18	7	11	1.09	.87	1.29
Cholera nostras (15)	36	9	27	2.18	1.12	3.17
Dysentery (16)	10	4	6	.61	.50	.70
Diseases of nervous system (acute):						
Cerebral hemorrhage and apoplexy (74)	15	5	10	.91	.62	1.17
Convulsions and cramps (79, 80)	13	11	2	.79	1.37	.23
Hysteria (part of 82)	7	1	6	.42	.12	.70
Diseases of the digestive system:						
Stomach trouble, indigestion, "biliousness," etc. (112)	955	398	557	57.82	49.74	65.41
Diarrhea −2 years (113)	79	38	41	4.78	4.75	4.81
Diarrhea +2 years (114)	123	50	73	7.45	6.25	8.57
Acute intestinal conditions (119)	25	12	13	1.51	1.50	1.53
Jaundice (part of 124)	45	18	27	2.72	2.25	3.17
Diseases of teeth and gums (part of 108)	136	50	86	8.23	6.25	10.10
Eye conditions:						
Conjunctivitis and other acute eye trouble (85)	125	67	58	7.58	8.37	6.81
Ear conditions:						
Otitis media (part of 86)	166	76	90	10.05	9.50	10.57
Earache and other unqualified ear trouble (part of 86)	71	23	48	4.30	2.88	5.64
Adenitis (part of 94)	57	28	29	3.45	3.50	3.41
Diseases of skin and cellular tissue:						
Furuncle (152)	77	56	21	4.66	7.00	2.47
Abscess (153)	31	12	19	1.88	1.50	2.23
Impetigo contagiosa (part of 154)	25	13	12	1.51	1.62	1.41
Scabies and itch (part of 154)	24	16	8	1.45	2.00	.94
Sores (part of 205)	67	36	31	4.06	4.50	3.64
Hives and rash (part of 205)	48	21	27	2.91	2.62	3.17
Other and unqualified skin conditions (part of 154)	49	25	24	2.97	3.12	2.82

observation for at least two years and that nine-tenths of them were observed for at least one year by a competent field assistant who took advantage of the opportunity to become fairly well acquainted with every family, should also be considered in appraising the completeness of the information collected and the accuracy of the rates in this table. In fact, we are inclined to place

TABLE IV   Prevalence of certain chronic conditions resulting in illnesses during a 28 months' period in a general population group in Hagerstown, Md.

Diseases or conditions (numbers in parentheses refer to those given in the International List of Causes of Death, 1920)	NUMBER OF PERSONS REPORTING SPECIFIED CONDITIONS			RATE PER 1,000 INDIVIDUALS OBSERVED		
	Both sexes	Males	Fe-males	Both sexes	Males	Fe-males
Tuberculosis, pulmonary (31)	49	15	34	5.71	3.60	7.69
Tuberculosis, nonpulmonary (33–36)	11	4	7	1.28	.96	1.58
Venereal diseases (38–40)	31	6	25	3.61	1.44	5.65
Cancer (43–49)	20	3	17	2.33	.72	3.85
Tumors, benign (50)	7	2	5	.82	.48	1.13
Rheumatism (51–52)	246	84	162	28.65	20.16	36.64
Lumbago, myalgia, myositis (part of 158)	46	23	23	5.36	5.52	5.20
Rickets (56)	4	3	1	.47	.72	.23
Diabetes (57)	12	2	10	1.40	.48	2.26
Anemia (58)	13	1	12	1.51	.24	2.71
Goitre, exophthalmic (60a)	9	1	8	1.05	.24	1.81
Paralysis (75)	27	9	18	3.14	2.16	4.07
Epilepsy (78)	8	6	2	.93	1.44	.45
Chorea (81)	16	4	12	1.86	.96	2.71
Neuralgia (part of 82)	113	25	88	13.16	6.00	19.91
Neuritis and sciatica (part of 82)	74	16	58	8.62	3.84	13.12
Neurasthenia and nervous exhaustion (part of 84)	192	28	164	22.36	6.72	37.10
Diseases of eye (chronic) (85)	14	6	8	1.63	1.44	1.81
Diseases of the heart (87–90)	182	57	125	21.19	13.68	28.27
Arteriosclerosis (part of 91)	29	16	13	3.38	3.84	2.94
Hemorrhoids (part of 93)	18	9	9	2.10	2.16	2.04
Varicose veins and phlebitis (part of 93)	9	3	6	1.05	.72	1.36
High blood pressure (part of 96)	22	7	15	2.56	1.68	3.39
Asthma and hay fever (105, part of 107)	61	27	34	7.10	6.48	7.69
Ulcers of stomach and duodenum (111)	8	6	2	.93	1.44	.45
Chronic indigestion, constipation, and other stomach or intestinal conditions (112, 114, 119)	85	29	56	9.90	6.96	12.67
Intestinal parasites (116)	23	14	9	2.68	3.36	2.04
Appendicitis (117)	85	25	60	9.90	6.00	13.57
Hernia (118)	21	14	7	2.45	3.36	1.58
Biliary calculi and calculi of the urinary passages (123, 132)	57	14	43	6.64	3.36	9.73
Cholecystitis (part of 124)	24	3	21	2.79	.72	4.75
Unqualified and other liver conditions (part of 124)	28	9	19	3.26	2.16	4.30
Nephritis (acute and chronic) (128, 129)	60	25	35	6.99	6.00	7.92
Unqualified and other kidney conditions (131)	84	23	61	9.78	5.52	13.80
Diseases of bladder (133)	41	14	27	4.77	3.36	6.11
Diseases of male organs (135, 136)	12	12		1.40	2.88	
Chronic diseases of female genital organs (137–142)	70		70	8.15		15.83
Menopause (part of 141)	37		37	4.31		8.37
Congenital malformation (159–161)	15	5	10	1.78	1.20	2.27
Number of persons	**8,587**	**4,166**	**4,421**			

slightly more dependence upon the data shown in Table IV than upon the records of not serious attacks of some of the more acute diseases shown in Table III.

Acknowledgments

The continuous field observations upon which the foregoing report is based were made by the following assistants: F. Ruth Phillips, Mrs. Mary King Phillips, Louise Simmons, Mrs. Clara

Bell Ledford, Clarice Buhrman, and Mrs. Alcesta Owen, under the immediate supervision of Passed Asst. Surg. R. B. Norment, jr., Acting Asst. Surg. A. S. Gray, and, later, Surg. C. V. Akin.

In the analysis of the data I am especially indebted to Associate Statistician S. D. Collins and Assistant Statistician Dorothy G. Wiehl, and other members of the statistical staff, as well as to several officers of the Public Health Service for constant advice on medical points.

Public Health Reports
September 24, 1926

4

Statistics of Morbidity[1]

EDGAR SYDENSTRICKER

I

"Morbidity" is one of the terms in the definition of which the dictionary resorts to vague synonyms. We are told that morbidity is a "diseased" or "abnormal," "not sound," "not healthy," "sickly" state, and are referred to our livers in order to illustrate its meaning. Further reflection might lead us to ask how much morbidity is "normal" reaction to environment, or what proportion of illnesses is merely an unavoidable concomitant of the wearing out of human clocks, to use Pearl's metaphor, some of which are set by heredity to run a shorter time than others. When is death "normal"? At threescore years and ten, or at the century mark, or even at Methuselah's reputed age? How much of Methuselah's life was occupied in dying?

I am afraid that purely philosophical attempts to define the term will lead to a state of obfuscation—which might well be regarded as a form of morbidity in itself. Let us concede at the outset that morbidity is not as precise a concept as the statistician would desire; that it is a relative term, since one person may feel ill, stay away from work longer, be a greater nuisance than another who has the same objective symptoms; and that morbidity is

[1]De Lamar Lecture in Hygiene at the School of Hygiene and Public Health, the Johns Hopkins University, December 15, 1931.

228

essentially a subjective phenomenon. But let us take cognizance of the fact that illness, to use the commoner and more expressive term, is an undeniable and frequent experience of every person except, of course, the favored nonagenarian who, after a career devoted to tobacco, hard liquor, and perhaps other gayer irresponsibilities, is alleged in newspaper interviews never to have been sick a day in his life. Unlike birth or death, which can come but once to an individual, illness may occur often, its frequency depending not only upon its nature, its causes, and upon the susceptibility of the person concerned, but also upon its duration in relation to the length of time considered. Obviously the calculus of probability can not be used in morbidity statistics in the same ways as in birth or death statistics. Yet, in spite of difficulties of reducing it to precise statistical unity, illness is a *datum* measurable in fairly exact terms of duration, degree of disability, symptoms, cause, and sequelae. From the point of view of diagnosis it has an obvious advantage over death since the ill person is still subject to observation whereas the dead are unable to give further data except through autopsies. Statistics of illness can afford an indication of vitality that is not less biologically significant and is more illuminating than mortality. They portray the condition of a people's health far more delicately than death rates. They reveal the prevalence and incidence of disease in a population in a manner that is as useful to the student of society as clinical observation of the individual patient is to the physician.

II

The development of morbidity statistics has been very slow, and they are yet in their infancy. Their tardy progress may be ascribed to three principal reasons. One is expressed by the truism that statistics of a given kind are not continuously collected on a large scale unless there is a sufficient demand for their use in some practical way. A second reason is that the demand has come for morbidity statistics of special kinds and for specific population groups; little, if any, standardization in morbidity statistics has been attained. A third reason follows in some sense from the second—a confusion as to the concept of morbidity arising from differences in the uses to which the statistics are put. In addition to this confusion, differences in methods of collecting data, variety in definitions of a "case" of illness, the existence of peculiar factors that affect the accuracy of the record, the time element involved, and similar difficulties, have been deterrents to the accumulation of a large body of homogeneous morbidity data. It will not be possible upon this occasion to review the history or to forecast the future of morbidity statistics, but the opinion may be ventured that it is doubtful that we shall ever need, and therefore shall ever have, continuous registration of illness in accordance with a standardized procedure such as has been established in the field of natality and mortality. On the other hand, the future development of morbidity data promises great usefulness in two main directions:

1) As an epidemiological method whereby population groups can be accurately observed continuously in order to ascertain how actual conditions of human society influence the incidence and spread of disease.

2) As a means of portraying from time to time and for various population groups and areas, the problems of disease in far better perspective than can be given by statistics of mortality or by any other data practicable in the near future.

Our discussion purposely will be centered on the beginnings of morbidity statistics in the second direction, although the greater opportunity for development seems to me to be in the first.

III

Although many kinds of morbidity statistics exist, their varieties may be classified in five general groups. I shall refer to each very briefly in order to present in somewhat greater detail some results of one study of illness.

1) *Reports of Communicable Diseases.* In a strict sense, these are not morbidity data since illness is not necessarily involved. They exist, or *should* exist, for a specific purpose,

namely the notification of those diseases for which reasonably effective methods of administrative control actually have been devised. Only to a limited extent are communicable disease reports useful for epidemiological studies. As Hedrich and I have shown,[2] not only are the reports of most diseases extremely incomplete but their incompleteness varies according to age.

2) *Hospital and Clinic Records.* These are of little use in determining the prevalence or incidence of illness in a population, either in terms of a gross rate or from any specific disease. Properly made, as they rarely are, they are valuable for clinical studies and may become more so as the tendency to hospitalization increases and as clinicians become trained in analytical methods.

3) *Insurance and Industrial Establishment and School Illness Records.* The outstanding examples are the sickness experience of European insurance systems and of absences on account of illness of workers in industrial establishments in the United States. It is essential to bear in mind that important conditions affect the content, meaning, and validity of the data, although the concept of illness is more than usually specific because of technical and arbitrary definitions imposed for administrative reasons. One condition is the inclusion of only persons well enough to be employed. Another is the exclusion of all cases except disabling illnesses. Another is the exclusion of illnesses of short durations by reason of regulations as to the "waiting period," or the period of disabling illness that must elapse before the patient begins to draw sick benefits and therefore before the record of illness begins. Thus the annual disabling illness rate among male industrial workers with a waiting period of one week was 104 per 1,000, whereas the rate for males in a large public service company without any waiting period was 1,044 per 1,000.[3] Again, "if wages are lost

[2]Sydenstricker, Edgar, and Hedrich, A. W.: Completeness of Reporting of Measles, Whooping Cough, and Chickenpox at Different Ages. *Public Health Reports,* June 28, 1929, lxiv, No. 26, pp. 1537–1543.

[3]Brundage, Dean K.: The Incidence of Illness Among Wage-Earning Adults. *Journal of Industrial Hygiene,* November, 1930, xii, pp. 342, 347.

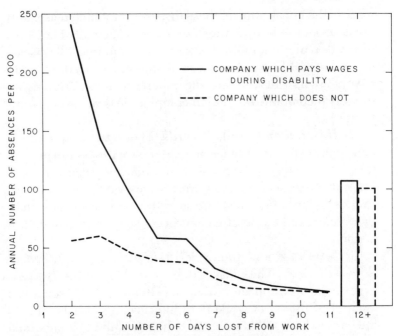

Figure 1 Frequency of absence due to disability among male employees of a company which pays wages during disability as compared with male employees of a company not paying during disability.

entirely when the worker is absent on account of sickness," as Brundage has shown, "the record usually shows a much lower rate of absences of relatively short duration than when full wages are paid during sickness" (Fig. 1), although malingering was not found to be an important factor in two establishments studied.[4] Malingering undoubtedly must be regarded as a condition affecting the accuracy of statistics based upon records of disability or absence. The lad who is too sick from a headache to remain in school but finds the fresh air of the baseball field beneficial, may or may not be malingering; at any rate he is often abetted by sympathetic parents. Yet the interesting suggestion has been made by Collins,[5] and illus-

[4]*Ibid,* p. 340.

[5]Collins, Selwyn D.: The Place of Sickness Records in the School Health Program. Transactions of the Fifth Annual Meeting of the American Child Hygiene Association, October, 1928.

trated by Downes,[6] that records of illness involving absence from school, if kept with some degree of specificity as to the nature of the illness, profitably could be used to complement the findings of the relatively infrequent and usually unsatisfactory physical examinations as a method of referring certain children for diagnosis and treatment.

4) *Illness Surveys.* These have been made, notably by the Metropolitan Life Insurance Company, to ascertain what the *prevalence* of illness is at a given date in sample populations. The method of these surveys is a simple house-to-house canvass. The results indicate that about 2 per cent of the population, including persons of all ages and at home or at work, are ill. The *incidence* of illness within a given period is not revealed by this method and, when the results are analyzed by cause, obviously the proportion of cases of long duration and of chronic type is much higher than is shown by records of incidence.

5) *Records of the Incidence of Illness in a Population Continuously or Frequently Observed.* Although this method was first employed on a considerable scale in the field of study of a single disease, pellagra, by Goldberger and myself and our associates,[7] the first attempt so far as I am aware to record all illnesses continuously in a typical population on any considerable scale was made by the United States Public Health Service in Hagerstown, Maryland, in 1921–1924. The same methods, with some elaborations, have been used in several subsequent morbidity and epidemiological studies. The two main purposes of the Hagerstown study were 1) to ascertain the annual illness rate in a representative population and 2) to develop an epidemiological method whereby human populations could be observed for as complete an incidence as possi-

[6]Downes, Jean: Sickness Records in School Hygiene. *American Journal of Public Health,* November, 1930, xx, pp. 1199–1206.

[7]Goldberger, J.; Wheeler, G. A.; and Sydenstricker, Edgar: A Study of the Relation of Diet to Pellagra Incidence in Several Textile Communities of South Carolina in 1916. *Public Health Reports,* 1920, xxxv, pp. 648–713, and later publications.

ble of various diseases, so far as they are manifested in illness, under actual conditions of community life.

IV

Before referring to some of the results of this study from the viewpoint of general morbidity, it is important to consider the nature of the data obtained by the method of frequent and continuous observation employed in this and later similar studies.

Experience has shown that the completeness of a record of illness depends upon at least three important conditions. One is its severity and nature; the second is the length of the period for which the informant is asked to report; the third is the subjectivity of the record itself. Nearly every adult will remember an illness due to typhoid fever incident upon himself or in his family if it took place within the preceding ten or twenty years; few will recall a brief illness due to a common cold unless it occurred within a very short period immediately preceding the date of inquiry. Illnesses of a minor kind are observed and remembered when incident upon the informant himself with a greater degree of completeness than when incident upon others, even in the same family.

A few illustrations may be given. The annual incidence of illness of respiratory nature in families reported upon every half month was two attacks per person,[8] whereas in families reported upon at intervals of six to eight weeks it was only about 0.7 attacks per person.[9] The annual illness rate for women reporting upon themselves was 70 per cent higher for respiratory conditions, 130 per cent higher for nervous conditions, and 8 per cent higher for digestive disorders than the rates for women reported upon by others in the same household.[10] On the other hand, respiratory

[8]Townsend, J. G., and Sydenstricker, Edgar: Epidemiological Study of Minor Respiratory Diseases. *Public Health Reports*, January 14, 1927, lxii, No. 2, p. 112.

[9]Sydenstricker, Edgar: A Study of Illness in a General Population Group. *Public Health Reports*, September 24, 1926, lxi, No. 39, p. 12.

[10]Sydenstricker, Edgar: The Illness Rate Among Males and Females. *Public Health Reports*, July 29, 1927, lxii, No. 30, p. 1952.

attack rates in families where adult males were the informants were higher for themselves than among adult females in the same families whereas all objective observations point to a higher rate among women than among men.[11] Such experiences as these point to the necessity for taking influencing conditions into account that only participation in the collection of the data can possibly reveal.

V

I would have liked very much upon this occasion to have been able to bring you fresh reports upon several field studies of morbidity using or involving the recording of illness by the method of continuous observation of population groups. Unfortunately these studies either are still under way or are as yet in the process of tabulation. One is the observation of a population group of 5,000 in a city of nearly 200,000 people and another is of a group of similar size in a rural area. The purposes of these studies are not merely to secure a record of the illnesses in order to depict the condition of a typical population's health in so far as it is revealed by illness, but to ascertain the extent to which illness is receiving medical service and the population itself is being served in various ways by the public health agencies, both official and unofficial. In these and other field inquiries under way, the reasons why health services of different kinds are not used by the families and individuals are being ascertained in order to learn the attitude of the public and to appraise the efficiency of educational efforts. Thus the underlying method of continuous observation of a population is being applied in these two studies as a mode of measuring the effectiveness, from an important point of view, of public and private medicine—using the term "medicine" in its broad sense. A third study, in which this method is being employed, was conducted on a large scale in the United States in order to find out, with far greater accuracy than ever before, the extent to which

[11]Sydenstricker, Edgar: Sex Differences in the Incidence of Certain Diseases at Different Ages. *Public Health Reports*, May 25, 1928, lxiii, No. 21, pp. 1269–1270.

families of different economic status actually availed themselves of medical, hospital, and other services and the actual costs of these services in detail for every illness during the period of a year. This inquiry extended into communities of different types and sizes and in many geographic areas of the country.

This particular method of the morbidity study—the continuous or frequent observation of a population—is thus being adopted for other purposes in the fields of public health and medical economics. It is essentially the method of the field zoologist, botanist, and the laboratory worker applied to the study of human populations living under conditions as they are found, but with far greater possibilities of precision in and completeness of observation than routine records made for other purposes can ever achieve. It will doubtless become a most valuable epidemiological tool as the technique of observation for specific diseases is divided and improved through experience. I need not refer here to the studies of respiratory affections conducted at the Johns Hopkins University which are notable examples of this use of the method. Epidemiological method, however, does not lie within our subject; I merely mention it in order to illustrate the fact that the study of morbidity is developing into an epidemiological mode that is both scientific and practicable.

VI

For an illustration of morbidity studies used to depict the health of a population we may turn to the one made in Hagerstown.

The Hagerstown morbidity study[12] included 16,517 "years of observation," or an equivalent of a population of 7,079 persons observed continuously for twenty-eight months beginning December, 1921. Illnesses were recorded as reported to experienced field investigators visiting each family every six to eight weeks, the reports being made by the household informant (usually the

[12]Sydenstricker, Edgar: Hagerstown Morbidity Studies. A Study of Illness in a Typical Population Group. Reprints 1113, 1116, 1134, 1163, 1167, 1172, 1225, 1227, 1229, 1294, 1303, and 1312 from the *Public Health Reports*.

wife) either as experienced by herself or as she observed them in her family.

The results of the study indicated that a fairly accurate record of real illnesses was secured. Less than 5 per cent of the illnesses of exactly stated durations recorded were one day or less in duration. Approximately 40 per cent were not only disabling but caused confinement to bed. It is evident, therefore, that in the main the illnesses recorded were more than trivial in their character, in spite of the fact that in some instances mere symptoms were given as diagnoses. The incidence of acute attacks of specific and generally recognizable diseases was, we believe, recorded with a satisfactory degree of completeness. On the other hand, the incidence of mild attacks, as for example, of coryza, was quite incompletely recorded as judged by data on minor respiratory attacks obtained later by more intensive methods for other population groups.

For this population 17,847 illnesses were recorded in the twenty-eight month period, an annual rate of 1,081 per 1,000 years of life observed, or about one illness per person per year. This illness rate was over 100 times the annual death rate in the same population.

Perhaps the most interesting results of this first morbidity study of a typical population related to the variations in the incidence of illness according to age. Up to the time the Hagerstown study was made the only data on adults came from "sickness" records of European insurance systems, English voluntary sick benefit societies, and a few American industrial employee funds. Nearly all of these records include only absences from work due to illness lasting a week or longer, and naturally indicate a rapid rise in the rate according to age because they reflected the serious illnesses only. The Hagerstown study showed that for a group composed of persons at work and at home the illness rate was high even in the younger adult ages and did not rise so quickly with age. The study also furnished data for the first time on children and adolescents with the surprising result that the peak of illness incidence was to be found in childhood and the lowest in the age period 15–24 years, a finding that has been confirmed by later studies employing similar methods (Fig. 2).

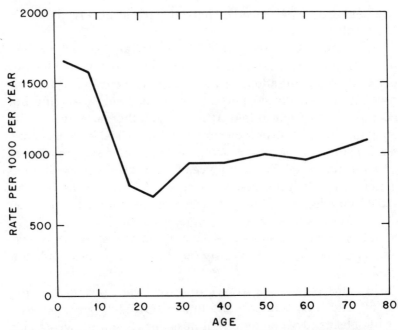

Figure 2   Age incidence of illness from all causes in Hagerstown, Maryland, as observed in a general population group, December 1, 1921–March 31, 1924.

This extraordinary age variation in the illness rate may be interpreted from various points of view, but before you venture any interpretations of it, certain other general considerations should be taken into account.

One is the fact that the proportion of persons suffering frequent attacks, four or more illnesses per year, was highest (45 per cent) in childhood (2–9 years), lowest at 20–24 years (11 per cent), rising gradually to a level of about 21 per cent beginning with the age of 35. Thus the age variation in illness was partly due to the age distribution of frequently sick individuals. The proportion of persons sick once a year was about the same in every age period. On the other hand, the proportion of persons free from illness during the period was lowest in childhood (5 per cent at 3–4 years), sharply rising through adolescence to a maximum of 30 per cent at 20–24 years, and thereafter declining until the end of the life span (Fig. 3).

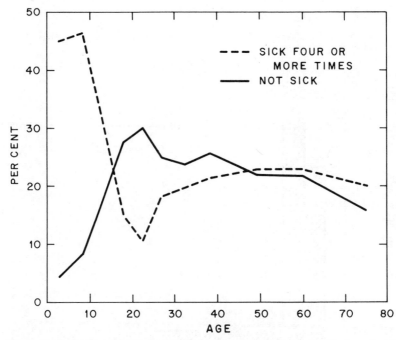

Figure 3   Proportion of persons at different ages who suffered a specified number of illnesses during twenty-six months.

A second consideration is the age variation in the severity of cases of sickness. Severity may be measured in various ways—by duration, degree of incapacitation, cause or nature of the attack, or by fatality. In order to suggest in a general way the ill person's resistance to death at different ages, a convenient mode of expression is the ratio for different age periods. The anticipated variations are clearly indicated, namely that his greatest resistance to death is in childhood, the age period 5–14; his lowest resistance is in infancy and early childhood (0–4 years) and toward the end of the natural life span. Ability to *survive* illness thus varies markedly from resistance to attacks of illness at different ages, particularly in childhood (5–14) when the average individual suffers from illness frequently but has a relatively small chance of dying, and in the older years when not only does his susceptibility to illness increase but also his chances of death. This is due partly, of

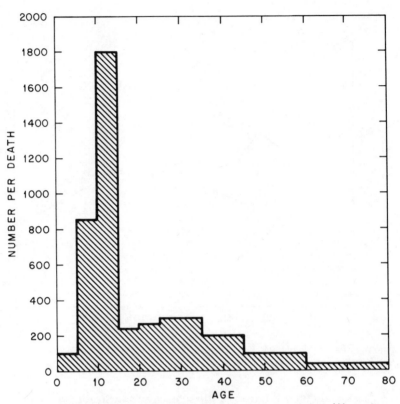

Figure 4   Illnesses per death at different ages in the white population of Hagerstown, Maryland, December 1, 1921–March 31, 1924.

course, to differences in the nature of illness occurring at these ages and partly to the diminished ability to resist the diseases which manifest themselves in morbidity (Fig. 4).

A third consideration is of basic importance—the cause or nature of illness at different ages. I can only summarize very briefly the data collected in the Hagerstown and subsequent studies. The generally known fact that each period of life is characterized by its own distribution of the causes of illness was more clearly and completely defined. In childhood, illness other than respiratory is caused chiefly by communicable diseases, diseases and conditions of the skin, ears, eyes, and teeth, and nervous and digestive disorders; in old age, illness other than respiratory is caused by the organic group of diseases and conditions, those of the circulatory system, nervous sytem, and kidneys. Illnesses resulting from all these causes are at their lowest level in adolescence and young adult ages. The only major cause which results in a higher rate of disability in young adult life than at any other age is the puerperal condition, and this, of course, relates to females only. Certain specific causes of illness do have their highest incidence in the young adult period of life, such as venereal diseases, typhoid fever, and pulmonary tuberculosis, except under conditions of special strain or hazard. But, by and large, this is the age most free from illness (Figs. 5, 6).

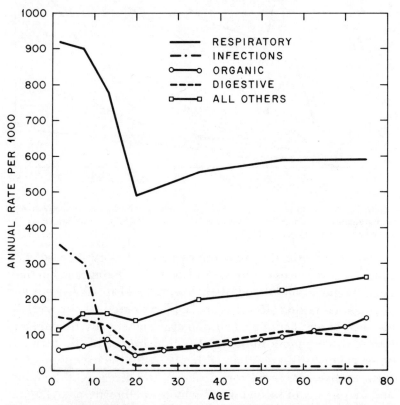

Figure 5   Causes of illnesses at different ages in a white population group in Hagerstown, Maryland, December 1, 1921–March 31, 1924. Under infectious diseases are included the "epidemic, endemic, and infectious diseases" and under "organic" the following: diseases of the eyes, ears, circulatory system, teeth and gums, kidney and genito-urinary system.

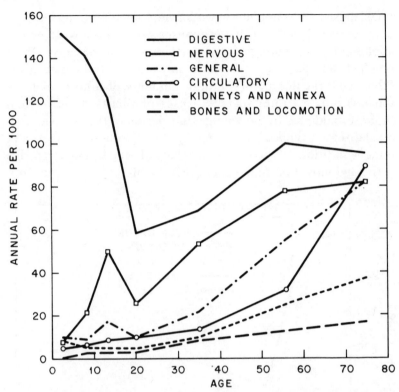

Figure 6 Variations, according to age, of certain groups of diseases which were primary causes of illness in a white population group in Hagerstown, Maryland, December 1, 1921–March 31, 1924.

The predominating importance of respiratory diseases and conditions as causes of illness at all ages is a striking fact, but their great height in childhood, their lowest level in adolescent and young adult period (15–24 years), and their gradual rise with the advance of age had not been depicted statistically. Respiratory illnesses were more frequent at both extremes of life than any other general disease group; although, with the exception of infectious diseases, circulatory diseases, and diseases of the bones and of "organs of locomotion," which so clumsily describe diseases that affect certain muscles, nearly all of the major groups of causes of illness tend to appear among the very young and among the old. In contrast to the organic troubles which so definitely begin to be manifested in middle life and which characterize old age, are the infections and the diseases and conditions affecting the skin, teeth, eyes, and ears that occur with greatest frequency in childhood.

A fourth consideration is the differential illness rates according to family economic status. After taking into account the differences in the age distribution of persons in different economic classes, the annual illness rates for Hagerstown were 991 per 1,000 for the highest economic class, 1,068 for the middle or "moderate circumstances" class, and 1,113 for the "poor." These differences are not of the same magnitude as those found previously for infant mortality, tuberculosis, or pellagra, for example. Doubtless one reason was that the classes were not so sharply defined since the classification was based on the general impression of the investigator over two years of observation rather than upon an exact appraisal of income. A somewhat detailed analysis of the data, however, revealed the facts that the association of illness with poor economic status 1) appeared for certain causes only, and 2) was indicated in adult life and not in childhood or adolescence. An association with poor economic status was indicated for respiratory diseases, rheumatism, nervous conditions and disorders, and accidents. The commoner infectious diseases—measles, whooping cough, and chickenpox, for example—were not respectors of economic class. The lack of an association with favorable economic status with respect to diseases and conditions of the eyes and ears and of the circulatory, digestive, and eliminatory organs, may reflect the fact that such cases were more frequently attended by physicians and therefore more accurately described for the higher economic class than for the lower.

VII

From the many interesting and suggestive data yielded by morbidity studies of this nature we may select one more fact. It is this: The general picture given by records of illness according to cause—or, more precisely, according to the *kind* of morbidity—is in sharp contrast to that given by mortality statistics. Respiratory diseases and disorders account for 60 per cent of illness as against about 20 per cent of deaths; the general group of "epidemic, endemic, and infectious" diseases accounts for 8 per cent of illnesses, whereas only about 2 per cent of the deaths were ascribable to this group; digestive diseases and disorders caused or characterized 10 per cent of the illnesses as against 6 per cent of the total mortality. On the other hand, the group of "general" diseases (which includes cancer), the diseases of the nervous and circulatory systems, and the diseases of the kidneys and annexa were relatively much more important causes of mortality than of morbidity. The diseases of the heart and circulatory system show the sharpest contrast, 24 per cent of deaths being ascribed to these conditions as against only 2 per cent of illnesses. In other words, these diseases manifest themselves in relatively few instances of illness, although undoubtedly they shorten life and make life less efficient and enjoyable while it lasts.

VIII

I hesitate to draw the most obvious conclusion from the facts so far yielded by all studies of morbidity because I do not like to close on a note that might be thought discouraging. I have confidence, however, in the stimulating challenge of facts. You may remember the soliloquy of *Faustus* upon the choice of a profession, written nearly 350 years ago by Christopher Marlowe, in which he weighed the success of medicine in these words:

> "Summum bonus medicinae sanitas
> The end of physic is our body's health.
> Why, Faustus, hast thou not attained that end?
> Are not thy bills hung up as monuments, whereby
> Whole cities have escap'd the plague, and
> Thousand desperate maladies been cured?"

So, today, we may apply to preventive medicine the test afforded by statistics of illness. It is true that some of the plagues and pestilences of Marlowe's day have been banished from a part of the world; that many more maladies have yielded to modern treatment; that millions of people have escaped certain diseases and have lived lengthened lives. These achievements are monuments indeed to scientific discoveries and to the unselfish art of medicine. Yet undeniable morbidity experience in the twentieth century is overwhelming evidence that the goal of preventive medicine, which is a healthy people, is far from being reached. It is impossible to escape the conclusion to which these statistics drive us, that public health and the practice of medicine have as yet barely touched the task of *preventing* the conditions which manifest themselves in actual illness and all that illness implies.

Milbank Memorial Fund Quarterly
April, 1932

5

EPIDEMIOLOGICAL STUDIES

COMMENTARY
ROBERT F. KORNS AND
PETER GREENWALD

Edgar Sydenstricker came to epidemiology at the opportune moment when it was shifting from a limited descriptive discipline to one which was more analytic. The study of disease incidence in comparison groups, as related to population and environmental characteristics, needed accurately defined and quantitated data. Detailed knowledge of both the numerators and denominators, from which comparison rates were derived, was essential. His background in economics, or more broadly, the social sciences, brought to epidemiology insights on the importance of the "way of life" as a complex of elements in disease causation, that many investigators, steeped in the tradition of single, specific etiologies, tended to forget.

What is amazing to the present day reader of his publications is the astonishing breadth of view exhibited, not only in the variety of problems tackled, but in his grasp of the complexities of human ecology. He had an uncanny knack of focusing on the pertinent epidemiologic variables and deleting the false leads. His logical thinking is always recorded and the evidence for or against the given hypothesis is presented in detail, usually from data generated by his own studies.

Pellagra

It was indeed a fortunate circumstance that his first assignment in epidemiology was with Joseph Goldberger, the "John Snow of American epidemiology." The brief paper on pellagra by Goldberger,[1] the first of the series which ultimately totaled 54 publications, stated clearly the epidemiologic rationale for discarding the hypothesis of an infectious disease etiology for the disease, and suggested a dietary one as a likely possibility. The sequence of studies set in motion at that time represents a remarkably thorough step-wise approach to proving this hypothesis and identifying the specific dietary deficiency. Sydenstricker joined this research team in 1915 and was author or co-author of nine of the early papers, one of which is reproduced in this section.

His primary contribution lay in the development and implementation of community surveys in the mill towns of South Carolina. These are classical examples of methodologic rigor and comprehensiveness. Although he had published an earlier paper on the prevalence of pellagra as related to the rise in cost of food,[2] that report had been based largely on a historical review of the problem and an analysis of published documents relevant to income and food consumption. The paper reproduced here was the first published report allowing comparison of pellagra incidence rates by economic status. One might ask why this tremendous effort in data collection and refined analysis was needed to reenforce the evidence presented in other papers in the series, which seemed to offer direct and definitive proof of the dietary deficiency hypothesis. These had included an intervention study[3] on institutional inmates where alterations in the diet clearly prevented pellagra and appeared to cure the disease, as well as a controlled human volunteer study in a prison population[4] where the disease was produced by specific dietary restrictions. It should be recalled, however, that just prior to these studies, the Thompson-McFadden Pellagra Commission report had appeared.[5,6] This represented an extensive investigation, by capable epidemiologists, that came to quite different conclusions. Furthermore, the populations studied included several of the South Carolina cotton-mill villages later surveyed by Sydenstricker. Among the conclusions reached was the following: "Pellagra is in all probability a specific infectious disease communicable from person-to-person by means at present unknown."[7] These investigators examined with great care the dietary intake of families with cases of pellagra. Several firm statements in their reports are difficult to reconcile with the subsequent Goldberger and Sydenstricker accounts, e.g., "observations on the habitual use of the more common foodstuffs failed to discover any points of difference between pellagrins and non-pellagrins in the county",[8] "those avoiding fresh meat contracted this disease least",[9] "that pellagra was, on the whole, somewhat less common in families using milk daily."[10]

The contemporary studies of Jobling and Peterson[11] in Nashville, Tennessee came to somewhat similar conclusions. Although their dietary explorations were extensive and detailed, they failed to show significant deficiencies in the diets of most pellagrins. In discussing the probable reasons for the faulty findings of these studies Goldberger, Wheeler and Sydenstricker highlighted the following points:

1) "that the data are again of a very general character;
2) that there is no evidence of appreciation on the part of these workers of the importance of the seasonal factor in relating diet to the incidence of the disease;
3) that the data relate to family, not to individual use of foods;
4) that the term 'pellagrin' is not defined, leaving one in doubt whether, in some of their analyses, this includes only active cases, or whether, as seems not improbable, it also includes some quiescent cases; and
5) that an error, the magnitude of which it is impossible to estimate from the data published, probably entered as the result of the relative incompleteness, for the purposes of such study, of the pellagra incidence data that is certain to arise unless cases are systematically and continuously sought for by personal canvass."[12]

In the studies in which Sydenstricker participated, these deficiencies were carefully avoided, either through changes in study design or through more meticulous collection of data. Thus cases were completely ascertained on clinical grounds, by a physician through bi-weekly house-to-house visits, and analyses were focused on the incidence of active disease. Studies of the seasonal incidence of pellagra demonstrated a pronounced peak in early summer, so that the assessment of economic status and diet were restricted to the immediately preceding period, April 16–June 15. The data on income for this time period were derived primarily from the records of the cotton mills which employed most of the study population, supplemented by careful inquiry of the housewife and others in the home. Diet, again for this two month period, was derived from these same sources, the records of purchases at the company store, other retail outlets, the hucksters of the area, nearby farm producers and family gardens and livestock. The thoroughness and completeness of this survey is indeed impressive. Since the numbers of persons in each household varied and the age/sex composition differed for different income groups, it was necessary to standardize the analysis in terms of adult male units based on the Atwater scale of food requirements. Sydenstricker carefully measured the impact of each of these refinements on the analysis and documented fully the justification for each step. His footnotes frequently include supplementary tables bearing on the point at issue. The range of bi-weekly income was remarkably small, classified as under $6, $6–7, $8–9 and $10 and more so that the dietary data needed to be accurately and completely collected to demonstrate the observed differences. It became apparent that income level did not correlate exactly with pellagra incidence. Comparison of the rates in the seven study villages suggested that food availability, apart from income, was an important variable. Data to document this were thoroughly studied and indicated that the critical food items (fresh milk and meat) were far less obtainable for the populations showing high pellagra incidence. This led to the observation that the geographic topography surrounding these villages and the related single-crop economy, namely cotton, was one of the basic underlying factors in the pellagra problem. This observation was further confirmed in Goldberger and Sydenstricker's later study of pellagra in the Mississippi flood area.[13] The details concerning specific items of diet clearly identified the significant deficiencies and exonerated the presumed excesses of carbohydrates, especially corn.

Sydenstricker and his colleagues marshalled all of these data and supplementary analyses in an admirably logical, step-wise manner that is impressive and entirely convincing. One can clearly see that the basic methodology, centering around data collected through biweekly household surveys, formed the pattern for his later Hagerstown studies (see Section 4), which in turn served as models for several subsequent local and national surveys.

It is perhaps fortunate that in the pellagra studies, the investigators were dealing with a disease, which although chronic and ill-defined, did show characteristic clinical signs rather promptly after the specific dietary deficiency had developed. Had this been otherwise, isolating the dietary deficiency as the specific etiological factor might have been far more difficult. Present studies of colon cancer, for example, face this dilemma. A dietary etiology hypothesis, based in part on international comparisons in cancer experience and the disease in migrant populations, is strongly suggested. In this instance, however, the epidemiologist is faced with the task of identifying the critical item of diet which may have produced its effect 20 years earlier. This is frequently complicated by the need to explore the diet through surrogate respondents, since most of the cases may be dead at the time of study. Perhaps the modern day epidemiologist should take his cue from Sydenstricker's pioneering efforts, and look for the proper study model that may shed light on this problem and then proceed to collect pertinent data in a methodologically rigorous manner. Undoubtedly the epidemiology of pellagra, at that time, was equally mystifying.

Influenza

The 1918 pandemic of influenza had an impact not only in terms of the recognizable cases and deaths from the disease (conservatively estimated at 200 million cases and over 10 million deaths), but on mortality statistics for most of the major causes of death. Epidemiologists and other scientists from many countries tackled the study of this disaster with vigor, in the hope of shedding some light on the precipitating factors, as a means of future prevention. It was in this setting that Sydenstricker and Wade Hampton Frost, both with the U.S. Public Health Service, carried out extensive surveys in late 1918 and early 1919. Most of the pertinent findings of these studies were published promptly. For that matter, Frost's paper, presented at the American Public Health Association meetings in New Orleans in October, 1919[14] includes much of the material which makes up Sydenstricker's more extensive analysis reproduced here, and first published in January, 1931. One can only speculate as to what motivated him to pick up these data again, after an interval of almost thirteen years in order to digest them more fully. The world was then in the midst of the 1929 depression which gave added cogency to Sydenstricker's lifetime passion for studying the relationship between disease and socio-economic variables. Despite the lapse of years, little had been added to the understanding of the influenza pandemic. This awaited the first demonstration of influenza Type A virus in 1933, Type B in 1940, and the multitude of laboratory-based studies which were to follow. It was characteristic of the man, not to allow a set of carefully collected data to lie fallow, without squeezing them for all meaningful analyses relevant to important epidemiological inferences.

The paper starts with the familiar comment about the pandemic "the flu hit the rich and the poor alike." Sydenstricker then attempts to document this generalization with data collected by survey, and finds that the general impression is true only in part. These surveys had been carried out in the wake of the pandemic wave in nine cities of over 25,000 population, scattered across the United States. By modern standards, the population sampling procedure was relatively unsophisticated, but was quite adequate for the purpose. Ascertainment of bonafide cases of influenza was of course without the support of modern laboratory tests, but undoubtedly was fairly accurate since the carefully supervised house-to-house interviews were made as the epidemic receded, when memories of recent acute illnesses would still be sharply in mind. Inapparent infections that have been shown, by serologic means, to make up a varying proportion of cases (e.g. 25 percent) in subsequent epidemics, probably were far less frequent in the 1918–19 episode. In San Antonio, for example, with 98 percent of the households involved and an overall clinical attack rate of 535 cases per 1,000 population, there was relatively little room for subclinical disease.

Sydenstricker approached the study of morbidity and mortality rates and case fatality ratios as related to socio-economic groups, in a detailed and systematic fashion. Both morbidity and mortality rates, standardized by age, were sharply higher in the poor than in the well-to-do. That the excess in mortality was not solely due to the excess in morbidity was shown by study of the case-fatality ratio, which was nearly twice as high in the very poor. This excess was most striking among the young and the old. From a long list, presented as possible reasons for these findings, Sydenstricker focused on three for which the meager data at his disposal offered some insight. The first deals with the influenza attack rate by household, by economic class, adjusted for age and sex and weighted appropriately to take account of the differences in family size by economic class. The excess of households with at least one case stands out among the poor. He then proceeded to study the secondary attack rate in these affected households, standardized as before. This showed a sharp excess of secondary case incidence among the poor households, and allowed him to draw the inference that economic status "was a relatively unimportant determinant of the extent to which the disease spread in a community but was of considerable importance as a determinant of the morbidity rate within the households attacked" (p. 324).

Finally, he explored the possibility that crowding, as defined by "the number of persons per room," accounted for this observed difference. He was forced to conclude that this factor, at least in the populations studied, did not seem to account for the differences in influenza rates in 1918, although it was clearly a concomitant of poverty.

Whooping Cough

The paper entitled "Effect of a Whooping Cough Epidemic upon the Size of the Non-immune Group in an Urban Community" reproduced here, is a gem of methodological refinement. Just as with the paper on influenza, this represents a return to data collected a decade earlier, for the purpose of making a specific point pertinent to the epidemiology of the disease, and, even more broadly, to the natural history of epidemics in general. At that time, whooping cough was still an important health problem in the United States, giving rise each year to approximately 7,000 deaths among two million children attacked by this debilitating acute disease. The subsequent advent of an effective vaccine and the antibiotics has, of course, changed this picture, with something less than 3,000 cases and 30 deaths reported in 1972, largely among unvaccinated individuals.

Sydenstricker may have been stimulated to explore this subject by the contemporary studies of measles by Reed and Frost in Baltimore[15] in which they attempted to construct a mathematical model for epidemics. For this purpose, they needed to define more clearly the critical level of population susceptibility that might allow an epidemic wave to develop. Sydenstricker's study was a spin-off from his classic morbidity surveys in Hagerstown in 1921–1924. Characteristically, he took advantage of the natural occurrence of a sizeable whooping cough epidemic in the midst of his carefully planned and executed surveys, involving household visits by trained investigators every six to eight weeks throughout the consecutive 28-month period. Since official reporting of the disease was estimated as being only 15 percent complete, this set of data offered a rather unique opportunity to shed light on this question.

After a lapse of twenty months without whooping cough, the epidemic came in two waves, striking different portions of the city on each occasion. Historical information of previous attacks of the disease had been collected on all persons at the first survey visit. These records showed that the percent of persons with a history of a prior attack increased continuously from birth to fifteen years of age, when it reached a plateau at about 75 percent. Thus, a quarter of the population over this age had no recognized history of the disease, raising the question as to whether they had been immunized through subclinical infection at some time in the past. He then proceeded to assess this possibility by studying age specific attack rates, during the epidemic, in persons without prior history, who were exposed to the disease as members of affected households. These data are presented in detail, showing that 85 of the 356 individuals without a history of whooping cough under 15 years of age, who were so exposed, failed to develop clinical disease. These presumably represented that portion acquiring immunity from subclinical infection. Finally, correcting his data for this factor, he proceeded to calculate the percentage of susceptibles, in the age group under 15 years, at six points during the twenty-eight month experience, comparing these points with the percentage of susceptibles that might have been expected had no epidemic of whooping cough occurred. The paper is a model of logical, clear presentation, with appropriate comment on the limitations of the data and cautious conclusions.

Although in the ensuing fifty years, since the data were collected, our knowledge of whooping cough has expanded, his observations remain secure. Case ascertainment through periodic house-to-house survey, supplemented by the clinical impressions of the attending physician, was about as complete and accurate as might be achieved today, with the added support of nasopharyngeal swabs. His epidemiological reasoning is crystal clear.

Sydenstricker evidently retained his interest in whooping cough, since one of his last papers, published posthumously[16] was entitled "Whooping Cough in Surveyed Communities."

Tuberculosis

The last two papers in this section deal with tuberculosis, a disease which seemed to intrigue Sydenstricker, perhaps because its natural history is linked so clearly to socio-economic variables.

Public health attention was focused strongly on tuberculosis at the time and various voluntary agencies, including the Milbank Memorial Fund, selected the disease for special attention. Frost, and many of his students at Johns Hopkins throughout this period, were devoting most of their efforts to methodological refinements in the study of tuberculosis. It is noteworthy that such pains were taken to assess whether the control program per se was having a favorable impact on morbidity and mortality. Evaluation of these efforts became more feasible with the advent of effective chemotherapy and chemoprophylaxis in 1952. However, despite the phenomenal decline in the U.S. from 79,000 deaths from the disease at a rate of 63 per 100,000 in 1932, to 4,000 at a rate of less than 2 per 100,000 in 1972, the major impediment to further progress in control is still sociological rather than technological. Today, for this country at least, the problem centers around motivating patients to stay on drug treatment for the requisite time after they have become completely asymptomatic.[17]

The first of these papers is a remarkably mature assessment of the multiple factors, which seemed to have contributed to the decline in mortality from tuberculosis which started in the late eighteenth century, and proceeded uninterrupted, except for the 1918 influenza pandemic period, up to the moment of his thoughtful presentation in 1927. One can sense the atmosphere of the meeting, which brought together dedicated tuberculosis workers from across the country. Sydenstricker had been assigned his topic and proceeded to serve as the epidemiological conscience of the gathering. It must have been a disheartening revelation to many of those present. Having reviewed the basic components of scientific evaluation, and pointing to the lack of definitive data which would allow such assessment, he was forced to "relinquish the task of analytical statistician and frankly assume the role of the historian who, with such understanding of the nature of the events as he may have, employs deductive rather than inductive processes in reaching a conclusion" (p. 348). The thesis he then pursued was "that the decline in the tuberculosis death rate ought to be viewed primarily as a social development" (p. 348).

The paper is full of pertinent commentary on relevant factors in our society. He admits frankly that accurate evaluation of the specific public health effort, called anti-tuberculosis work, was not possible, short of carrying out a heroic, coldly planned and delicately conducted experiment in human populations. His final sentence softens the blow somewhat: "Until that is done (the controlled experiment) it seems to me that we ought to be satisfied with a real and vitally important participation in the forces that are guiding and making mankind to progress" (p. 367).

The last paper represents an attempt at such evaluation in a specific tuberculosis control program in Cattaraugus County, New York. This program had been sharply expanded and intensified, starting in 1925, with financial support from the Milbank Memorial Fund. It brought to this semi-rural county all of the recommended control technics then available, with thorough combing of the population for evidence of the disease. Sydenstricker approached the evaluation cautiously, realizing full-well the limited experience (1925 through 1927) being examined, and the crude end-point available, namely, mortality. The analyses are fairly simple and straightforward, but it is in the careful handling of the data and sage comment that we see his special talents exhibited. The statistical analyses are of three sorts: 1) The trend of tuberculosis mortality established in Cattaraugus County 1900–1924 and the expected death rates compared to those observed in 1925–1927. The observed rates were significantly lower ($p = 0.000004$) than the trend line. 2) A comparison with the mortality trends for the same time period in twelve other similar counties in upstate New York. Here again, Cattaraugus County stands out as being the only one with significant declines from the expected during this three-year period. 3) The shift in the age-specific mortality rates in 1925–1927 compared to 1916–1924. To Sydenstricker this change appeared to be a better index of the effect of the control program. It showed that the sharp decline in mortality was manifest primarily in the age groups 5–39 years, amounting to 50 percent of the mean rate for the preceding nine years, and of itself statistically significant.

This brief paper has an important though limited objective, which Sydenstricker fulfilled nicely. As an historical exercise, the present writers attempted to collect from the files of the New York State Department of Health the tuberculosis mortality rates for Cattaraugus and the comparison counties through 1936, in order to determine whether Sydenstricker's projections were confirmed by later experience. As might be expected, the differences which he demonstrated were lost in the rapid declines in mortality noted in all the counties, and for upstate New York as a whole, during this period. Unfortunately, age–specific tuberculosis mortality rates by county, for that time period, were not available and could not be calculated, since the original reports had been discarded.

Over all, Sydenstricker's contribution to epidemiology was sizeable. Relatively little of his work was aimed directly at uncovering specific etiologies of disease, but he brought into prominence the role of "socio-economic status" as a complex of factors associated with disease incidence and mortality. Of course, we still face the difficult problem in the epidemiologic study of many diseases of identifying the specific factors within this complex that may be of critical importance. However, Sydenstricker forcefully led the way to their exploration. Although his teaching role was not formalized in a classroom, his influence on epidemiologist and statistician colleagues was pervasive. As organizer and first Chief of the Office of Statistical Investigations of the U.S. Public Health Service, he played the primary role in studies covering a wide range of subjects, e.g., epidemiology, maternal and child hygiene, industrial hygiene and general morbidity and mortality. His pioneer work in developing the methodology of periodic morbidity surveys may be the most enduring. At the time they were carried out and for the following decade, they represented a unique record of total morbidity and physical impairment in the population studied, which was, of course, eventually superseded by later surveys. As one scans modern textbooks on public health practice or published papers of the last few years on subjects as widely divergent as: community air pollution, socio-cultural factors in duodenal ulcer, morbidity in rural areas, psychiatric illness in the general population, measurement of physical health (as only a few examples) one sees his papers among the references cited, especially those from the Hagerstown series.

Notes and References

1. Goldberger, J., "The Etiology of Pellagra. The Significance of Certain Epidemiological Observations with Respect thereto," Public Health Reports 29:1683–86. June 26, 1914.
2. Sydenstricker, E., "The Prevalence of Pellagra. Its Possible Relation to the Rise in the Cost of Food," Public Health Reports 30:3132–48. October 22, 1915.
3. Goldberger, J., Waring, C. H. and Willets, D. G., "The Prevention of Pellagra: a Test of Diet among Institutional Inmates," Public Health Reports 30:3117–3131. October 22, 1915.
4. Goldberger, J. and Wheeler, G. A., "Experimental Pellagra in the Human Subject Brought about by Restricted Diet," Public Health Reports 30:3336–3339. November 12, 1915.
5. Siler, J. F., Garrison, P. E. and MacNeal, W. J., "Pellagra, a Summary of the First Progress Report on the Thompson-McFadden Pellagra Commission," Journal of the American Medical Association 62:8–12. January 3, 1914.
6. Siler, J. F., Garrison, P. E. and MacNeal, W. J., "Further Studies of the Thompson-McFadden Pellagra Commission. A Summary of the Second Progress Report," Journal of the American Medical Association 63:1090–93. September 26, 1914.
7. Siler, J. F., Garrison, P. E. and MacNeal, W. J., op. cit. p. 12.
8. Ibid, p. 10.
9. Goldberger, J., Wheeler, G. A. and Sydenstricker, E., "A Study of the Relation of Diet to Pellagra Incidence in Seven Textile-Mill Communities of South Carolina in 1916," Public Health Reports 35:654. March 19, 1920.
10. Siler, J., Garrison, P. E. and MacNeal, W. J., "A Statistical Study of the Relation of Pellagra to Use of Certain Foods," Archives of Internal Medicine 14:357. September, 1914.
11. Jobling, J. W. and Peterson, W., "The Epidemiology of Pellagra in Nashville, Tenn. (II)," Journal of Infectious Diseases 21:109–131. August 1917.
12. Goldberger, J., Wheeler, G. A. and Sydenstricker, E., op. cit. p. 655.
13. Goldberger, J. and Sydenstricker, E., "Pellagra in the Mississippi Flood Area," Public Health Reports 42:2706–2725. November 4, 1927.
14. Frost, W. H., "Statistics of Influenza Morbidity, with Special Reference to Certain Factors in Case Incidence, and Case Fatality," Public Health Reports 35:584–597. March 12, 1920.

15. Lowell J. Reed and Wade Hampton Frost presented their "Epidemic Theory" about 1930, but never published their work. They utilized some of the material for laboratory exercises in courses in epidemiology and biostatistics at the Johns Hopkins School of Hygiene and Public Health.
16. Sydenstricker, E. and Wheeler, R. E., "Whooping Cough in Surveyed Communities," Journal of the American Public Health Association 26:576–585. June 1936.
17. Edwards, P. Q., "Is Tuberculosis Still a Problem?" Health Services Reports 88:483–485. June-July, 1973.

Robert F. Korns, M.D.
Research Consultant
Bureau of Cancer Control
New York State Department of Health

Peter Greenwald, M.D.
Director
Bureau of Cancer Control
New York State Department of Health

1

A Study of the Relation of Family Income and Other Economic Factors to Pellagra Incidence in Seven Cotton-Mill Villages of South Carolina in 1916

JOSEPH GOLDBERGER, G. A. WHEELER
AND EDGAR SYDENSTRICKER

In the spring of 1916 we began a study of the relation of various factors to pellagra incidence in certain representative textile-mill communities of South Carolina. On a varying scale the study was continued through 1917 and 1918. The results of the first year's (1916) study with respect to diet,[1] to age, sex, occupation, disabling sickness,[2] and to sanitation[3] have already been reported. At the present time we wish to record the results of the part of the study dealing with the relation of conditions of an economic nature to the incidence of the disease.

I. Review of Literature

A close association of pellagra with poverty has been repeatedly remarked upon since the time of the first recognition of the disease. In the earliest account, Casal (1870, p. 93), discussing

[1]Goldberger, Wheeler, and Sydenstricker, 1918 and 1920a.

[2]Goldberger, Wheeler, and Sydenstricker, 1920b; Sydenstricker, Wheeler, and Goldberger, 1919.

[3]Goldberger, Wheeler, and Sydenstricker, 1920c.

the diet of those persons attacked by the disease, remarks that "they eat meat very rarely since most pellagrins are poor field laborers, and this circumstance does not permit them to eat meat daily nor even from time to time." Continuing, he says: "Their only beverage is water. Their clothes, beds, habitations, etc., are strictly in keeping with their extreme poverty." Further along, discussing the treatment of the disease, Casal states that "milk, thanks to the butter it contains, is certainly capable of supplying the nutritive lack of the other foods; they use it but rarely without having first removed the butter, since these poor people sell the butter in order that they may be able to buy other necessaries, thus using in their own diet what remains in the milk after having thus treated it."

Much more definite and direct is Strambio (1796) who states that "thus much is certain, that pellagra is most at home where poverty and misery reign and increases as they increase."

Very interesting and significant is Marzari's observation.[4] "I have several times observed," he states, "that if a villager falls into poverty, as happens so often as a result of a storm, drought, or other calamity, pellagra does not fail to crown his misfortune and put an end to his miserable existence."

Holland (1820), in introducing his discussion of the cause and symptoms of pellagra in a paper read in 1817, based on observations of his own and on information secured from Italian physicians in the course of a journey to Italy, remarks: "The pellagra is a malady confined almost exclusively to the lower classes of the people, and chiefly to the peasants and those occupied in the labors of agriculture." He repeats this two or three times in other connections. In his discussion of the etiology of the disease (p. 322) we find the following highly suggestive statements: "Though I have spoken of Lombardy as one of the most fertile portions of Europe, yet to those who consider the little certain relation between mere productiveness of soil and the prosperity or comforts of the population dwelling upon it, it will not appear very extraordinary that the peasants of this district should be subject to various physical privations unknown to the people of

[4]Cited by Russell, 1845, p. 167.

countries which are much less favored by nature. The fact unquestionably is, whatever be our speculations as to the cause, that the peasants of Lombardy do for the most part live in much wretchedness, both as regards the quantity and quality of their diet and the other various comforts of life. It further seems probable, if not certain, that this evil has been progressively augmenting within the last 50 years; partly, perhaps, an effect of the wars which have so often devastated the country by marches and military contributions; partly a consequence of the frequent changes of political state; together with the insecurity, the variable system of government, and the heavy taxes and imposts attending such changes. To these causes may be added a decaying state of commerce and a faulty system of arrangement between landlords and the cultivators of the soil, all tending to depress agriculture and to reduce the peasantry at large to a state of much misery and privation." Continuing this discussion, Holland remarks further (p. 333): "Animal food rarely forms a part of their diet, and although living on a soil which produces wine their poverty almost precludes the use of it, even when sickness and debility render it most needful. The same condition of poverty is evident in their clothing, in their habitations, and in the want of all the minor necessaries and comforts of life. The immediate effect of these privations is obvious in the aspect of squalid wretchedness and emaciation which forms so striking a spectacle at the present time throughout the greater part of Lombardy. I say particularly *at the present time*,[5] because whatever may have been the progress of misery among the peasants of this country during the last half century it appears to have increased in a tenfold ratio during the last two years, the effect of bad harvests added to the preceding wars and political changes which have distressed this part of Italy."

Hameau (1829), in the first recorded observations of pellagra in France, reported that "this disease attacks individuals of both sexes and all ages, but I have not yet seen it in any but the poor and uncleanly who subsist on coarse food."

Lalesque (1846), in his account of pellagra of the Landes, cites a number of instances illustrating the conditions of misery under

[5]Italics in original.

266   The Challenge of Facts

which pellagra occurred, finally exclaiming (p. 421): "These are the individuals attacked by pellagra, for it attaches itself to poverty as the shadow to the body."

In a discussion of pellagra in Gorz-Gradisca, Berger (1890) very significantly observes: "The appearance during the last decennium of diseases of the vine, the reduction in value of the product of the soil because of foreign competition, crop failures, increase in taxes, increasing living costs, all operated to undermine economic conditions, particularly of the poorer country folk, and thus prepared favorable conditions for the spread of the disease."

Discussing the therapy and prophylaxis of pellagra in Bessarabia, V. Rosen (1894) bewails the attendant difficulties "in that, on the one hand, the alimentation with cornmeal porridge is a deeply rooted national custom, and, on the other, that the disease attacks the poorest class of the population; 'N'am vaca, n'am lapte a casa' ('I have no cow and no milk in the house') is uniformly the reply of the patient to questions in relation to this subject," and Sofer (1909, p. 219), discussing the economic status of pellagrins (in Austria), remarks that "89.9 per cent haven't even a cow."

The extremely unfavorable economic conditions of those subject to pellagra (in Austria-Hungary, at least), is further strikingly suggested by the character of some of the recommendations for its control. Thus Von Probizer (1899, p. 141) urged, as a necessary measure, "pecuniary aid by the Government in view of the deplorable condition of the peasantry in the affected localities."

V. Babes (1903), writing on pellagra in Roumania, remarks (p. 1187) that "practically all pellagrins are very poor;" and goes into some detail in describing the unfavorable economic condition of the Roumanian peasant, which leaves him in debt to the landowner and the tax collector.

In modern Spain we have Calmarza (1870) remarking (p. 66) that although he had seen cases in well-to-do individuals, the disease only exceptionally occurred in those of this class. He adds (p. 67) also that in his experience, unlike the reported observations of others (Roussel, 1866, p. 431), pellagra is quite common in beggars. In discussing the etiological role of widowhood, this keen observer expresses the opinion (p. 68) that this plays a part only in proportion as it tends to bring about a depression in economic well being and a consequent insufficient alimentation. Huertas (1903) describes the disease as occurring among the most miserable class of the population of Madrid, who live on the food picked from the city's garbage.

In Egypt, Sandwith (1903) found the disease highly prevalent among the poorer peasants of Lower Egypt. "In one village," he reports, "where the inhabitants are especially well-to-do because they get regular pay throughout the year from the Domains administration, there were only 15 per cent of pellagrous men, while among the men of the village, which has the reputation of being the poorest, the percentage rose as high as 62."

Gaumer (1910), discussing pellagra in Yucatan, states that the disease did not become epidemic in that State until 1884, two years after a destructive invasion by locusts or grasshoppers. "Among the better classes the disease seldom made its appearance. * * * It was the middle and lower classes who, from reduced circumstances, were obliged to purchase the cheapest corn in the market that suffered most from the ravages of the disease.

"From 1891 to 1901 Yucatan produced sufficient corn for home consumption, and new cases of pellagra were no longer to be found, * * *.

"From 1901 to 1907 the corn crops were almost total failures and corn was again imported in greater quantities than ever before * * *.

"Pellagra again became epidemic, but was not then confined to the middle and lower classes, as in the former invasion. The wealthy hemp owners, on account of the exorbitant prices paid for hemp, found it was more profitable to import than to raise corn for home consumption, thus compelling even well-to-do people to consume the imported article," which was believed to have been spoiled in transport from the United States. "Pellagra then spread alike among the rich and the poor, until by the close of 1907 about 10 per cent of the inhabitants were victims of the disease * * *."

In Barbadoes, B.W.I., the disease, according to Manning (1907), is "confined to the laboring classes and is most prevalent among those who are badly off or poverty stricken. It is very seldom found among the whites, but cases do occur among those in straightened circumstances." In the pioneer reports on pellagra in the United States such references as are made to the relation of economic status to the disease are of a very general character and appear for the most part to be echoes of European opinion. So far as we are aware credit for the first study of this relationship is due to Siler and Garrison (1913). This study was made in South Carolina in 1912 and relates to pellagrins alone. In recording their data relating to the economic conditions under which the patients lived, Siler and Garrison adopted five classes, namely, squalor, poverty, necessities, comfort, and affluence. Of the 277 cases so classified, the economic conditions were reported as poor (squalor, poverty, necessities) in 83 per cent, within the average (comfort) in 15 per cent, and well above the average (affluence) in 2 per cent.

Jobling and Petersen (1917) in their second year's study of the epidemiology of pellagra in Nashville, Tenn., "endeavored to make a most accurate study of the economic condition of pellagrous patients." "In order to do this," they state that their examiners "ascertained the average rentals for the entire city, the weekly income of the pellagrin when a wage earner, and the total income of the pellagrous family." From these data the amount of money available for each pellagrin per week was computed by dividing the total income by the number of individuals, children being accorded the same value as adults.

They found that 70 per cent of their white adult male pellagrins were wage earners, more than 60 per cent of whom earned $10 or more per week. Of the white adult females, 22 per cent were wage earners, and of these, 56 per cent earned less than $10 per week. Of the colored wage earners, 66 per cent of the males earned less than $10 per week, while a similar per cent of the females earned under $8 per week.

When the amount of money available for each pellagrin per week was estimated, Jobling and Petersen found that of the whites 56.5 per cent and of the colored 24 per cent had an available income of $2.50 or more per week.

These workers also made an estimate of the economic status of the pellagrous class on the basis of rentals, which they considered a "fairly reliable basis" for this purpose. They found that of the whites 11 per cent and of the colored 16 per cent owned their own homes or were buying them on the installment plan. "The rentals paid by the balance were practically all under $15 per month, only 3 per cent of the cases occurring in families paying more than this amount. Of the colored families few pay more than $8 per month."

It will be observed that the study of Jobling and Petersen, like that of Siler and Garrison, concerns itself exclusively with the pellagrin. Neither study affords any basis for a comparison with the economic distribution of the general population so that neither these nor, so far as we are aware, any previous observations give us any means of measuring in a definite objective manner the degree of association between economic status and pellagra incidence. This deficiency we have endeavored to repair by the study that we shall now proceed to detail.

II. Plan and Methods of Present Study

Locality

The study was made in seven representative cotton-mill villages situated in the northwestern part of South Carolina.

Population

The villages were of about average size; none had over 800 or less than 500 inhabitants. Each constituted a distinct, more or less isolated community in close proximity to a cotton-cloth manufacturing plant and was composed practically exclusively of the mill employees and their families. The few Negro families present and living somewhat apart were not considered, so that our study deals with an exclusively white population, which, with hardly a single exception, was of Anglo-Saxon stock born in this country of American-born parents. Besides the Negroes, there were also excluded from this study the mill executives, store managers, clerks, and their households, so that we had left for study an exceptionally homogeneous group with respect to racial stock, occupation, and general standard of living, including dietary custom. An enumeration of the population was made in May and June in connection with the collection of our dietary and economic data, and totaled about 4,160 people, included in about 750 households.

Pellagra Incidence

The procedure adopted for determining the incidence of pellagra in this population has been described at length in a previous paper of this series.[6]

Briefly, in order to ascertain the incidence of the disease as completely as possible, the expedient of a systematic biweekly house-to-house search for cases was employed and practically exclusively depended on.

Only cases with a clearly defined, bilaterally symmetrical dermatitis were recorded as pellagra; cases with poorly defined eruptions, or those with more or less suggestive manifestations but without clearly marked eruption, were recorded at most as "suspects" and are excluded from present consideration.

Just as in our study of pellagra incidence in relation to diet, so here, in relating pellagra incidence to economic conditions, no distinction is made between first and recurrent attacks, but all active cases as above defined are considered. So-called inactive or quiescent cases, that is, individuals who had had the disease in a previous year but during 1916 presented no definite eruption or evidence sufficient to be classed as "suspects," are considered as nonpellagrous.

As a considerable proportion of the population of any village is of transient character,[7] and as much of the pellagra occurs in this

[6]Goldberger, Wheeler, and Sydenstricker, 1920a.
[7]See in this connection Goldberger, Wheeler, and Sydenstricker, 1920b.

class,[8] some assumption was necessary on the basis of which cases might be assigned to households and villages. Accordingly the rule was adopted that a case was to be charged to a household or village only if the affected individual had been a member of that household or had resided in the village not less than 30 days immediately preceding the beginning of the attack (as above defined).

Season

It would seem reasonable to expect, if diet, economic status, or other factor has any influence in relation to the seasonal rise in incidence of the disease, that this influence is most effective during a period immediately anterior to the sharp rise and peak of incidence. Such statistics of pellagra morbidity as were available to us at the beginning of our study indicated that the rise of the seasonal curve of pellagra incidence in the southern States began in the late spring and reached its peak in June. It was assumed, therefore, that the factors favoring the production of pellagra were most effective during the season beginning some time in the late winter or early spring and continuing up to or possibly somewhat into June. The period actually selected by us as representative of this season extended from April 16 to June 15, 1916. Information

[8]This is clearly suggested by the following table, length of residence being assumed to be a fair index of the moving habit of the houshold.

Pellagra incidence in families, according to length of residence, in seven cotton-mill villages of South Carolina during 1916

Length of residence in village	FAMILIES CLASSIFIED ACCORDING TO LENGTH OF RESIDENCE IN VILLAGE		PELLAGRA INCIDENCE IN FAMILIES RESIDING SPECIFIED PERIODS IN VILLAGE	
	Number considered	Per cent residing specified periods	Number of pellagrous families	Per cent of families pellagrous
Any period	753	100.0	56	7.4
Less than 1 year	297	39.5	32	10.8
1 year	74	9.8	5	6.8
2–4 years	189	25.1	9	4.8
4 years or more	193	25.6	10	5.2

relating to family income, household food supply, and the composition of the households, etc., for sample sections of this period
was secured by trained enumerators who canvassed the village in
successive 15-day periods under the immediate direction and
supervision of one of us (E.S.).

Dietary Data

The methods adopted for securing data relating to diet have
been described fully in a previous communication (Goldberger,
Wheeler and Sydenstricker, 1920 a). It will suffice in the present
connection to recall that these data relate to the food supply of the
household, not to that of the individual, and so do not indicate the
differences that may have existed in the diets of the individual
members. It being impracticable to secure our dietary data simultaneously in all villages, the record of household food supply
secured in the several villages was for successive 15-day periods
between April 16 and June 15. It was assumed that an accurate
record for a 15-day period would be a sufficiently representative
sample of the supply of the season immediately anterior to the
peak of seasonal incidence of the disease, that is, of what may be
considered as the pellagra-producing season.

Data Relating to Economic Conditions

Since nearly 90 per cent of the individuals composing the
population studied were found to be dependent upon the income
of family groups composed of more than one person, family income was adopted as the basis for classifying the population
according to economic status.

Family income.—The data relating to family income were
secured by inquiries of the housewife or of some other responsible member or members of each family, supplemented by data
from the mill pay rolls. For the latter we are greatly indebted to the
willing cooperation of the administrative officials of the mills.

The information obtained from the families covered *(a)* the
rate of daily earnings of each member earning wages during the

half month preceding the week of the canvass and the various rates of daily earnings of all members who had been employed during the 12 preceding months; (b) the days not at work for all members who had worked for wages during the 12 preceding months; (c) the income from all other sources during the preceding half month as well as during the preceding 12 months, this information being secured in detail for each source of income. On the basis of this information it was possible to approximate the total income of each family for the half month preceding the visit of the enumerator, and, roughly, for any part or all of the preceding year.

Finding that approximately 90 per cent of the total income of the families studied came from the earnings of wage-earning members, the family statements of earnings during this half-month period were compared with the records on the mill pay rolls, and, in the great majority of instances, were found to agree closely with them; but in order to reduce the error arising from even slightly inaccurate statements as to wages, the pay-roll records instead of the family statements have been used to supply the earnings data. For that small proportion of family income made up of wages earned in employment outside of the mills and of the amounts derived from other miscellaneous sources, the family statement was necessarily accepted.

On the basis of the results of some preliminary tabulations it was decided that the family income during the half month preceding the week of the enumerator's canvass would be a fairly accurate indication of family income during the season selected as most significant in relation to the occurrence of pellagra. The basis for classifying families with respect to income was, therefore, the total cash income of each during a 15-day period between April 16 and June 15, 1916. A half-month sample period was used, partly because it corresponded to the sample period for which dietary data were secured and partly because a majority of the mills in the villages paid at semimonthly intervals. The pay-roll data from other mills were adjusted to a half-month basis.

In the course of the canvass of the homes of the mill workers' families other data affecting the economic status of the families were also collected. These related principally to length of experience in mill work, occupational status of wage earners, and the amount and incidence of disabling sickness[9] among wage-earning and other members of the household.

Availability of food supply.—With the view of studying the relation of food availability to pellagra incidence, information was collected under the immediate direction of one of us (E.S.), relating to conditions that might effect the supply of a given food or foods. In collecting and recording this information a uniform method was followed as closely as possible except where specific points suggested the advisability of special inquiry. The principal sources of information and the nature of the information sought were as follows:

1) Statements were obtained from households as to the immediate source of every article of food entering into their half-month's supplies. Thus it was ascertained, for example, whether the fresh milk used by the household was produced at home, purchased from another mill worker's household in the village, or from some specific farmer, dairy, or store, or donated by a relative, neighbor, or other person. In the event that a household had a source of supply not common generally to households in the village, inquiries were directed with a view of ascertaining the length of time the household had had such a supply, particularly, with respect to the period after January 1, 1916.

2) From farmers, hucksters, or "peddlers" selling from house to house, statements were secured relating to the quantities sold, prices, frequency of selling, and character of produce sold since January 1, 1916.

3) From managers and clerks in the stores, markets, and other retail establishments at which mill workers' households largely dealt, data were secured relating to (*a*) prices during the 15-day period and price changes during 1916; (*b*) sources of each food sold, whether direct from near-by farms or through middlemen from local agricultural territory or from sections of the United States; (*c*) names of brands and quantities of the foods sold; (*d*)

[9]See Sydenstricker, Wheeler, and Goldberger, 1918.

practices with respect to credit to mill workers' households, especially as affected by the amount of earnings by the mill workers.

Economic Classification

Method of classification according to economic status.—As has already been mentioned, the great majority of the individuals composing the population studied were members of families who subsisted on the income of families composed of several persons; the small proportion not subsisting on such family income were boarders living under substantially the same conditions as the families with which they boarded. It would seem permissible, therefore, to classify these economically with the members of the family with which they boarded, although it is fully recognized that in so doing a certain, though, for the present purpose, unimportant, error is involved.

In classifying this population according to economic status on the basis of family income the conventional method of using total family income for a given period was found to be so inaccurate in many instances as to be misleading. The average total annual cash income of all of the families for which income data were secured was about $700, and relatively few had annual incomes of over $1,000. Thus the range of total income was relatively small and the families were, from this point of view, fairly homogeneous. They differed, however, very markedly in size and with respect to the age and sex of their members. Manifestly it was improper to classify, for example, a family whose half-month's income was $40, and was composed of only a man and his wife, with one whose half-month's income was also $40, but was composed of a man, his wife, and several dependent children. Since family income, for the purpose of this study, was used as an index of the economic status of individuals who composed the family group, it was necessary to take into consideration the number of such individuals in comparing one family with another. A per capita statement of income, however, while more accurate than the statement of total income, was subject to the inaccuracy arising from differences in the age and sex of members of the families to be compared. It appeared advisable, therefore, to employ a common denominator to which the individuals of both sexes and of all ages could be reduced in order to obtain a more accurately representative method of expressing the relative size of the families to be compared.

In the absence of a better common denominator for this purpose, the Atwater (1915) scale of food requirements was employed, and the size of each family was computed according to this scale and expressed in terms of "adult male units."[10] The assumption in the use of this scale was that the expenditures for total maintenance for individuals varied according to sex and age in the same proportion as did their food requirements. The assumption is by no means as accurate as could be desired; in its favor, however, it may be said that since family expenditures in the great majority of cases equaled total family income, and since food expenditures were nearly half (among poorer families considerably more than half) of total expenditures, a scale based on food requirements alone is obviously very much more accurate than one omitting any consideration whatsoever of the number, sex, and age of the individuals composing the families to be compared with respect to income.[11] For the present purpose, therefore, the

[10]The scale used was as follows:

Age	EQUIVALENT ADULT MALE UNIT	
	Male	Female
Adult (over 16)	1.0	0.8
15 to 16	.9	.8
13 to 14	.8	.7
12	.7	.6
10 to 11	.6	.6
6 to 9	.5	.5
2 to 5	.4	.4
Under 2	.3	.3

[11]In order to establish a more accurate basis for computing the size of families in comparing their incomes, a detailed study of expenditures for individuals in a number of representative families in cotton-mill villages was undertaken during 1917. While the tabulations of these data were not completed in time for use in the study of the data collected in 1916, it appears that the Atwater scale is roughly indicative of the variations, according to sex and age, in the consumption of all articles for which there are individual expenditures. It should be noted that before using the Atwater scale in the preliminary computations of family income, several published estimates of the cost of maintenance for individuals of various ages were

TABLE I   Number of families and members of families and their equivalents in adult male units in seven cotton-mill villages of South Carolina, classified according to family income during a 15-day period between Apr. 15 and June 16, 1916

Half-month family income per adult male unit	Families	Persons[a]	Equivalent adult male units[b]
	Number	Number	Number
Less than $6.00	217	1,289	866.2
$6.00–$7.99	183	972	675.9
$8.00–$9.99	139	704	529.2
$10.00 and over	208	800	607.1
All incomes	747	3,765	2,678.2
	Per cent	Per cent	Per cent
All incomes	100.0	100.0	100.0
Less than $6.00	29.1	34.2	32.4
$6.00–$7.99	24.5	25.8	25.2
$8.00–$9.99	18.6	18.7	19.8
$10.00 and over	27.9	21.3	22.6

[a]Exclusive of persons paying board and including only those dependent upon family income.   [b]According to the Atwater scale for food requirements.

examined. These estimates were based, in several instances, upon the results of investigation of actual expenditures of individual members of families. Using the estimated expenditures for an adult male as 100, the estimates for individuals of other ages of either sex were expressed relatively and compared with the Atwater scale. It appeared that, in most instances, the scales were fairly similar. The following table, computed from probably the most pertinent data available, indicates the relative cost of maintenance (at a "fair standard of living") for a year of individuals of various ages as estimated for Southern cotton-mill workers by the United States Bureau of Labor in 1911, in comparison with the Atwater scale for food requirements.

Comparison of the relative variations in individual expenses for all purposes with variations in individual food requirements according to age and sex

	MALE		FEMALE	
Age	Individual expenses (U.S. Bureau of Labor)	Food requirements (Atwater)	Individual expenses (U.S. Bureau of Labor)	Food requirements (Atwater)
Adult (over 16)	100	100	89	80
15 to 16	85	90	79	80
13 to 14	72	80	67	70
12	61	70	57	60
10 to 11	56	60	59	60
6 to 9	45	50	46	50
2 to 5	34	40	35	40
Under 2	26	30	26	30

The individual expenses estimated were for food (estimated by the U.S. Bureau of Labor, according to the Atwater scale), clothing, medical attendance, and medicines, insurance, amusements, tobacco, and school books. See report on Conditions of Women and Child Wage Earners in the United States, Vol. XVI, Family Budgets of Typical Cotton-Mill Workers by Wood F. Worcester and Daisy Worthington Worcester, Sen. Doc. 645, 61 Cong., 2d sess., 1911, p. 150.

TABLE II Average half-month family income, computed in terms of "per family," "per person," and "per adult male unit,"[a] for various income classes of the population in seven cotton-mill villages in South Carolina

Half-month family income per adult male unit	All family income during a half month	AVERAGE INCOME DURING A HALF MONTH		
		Per family	Per person[b]	Per adult male unit[b]
Less than $6.00	$3,990.45	$18.38	$3.09	$4.61
$6.00–$7.99	4,780.85	26.12	4.92	7.67
$8.09–$9.99	4,642.29	33.40	6.55	8.77
$10.00 and over	7,777.99	37.39	9.72	12.81
All incomes	**21,191.58**	**28.36**	**5.63**	**7.92**

[a]According to the Atwater scale for food requirements.   [b]Exclusive of persons paying board and including only those dependent upon family income.

total income of each family as defined above, has been divided by the number of "adult male units" subsisting on the family income, and the resulting figure has been termed the "family income per adult male unit."

Results of classification.—The 747 families for which income data were sufficiently accurate and complete for consideration have been classified by this method and grouped into four convenient classes, each containing a fair proportion of the total number. Table I presents this classification and also the resulting distribution of individuals and their equivalent "adult male units."

The differences in income are also indicated in Table II, which permits of a comparison of the results of classification on the basis of the average income during the half-month period per family, per person, and per "adult male unit." Table III, based on

TABLE III Ratio of the average income for each income class to that of all income classes of the population of seven cotton-mill villages of South Carolina

[*The average income is computed in terms of "per family," "per person," and "per adult male unit"*]

Family income per adult male unit	RELATIVE AVERAGE INCOME DURING A HALF MONTH PER—		
	Family	Person	Adult male unit
All incomes	100	100	100
Under $6.00	65	55	58
$6.00–$7.99	92	87	89
$8.00–$9.99	118	116	112
$10.00 and over	132	173	162

Table II, permits of the same comparison and perhaps expresses these differences more clearly. It will be noted that the same *general* differences in *average* incomes for the four groups are indicated by any of the three methods of classification. For reasons already stated, however, the "adult male unit" method is believed to be more accurately representative of actual conditions than either of the others and, therefore, to be preferred for the classification of individual families; it is the method hereinafter employed.

Before entering upon a consideration of the relation of family income to pellagra incidence it will be desirable to make brief reference to the factors affecting family income. An analysis of our data with a view of determining, so far as practicable, what these were, showed the principal ones to be as follows: (a) supplemental income, chiefly from boarders; (b) the number of dependent persons, principally children, in proportion to the number of wage-earning persons in the family; and (c) the earning capacity of the wage earners, including chiefly the factors of natural ability, length of training, and state of health. In the classification of this population according to "family income per adult male unit," those persons in the higher income classes appeared distinctly to have the advantage in each of these respects over those in the lower income classes.

III. Pellagra Incidence According to Economic Status

Having considered the methods employed for securing the basic data relating to the occurrence of the disease and for securing those relating to the classification of the population with respect to economic status, we may now proceed to determine the relationship existing between the economic status of the family and the degree of incidence of the disease.

We have in all 747 households for which our data are sufficiently complete and accurate to permit of classification according to income. There were recorded among the members of these households 97 definite cases of pellagra. In Table IV we have

The Challenge of Facts

TABLE IV   Number and per cent of households of different income classes affected with pellagra in seven cotton-mill villages of South Carolina in 1916

Half-month family income per adult male unit	All house-holds	PELLAGROUS HOUSEHOLDS IN WHICH WERE—		
		One or more cases of pellagra	Two or more cases of pellagra	Three or more cases of pellagra
NUMBER				
Less than $6.00	217	28	17	7
$6.00–$7.99	183	21	3	1
$8.00–$9.99	139	8	4	0
$10.00–$13.99	144	3	0	0
$14.00 and over	64	1	0	0
All incomes	**747**	**61**	**24**	**8**
PER CENT				
Less than $6.00	100.0	12.9	7.8	3.2
$6.00–$7.99	100.0	11.5	1.6	.5
$8.00–$9.99	100.0	5.8	2.9	0.0
$10.00–$13.99	100.0	2.1	0.0	0.0
$14.00 and over	100.0	1.5	0.0	0.0
All incomes	**100.0**	**8.2**	**3.2**	**1.1**

distributed these households in accordance with the family income per adult male unit during the sample half-month period and have indicated therein also the number and per cent of the households in each of the resulting five income classes that were affected with pellagra to the extent of *(a)* one or more cases, *(b)* two or more' cases, and *(c)* three or more cases.

It will be observed that the proportion of families affected with pellagra declines with a marked degree of regularity as income increases. This inverse correlation is even more clearly shown when weight is given to households with more than one case of the disease,[12] as is done in Table V, in which the incidence of pellagra is expressed as a rate per 1,000 persons in each income class.

The occurrence of multiple-case families, especially from the point of view of difference in income, invites special comment. The 97 cases of pellagra occurred in 61 families. In each of 24 of

[12]Upon the basis of the average half-month income per adult male unit for each of the income classes and the corresponding pellagra rate per 1,000 persons, the Pearsonian coefficient of correlation is -0.91 ± 0.05. While the small number of classes considered must, of course, be taken into account, the expression indicates high degree of correlation (-1.0 being perfect inverse correlation).

TABLE V   Number of definite cases of pellagra and rate per 1,000[1]
among persons of different income classes in seven cotton-mill
villages of South Carolina in 1916

Half-month family income per adult male unit	TOTAL			MALES			FEMALES		
	Number of persons	Number of cases	Rate[1] per 1,000	Number of persons	Number of cases	Rate per 1,000	Number of persons	Number of cases	Rate per 1,000
Less than $6.00	1,312	56	42.7	650	20	30.8	662	36	54.4
$6.00–$7.99	1,037	27	26.0	521	6	11.5	516	21	40.7
$8.00–$9.99	784	10	12.8	376	4	10.7	408	6	14.7
$10.00–$13.99	736	3	4.1	363	0	0.0	373	3	8.0
$14.00 and over	291	1	3.4	161	1	6.2	130	0	0.0
All incomes	**4,160**	**97**	**23.3**	**2,071**	**31**	**14.9**	**2,089**	**66**	**31.6**

[1]Since a marked variation in the pellagra rate according to age and sex was found for the population studied (Goldberger, Wheeler, and Sydenstricker, 1920 b), and since, ordinarily, differences in the distribution of persons according to age occur in different economic groups, computation of rates adjusted to a standard population was made. The influence of differences in the sex distribution in any age group was insignificant, and practically the same incidence rates were obtained after making adjustments to a standard age distribution, as is shown in the following table:

TABLE Va   Comparison of crude pellagra rates and of rates after
adjustment for age to standard population for each income class

[Standard population = total population, all incomes]

Family income per adult male unit	CASE RATE PER 1,000	
	Crude	Adjusted
Less than $6.00	42.7	41.0
$6.00–$7.99	26.0	24.8
$8.00–$9.99	12.8	14.2
$10.00–$13.99	4.1	5.2
$14.00 and over	3.4	2.5

these families, two or more cases occurred, while in each of 8, three or more cases developed. Taking into consideration the size of the families and assuming that all individuals were equally susceptible to the disease,[13] a computation of the probability of the occurrence of multiple-case families according to purely chance distribution indicated that in the 747 families we should expect about 90 families with one case each, about 8 families with two or more cases, while the probability of households each with three or more cases would be less than 2 in 10,000. The actual occurrence of 24 families with two cases each and of 8 families

[13]So far as sex and age are concerned, all families (with but few exceptions) contained fairly comparable proportions of "susceptible" individuals.

with three or more cases would thus seem to be far in excess of the result of chance.[14] The fact that multiple-case families occurred only in the lower-income classes and that families with three or more cases occurred practically only in the lowest-income class plainly shows that the tendency toward concentration of cases in certain families increases as income diminishes. Pellagra incidence in the population studied therefore not only varied inversely according to family income, but with decreasing income it seemed to show an increasing tendency to affect members of the same family.

Discussion

The very marked inverse correlation between low income and pellagra incidence naturally calls for explanation. Under the conditions of the study the following possibilities in this regard suggested themselves for consideration:

    a) Bad hygiene and sanitation;

    b) Difference in sex and age composition of the population in the several income classes; and

    c) Difference in diet.

    a) Bad hygiene and sanitation are in general closely associated with poverty so that the incidence of a disease, the dissemination of which is favored by such conditions, may be expected to be unusually high in the lower economic strata. Consequently it is natural to suspect that a disease found to be highly prevalent in an environment of poverty is dependent on the almost inevitably attendant unhygienic and insanitary conditions for its propagation, and to assume that it is of microbial origin. The possibility of an essential infective etiological factor in this disease has therefore been given careful consideration, and in a previous paper (Goldberger, Wheeler, and Sydenstricker, 1920 *c*) we reported the results of our study of the relation of certain factors of a sanitary character to the incidence of pellagra in these villages. No consis-

[14]Acknowledgment is made to Associate Statistician F. M. Phillips, United States Public Health Service, for assistance in this computation.

TABLE VI   Number and per cent of persons in each income class, classified according to age, in 7 cotton-mill villages of South Carolina in 1916

[The classes being divided from each other at those ages at which the pellagra incidence rate for the whole population varies most sharply[a]]

Half-month family income per adult male unit	All ages	Under 5 years	5–9	10–19	20–29	30–44	45–54	55 years and over
				AGE GROUP				

NUMBER

Half-month family income per adult male unit	All ages	Under 5 years	5–9	10–19	20–29	30–44	45–54	55 years and over
Less than $6.00	1,312	260	251	317	162	217	49	56
$6.00-$7.99	1,037	162	166	270	172	166	60	41
$8.00-$9.99	784	104	108	229	149	114	48	32
$10.00-$13.99	736	95	69	173	215	102	46	36
$14.00 and over	291	27	15	71	91	63	9	15
All incomes	**4,160**	**648**	**609**	**1,060**	**789**	**662**	**212**	**180**

PER CENT

Half-month family income per adult male unit	All ages	Under 5 years	5–9	10–19	20–29	30–44	45–54	55 years and over
Less than $6.00	100	19.8	19.1	24.2	12.4	16.5	3.7	4.3
$6.00-$7.99	100	15.7	16.0	26.0	16.6	16.0	5.8	3.9
$8.00-$9.99	100	13.3	13.8	29.2	19.0	14.5	6.1	4.1
$10.00-$13.99	100	12.9	9.4	23.5	29.2	13.9	6.2	4.9
$14.00 and over	100	9.3	5.2	24.4	31.3	21.6	3.1	5.2
All incomes	**100**	**15.6**	**14.6**	**25.5**	**19.0**	**15.9**	**5.1**	**4.3**

[a]See Goldberger, Wheeler, and Sydenstricker, 1920 b.

tent correlation was found.[15] This, coupled with the results of the other of our own studies (see discussion by Goldberger and Wheeler, 1920, pp. 36–41) and of the studies of other investigators (White, 1919; and Boyd and Lelean, 1919), and with the fact of the complete absence of any unequivocal evidence in support of an essential infective etiological factor in this disease, not only renders discussion of hygienic and sanitary factors in the present connection unnecessary but, we believe, permits of their dismissal from further serious consideration.

b) Differences in sex and age composition of the population in the several income classes.—We have shown in a previous communication (Goldberger, Wheeler, and Sydenstricker, 1920 b) that the incidence of the disease in the population of these villages differs markedly in the sexes and at certain age periods; it is conceivable, therefore, that differences in the sex and the age distribution in the different income classes might give rise to the

[15]The data collected during 1916 were not in a form to permit the study of the relation of crowding in the home to pellagra incidence. We may state, however, that a preliminary analysis of a considerable mass of data bearing on this point, collected during 1917, shows very little, if any, correlation between them when the effect of income is minimized.

phenomenon under discussion. That this is not the case, however, is evident 1) when it is recalled that we are dealing with a population composed of family units and 2) when we compare the indications afforded by Tables V and VI, showing, respectively, the sex and the age distribution of the population of each economic class, and note the agreement in the indications afforded by the crude rates and by the rates after adjustment to a standard population (footnote to Table V).

c) *Differences in diet.*—The results of budgetary investigations have repeatedly demonstrated the association of marked variations in diet with variation in family income.[16] It seemed doubly pertinent, therefore, to inquire what, if any, variations in diet were associated with variations in income among the families of our cotton-mill villages. Accordingly, we prepared Table VII, showing the average food supply of the households of the several income classes. To facilitate comparison between the averages thus presented, indices have been computed, the figures for the households with the highest income being used as the base. It will be noted that, from the point of view of income, the following general tendencies are suggested:

1. The smaller the income the smaller were the supplies purchased of all meats (except salt pork), green vegetables, fresh fruits, eggs, butter, cheese, preserved milk, lard, sugar (including sirup), and canned foods.

2. The smaller the income the larger were the supplies purchased of salt pork and corn meal.

3. In the households of the various income classes the quantities of the purchased supplies[17] of dried peas and beans, potatoes, dried fruits, wheat flour and bread, fresh milk, and rice appeared without any consistent trend.

----

[16]In this connection see Sydenstricker, 1915.

[17]Practically all food supplies, with the exception of fresh milk, were purchased (i.e., not home-produced) during the season (the late spring) of the year under consideration. Households securing supplies of milk from home-owned cows have not been included in the next table (Table VII), since supplies of food from this source constitute a factor affecting the diet of the population apart from the factor of family income. They are considered in another connection.

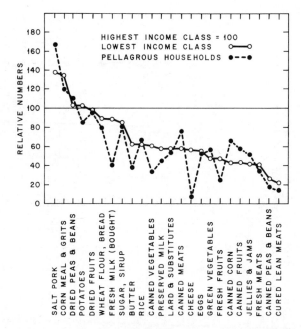

Figure 1   Comparison of the supply of certain articles of food in households with lowest incomes and in households having at least two cases of pellagra with that in households with highest incomes. (See Table VII)

Thus it appears that there were associated with differences in family income quite definite differences in household food supplies. In order to determine the outstanding differences more clearly, the households with intermediate incomes were disregarded and comparison was made of the food supplies in households presenting the greatest contrast from an economic standpoint (i.e., those households representing the respective extremes of family income), with the result that not only did the differences already noted stand out more clearly, but, in addition, it appeared that the supplies of wheat flour and bread and of fresh milk were appreciably smaller in the poorest households.

In that part of our study dealing with the relation of household food supply to pellagra incidence (Goldberger, Wheeler, and Sydenstricker, 1920a) a very definite significant relationship between the character of the diet and the incidence of the disease

TABLE VII Average supply (per adult male unit) during a 15-day period between Apr. 15 and June 16, 1916, of various purchased articles of food[a] in households of different income classes and in the group of those households in each of which two or more cases of pellagra occurred prior to Aug. 1, 1916

GRAMS PER ADULT MALE UNIT PER DAY

Half-month family income per adult male unit	Salt pork	Corn meal and grits	Dried peas and beans	Potatoes	Dried fruits	Wheat flour, bread	Fresh milk (bought)	Sugar sirup	Butter	Rice	Canned vegetables	Preserved milk	Lard & lard substitutes	Canned meats	Cheese	Eggs	Green vegetables[b]	Fresh fruits	Canned corn	Canned fruits	Jellies and jams	Fresh meats	Canned peas & beans	Cured lean meats
$14.00 and more	39	126	31	71	10	447	319	59	30	8	58	4	63	20	3	59	105	41	9	27	11	47	9	53
$10.00–$13.99	49	152	31	107	9	434	302	61	35	6	36	4	54	12	2	57	63	33	10	26	10	32	6	28
$8.00–$9.99	54	151	35	97	9	410	342	67	14	5	37	3	49	16	3	44	60	31	8	24	8	30	4	24
$6.00–$7.99	56	174	33	88	9	460	317	55	19	4	46	1	49	14	2	38	61	30	6	14	9	21	5	20
Less than $6.00	54	169	31	78	10	399	282	50	19	5	35	2	37	12	2	33	49	19	4	12	5	19	2	12
Pellagrous households	65	150	34	60	10	361	127	48	11	6	20	2	35	16	(c)	31	61	10	6	16	6	16	2	8

RELATIVE NUMBERS. BASE: SUPPLY PER ADULT MALE UNIT PER DAY IN HOUSEHOLDS WITH HIGHEST INCOMES

Half-month family income per adult male unit	Salt pork	Corn meal and grits	Dried peas and beans	Potatoes	Dried fruits	Wheat flour, bread	Fresh milk (bought)	Sugar sirup	Butter	Rice	Canned vegetables	Preserved milk	Lard & lard substitutes	Canned meats	Cheese	Eggs	Green vegetables	Fresh fruits	Canned corn	Canned fruits	Jellies and jams	Fresh meats	Canned peas & beans	Cured lean meats
$14.00 and more	100	100	100	100	100	100	100	100	100	100	100	100	100	100	100	100	100	100	100	100	100	100	100	100
$10.00–$13.99	126	121	100	151	90	97	95	103	117	75	62	100	86	60	67	97	60	81	111	96	91	68	67	53
$8.00–$9.99	138	120	113	137	90	92	107	114	47	63	64	75	78	80	100	75	57	76	89	89	73	64	44	45
$6.00–$7.99	144	138	107	124	90	103	99	98	63	50	79	25	78	70	67	64	58	73	67	52	82	45	56	38
Less than $6.00	138	134	100	103	100	89	88	85	63	63	60	50	59	60	67	56	47	46	44	41	45	40	22	23
Pellagrous households	167	119	110	85	100	81	40	81	37	75	34	50	55	80	…	52	58	24	67	59	55	34	22	15

[a] For explanation of terms, see Goldberger, Wheeler, and Sydenstricker 1920a, appendix.　[b] Includes string beans.　[c] Less than 0.5 of a gram.

was demonstrated, and since, as we have seen above, a marked inverse correlation exists between the amount of family income and the degree of incidence of the disease, it follows that the character of the diet of the population under consideration may be expected to vary with the amount of family income, in the sense at least that the lower the income the more the character of the diet will tend to approach that associated with pellagra. This is confirmed by the quite definite differences in food supply above actually shown to be associated with differences in family income, and further by the fact that when comparison is made, such as Table VII and Fig. 1 permit, it is found that in a general, but quite definite, way the food supply of the households of the lowest-income class tends to be similar to that of the group of pellagrous households in each of which at least two cases of pellagra occurred prior to August 1, 1916; that is, similar to that of the group whose food supply more closely approximates a representative sample of a pellagra-producing diet than does any other afforded by our study.

Differences in Incidence Among Households

From the foregoing considerations the conclusion would seem to be suggested that the inverse correlation between pellagra incidence and family income depended in large measure, if not entirely, on the unfavorable effect of a low income on the character of the diet. In this connection, however, it must be noted and consideration must be given to the fact that a large proportion of households with low incomes were not affected with the disease.[18] Thus, in the village of *In*, where the highest of the incidence rates observed by us in 1916 occurred and where the

[18]Similarly, a large proportion of the members of pellagrous households were apparently unaffected by the disease. As has already been stated, the present study deals with the household, not with the individual, excepting only as to pellagra incidence. We have, therefore, no special data on which an explanation of the exemption of the unaffected members of a household might be based. Nevertheless, in the light of (a) certain general observations and (b) of analogies to such food deficiency diseases as scurvy and beriberi, together with (c) the knowledge gained as the result of the newer work of many students in the field of diet and nutrition,

rate among persons constituting the households with incomes under the average was 90 per 1,000, over 65 per cent of these poorer households appeared not to be affected, and, in varying degree, this was true of each of the seven villages studied. That the exemption of these families from pellagra was not due to a lack of subjects of "susceptible" sex is evident from what has already been said on this point; and that it could not be attributed to lack of human material of "susceptible" age appears very clearly when the distribution of the population according to age is compared for the pellagrous and for the poorer nonpellagrous households in a representative village, as is done in Table VIII. Manifestly, therefore, the amount of family income—that is, money income (in the sense here used), such as wages, cash payments from boarders, cash receipts from sales of supplies, and other sources—was not the sole factor determining the character of the household diet.

the following suggestions may properly be submitted for consideration in this connection:

1. *Differences in diet consumed among individuals of the household.*—Although all members of a household presumably have the same diet available, as the result of individual likes and dislikes, observable at almost any table, slight differences in diet actually consumed are common and marked differences, amounting in some instances to outstanding individual eccentricities, are not rare. Furthermore, differences in diet actually consumed may arise from, or be accentuated by, food eaten between meals and by supplemental foods of one kind or another in respect to which individuals of the same household may differ considerably. Clearly, then, a knowledge of the exact composition of the diet of a household or other dietary group does not necesarily justify the assumption of a knowledge of the composition of the diet consumed by an individual member of such household or group. Failure to appreciate this, it may be noted, has been a frequent cause of serious error and consequent confusion in connection with studies of food-deficiency diseases.

2. *Differences in individual susceptibility or resistance.*—Assuming identity of diet actually consumed, differences in incidence among individuals of the same household or other dietary group may result from individual variation in resistance or susceptibility, which may conceivably be related to (a) an inherent individual characteristic, (b) the age or sex of the individual, (c) the existence of some exhausting underlying disease or condition (hookworm, dysentery, duodenal fistula), or (d) to unlike physical strain or exertion.

3. *Combinations of factors 1 and 2.*

TABLE VIII   Age distribution constituting the nonpellagrous
households with low family income[a] and the pellagrous
households of the mill village of In

		AGE GROUPS						
Households	All ages	Under 5	5–9	10–19	20–29	30–44	45–54	55 and over
	NUMBER OF PERSONS							
Nonpellagrous	265	52	53	61	33	45	14	7
Pellagrous	168	31	32	49	19	31	5	1
All households	**433**	**83**	**85**	**110**	**52**	**76**	**19**	**8**
	PER CENT							
Nonpellagrous	100.0	19.6	20.0	23.0	12.5	17.0	5.3	2.6
Pellagrous	100.0	18.5	19.0	29.2	11.3	18.5	3.0	.6
All households	**100.0**	**19.2**	**19.6**	**25.4**	**12.0**	**17.5**	**4.4**	**1.8**

[a]That is, under $8 per adult male unit during a half-month period in the late spring of 1916.

This is quite in accord with common experience, which teaches that there are many factors that, singly or in varying combination, may have an important influence on the character of the diet and that may vary among and thus may distinguish different households of the same income. In illustration of this, reference may be made to the group of factors that tend to determine the amount and proportion of family income available for the purchase of food, an example of which is the occurrence of sickness or injury, making an unusual draft on the family income. Related to such factors are the general spirit of the household with respect to thrift (which, when unwisely directed, may be harmful) and the intelligence and ability of the housewife in utilizing the available family income.

More tangible than these, and perhaps of more immediate practical importance in its effect on the household diet, is the difference among households with respect to the availability of food supplies. We found that, among households with similar incomes and of the same village and thus with access to the same markets, there were some more favorably situated in having sources of food supplies that others either did not possess or possessed in a lesser degree. Such sources frequently were gardens, home-owned cows, swine, poultry, and the like.

Differences in Incidence Among Villages

Besides differences among households with similar incomes and of the same village, quite marked differences in pellagra incidence were also observed, as has already been pointed out, among the villages themselves. We have sought to determine the explanation of this by considering in order the various possibilities that suggested themselves.

a) The general environment (except as to condition of sanitation and food supply), the origin and type of the population, the character of work, and the general habits of living among these populations being, as we have already stated, strikingly similar, do not call for consideration in the present condition.

b) Differences in sanitary conditions among villages were noted and their relation to differences in the incidence of the disease was studied without, however, discovering any consistent correlation among them. Reasons have been given why hygienic and sanitary factors might be dismissed from consideration in the attempt to explain the inverse correlation between family income and the incidence of pellagra.[19] Further discussion of these factors in the present connection would therefore seem to be unnecessary.

c) The marked association between low family income and pellagra incidence suggested the possibility that the difference in incidence among villages might be associated with a difference in the proportion of families of low incomes included in the populations of the several villages. But if the differences in the proportion of the population which had low incomes in the various villages be compared with the difference in pellagra incidence, as is done in Table IX, no consistent correlation is disclosed. Clearly the differences in pellagra incidence among these villages can not be accounted for by differences in the economic status of the populations concerned.

d) As family income is simply an index of the power to buy, and as this power is obviously limited by the cost of the thing desired

[19]See pages 282 and 283.

TABLE IX   Comparison of the relation of rate of pellagra incidence to proportion of population of low family income in seven mill villages of South Carolina in 1916

Village	PERCENT OF POPULATION WHOSE HALF-MONTH FAMILY INCOME PER ADULT MALE UNIT WAS LESS THAN—		Pellagra rate per 1,000 population (all incomes) in 1916
	$6.00	$8.00	
All villages	31.5	56.5	23.4
At	37.0	64.3	20.7
In	40.9	66.6	64.6
Ny	26.2	45.7	0.0
Rc	13.2	23.7	24.9
Sn	38.3	58.1	10.9
Sa	28.3	57.4	25.7
Wg	31.0	64.0	18.7

Pearsonian coefficient of correlation: $r = 0.33 \pm 0.23$

(in this instance food), the thought naturally suggests itself that differences in prices in the different villages might be of importance in the present connection. That this was a negligible factor, however, is shown by the fact that we found no significant differences in food prices in the different villages.

e) That individuals of "susceptible" ages may have been present in relatively insignificant numbers in the villages among whose poorer households few if any were affected by the disease, and that this may account for the differences, is an explanation that may be dismissed from consideration when the age distribution of the population is compared according to village, as may be seen by reference to Table X.

f) We thus come to a consideration, finally, of differences among villages with respect to availability of food supplies on the local markets or from home production. More or less marked differences in this respect were found to exist. In relating these to differences in pellagra incidence it should be borne in mind that the availability to a consumer of a supply of a given article or group of articles of food is often involved in a number of interrelated conditions, the influence of any one of which may be difficult to measure. Therefore, in analyzing community conditions affecting the supply of any article or articles of food, only the outstanding and clearcut differences between localities can be considered. Furthermore, since even considerable differences in pellagra in-

TABLE X   Comparison of the age distribution of the population constituting the households with low family incomes[a] of seven cotton-mill villages of South Carolina

CLASSIFIED BY AGE PERIODS (YEARS)

Villages	All ages	Under 5 years	5–9	10–19	20–29	30–44	45–54	55 and over
			NUMBER OF PERSONS					
At	367	65	65	82	63	59	18	15
In	433	83	85	110	52	76	19	8
Ny	331	60	56	87	45	57	15	11
Rc	206	37	42	50	34	32	5	6
Sn	338	65	46	69	61	52	14	31
Sa	268	51	51	68	40	34	14	10
Wg	407	62	72	120	39	73	24	17
All villages	2,350	423	417	586	334	383	109	98
			PER CENT					
At	100.0	17.5	17.5	22.3	17.2	16.1	4.9	4.1
In	100.0	19.2	19.6	25.4	12.0	17.5	4.4	1.8
Ny	100.0	18.1	16.9	26.3	13.6	17.2	4.5	3.3
Rc	100.0	18.0	20.4	24.3	16.5	15.5	2.4	2.9
Sn	100.0	19.2	13.6	20.4	18.0	15.4	4.1	9.2
Sa	100.0	19.0	19.0	25.4	14.9	12.7	5.2	3.7
Wg	100.0	15.2	17.4	29.5	9.6	17.9	5.9	4.2
All villages	100.0	18.0	17.7	24.9	14.2	16.3	4.6	4.2

[a] That is under $8 per adult male unit during a half month in the late spring of 1916.

cidence among localities of small population are not necessarily a reflection of community conditions, it seemed desirable to select for the study of the relationship under consideration villages presenting the most marked contrast in the incidence of the disease, thereby avoiding the possibly confusing effects of irregularities likely to arise in attempts to relate community conditions of food availability to pellagra rates for which community conditions were possibly responsible only in part or not at all. There was, moreover, the compelling practical consideration to thus restrict ourselves in the fact that the amount of labor involved in a detailed study of conditions in each of our villages was beyond the physical capacity of the available personnel to perform. Accordingly we selected for study *Ny* village, with no pellagra, and *In* village, with a rate of not less than 64.6 per 1,000 during 1916. The facts, as we were able to determine them relating to the availability of supplies of various foods in these two villages, are briefly summarized in the following:

1) *Retail grocery establishments.*—In both villages the mill workers' households purchased their supplies of all foods from

the company stores and from grocery stores in adjacent communities, with the exception of fresh meats, fresh milk, and varying proportions of their supplies of eggs, butter, green vegetables, and fresh fruits. Exclusive of the articles named, the availability of supplies of all foods appeared to be the same in both villages for the reasons that (a) in both villages there existed company stores which carried in stock practically the same kinds of foods and were operated along similar lines from the point of view of credit allowances to mill workers, and (b) within a mile of either village were general grocery stores carrying in stock the same kinds and varieties of foods as those sold at the company stores. The company stores at Ny, however, did not sell fresh vegetables, potatoes, and fresh fruits, there being an agreement with the lessee of the village market to the effect that the latter should have the exclusive store privilege of selling these articles. A much more regular and abundant supply of fresh vegetables and fruits was available at the Ny market than at the In company store.

It is of interest to note that the In households, whose incomes were less than the average income for the two villages, relied to a greater extent upon the company store than the Ny households with similar incomes. This is indicated by the purchase and food supply records during the 15-day period from May 16 to May 30, 1916, which show that 60 per cent of the In households purchased all of their groceries (exclusive of home produce and produce from near-by farms) from the company store as compared with only 13 per cent of the Ny households.

2) *Fresh-meat markets.*—In Ny there was a fresh-meat market which had been open seven days in the week the year round for several years. This market, as already noted, also sold fresh fruit and vegetables. The nearest other market was 1 mile away, and this market operated a wagon which regularly had taken orders and delivered fresh meat in the village at the doors of the mill workers' households during the spring and the preceding fall and winter. At the town of Seneca, 4 miles away, there were two other fresh-meat markets which were occasionally patronized by Ny mill workers. In In village there was no fresh-meat market, and there had not been any since the last of February, 1916. In Oc-

tober, 1915, a privately operated market was opened in the basement of the company store building. This market was kept open every week day until about January 1, 1916, but, from all accounts, it was poorly managed. For this reason and for the reason that locally produced fresh meats became scarce after January 1, the market was open only one or two days a week during January and February and its credit trade was severely curtailed, being now limited to those households which had been prompt in settlements. In the latter part of February the market ceased to be operated. In the town of Inman, a mile or more from the mill village, there was a market selling fresh meat for cash only, which had a few regular customers among the mill workers. No other market was accessible except in the city of Spartanburg, 13 miles away.

With the exception of a small amount of poultry purchased at home or purchased from near-by farmers, the sole sources of fresh meats in the two villages during the late spring of 1916 were these fresh-meat markets. The difference in availability of a fresh meat supply in the two villages is clearly reflected in the records of actual purchases during the 15-day period May 16–30, 1916, illustrated in Table XI, thereby suggesting a marked contrast in fresh-meat consumption between the two villages for households of similar incomes. (See also Table XIII.)

3) *Produce from adjacent farm territory.*—The two villages

TABLE XI   Comparison of availability of fresh meat as shown by the number of purchases and the average daily supply of this food during the period May 16–30, 1916, in households, with family incomes less than the average, of two mill villages of South Carolina

Number of purchases during 15-day period	VILLAGE OF NY. (AVERAGE DAILY SUPPLY PER ADULT MALE UNIT, 31.2 GRAMS)		VILLAGE OF IN. (AVERAGE DAILY SUPPLY PER ADULT MALE UNIT 7.0 GRAMS)	
	Number of households purchasing	Per cent of total households	Number of households purchasing	Per cent of total households
None	17	31.0	46	65.8
1	6	10.9	18	25.7
2	7	12.7	4	5.7
3	7	12.7	1	1.4
4	6	10.9	1	1.4
5	6	10.9	0	0.0
More than 5	6	10.9	0	0.0

presented a striking contrast with respect to the availability of food supplies from adjacent farm territory.

In the mill village of *In* there were no regular sellers of farm produce during the spring of 1916; farmers visited the village only occasionally and then practically solely in order to dispose of such goods as they had been unable to sell in the near-by town of Inman. The absence of hucksters was so marked that repeated and detailed inquiries were made of mill workers' households and of other persons living in or in close touch with the village, and the village was several times canvassed in order to secure as complete and accurate information as possible in relation thereto. *Ny*, on the other hand, appeared to be a center for marketing produce from near-by farms. In addition to a number of farmers who marketed their produce in that village occasionally, not less than 22 farmers who habitually sold in the village at retail were found and interviewed in a single canvass of the adjacent territory. These regular hucksters came to the village once a week or oftener practically the year round. Of the 22 who were interviewed, 15 sold fresh milk and butter, 10 sold eggs, 7 sold poultry, 5 sold fresh pork, 2 sold fresh beef, and practically all of them sold potatoes and vegetables. Those selling milk and butter delivered regularly throughout the year and marketed other produce in different seasons. Thus, eggs were sold principally in the spring, poultry in the summer, autumn, and winter, fresh beef and pork in the autumn and winter, and green vegetables in the spring, summer, and autumn. On the basis of statements made by those selling produce regularly, not less than 41,000 quarts of fresh milk (about 790 quarts weekly), 12,000 pounds of butter (about 230 pounds weekly), 1,800 dozen eggs, and 4,200 pounds of live poultry, fresh beef, and fresh pork were sold during the 12 months ending May 30, 1916. These totals do not include quantities sold by other farmers or by stores and markets.

This contrast in available sources of farm produce is indicated also by the statements of actual purchases by the households in the respective villages, secured in the course of the dietary canvass. These statements have been summarized for households of similar incomes in Table XII. A striking difference is shown in the

TABLE XII   Comparison of availability of certain foods in two cotton-mill villages of South Carolina, as indicated by the proportion of the households with family incomes under the average of the contrasted villages purchasing the specified articles from nearby farms during the period May 16–30, 1916

	Ny.			In.		
		HOUSEHOLDS PURCHASING			HOUSEHOLDS PURCHASING	
Article purchased	Average quantity per household purchasing	Number	Per cent of total households	Average quantity per household purchasing	Number	Per cent of total households
Fresh milk	22.5 qts.	24	51.0	29.3 qts.	3	4.5
Butter	3.4 lbs.	23	49.0	4.0 lbs.	1	1.5
Eggs	2.9 doz.	19	40.5	6.0 doz.	1	1.5
Fresh vegetables	. . . . .	31	66.0	. . . . .	1	1.5
Fresh fruit	. . . . .	8	17.0	. . . . .	0	0.0
Poultry	4.0 lbs.	1	2.1	3.0 lbs.	1	1.5
Any of the above articles	. . . . .	40	83.3	. . . . .	6	9.0
None	. . . . .	8	16.7	. . . . .	61	91.0

extent to which the households in Ny and In relied upon near-by farms for supplies of certain foods.

The difference between Ny and In in availability of food supplies from adjacent farm territory was so pronounced that further inquiries were made into some of the underlying conditions in order to discover, if possible, what other economic factors were responsible for bringing this about. From these inquiries it appeared that at least two conditions were important in causing the difference in availability of the supply of the foods in question: namely (a) differences in the kind of agriculture in the territory adjacent to the villages, and (b) differences in marketing conditions. The two are closely related, but for the sake of clearness it will be advantageous to discuss them separately.

a) Contrast in the kinds of agriculture near the two villages.—A census of the farm products in the agricultural territory adjacent to the two villages was not undertaken, but from observation in the course of several trips and canvasses in the sections in question it was quite clear that a marked contrast existed in the kinds of agriculture pursued. The territory around In was planted principally in cotton, and relatively little diversification in crops existed. Truck farming on any considerable scale was not engaged in. Few beef cattle were raised and milch cows apparently were usually not more than sufficient to supply the household needs of the farmers. Many farmers had no cows or pigs or even poultry. The agriculture in the *In* section seemed rather typical of the cotton areas in South Carolina. Cotton was the predominant crop; all other products were incidental, none of them constituting the principal output of any farm, so far as was observed. The territory around *Ny*, on the other hand, was exceptional for South Carolina in that a considerable amount of diversified farming was carried on, although not fully comparable in this respect with the farming sections in States where one-crop agriculture has not been the rule. Cotton was a relatively less important crop, and beef cattle, swine, poultry, and milch cows seemed much more abundant than in the *In* section. Apparently greater emphasis was given to gardens, and the amount of truck produced was noticeably larger. The physical character of the section apparently was one cause of this difference in products. The land around *In* is almost level, lies well below the foothills of the Blue Ridge Mountains, and is well suited for the growing of cotton. The land around *Ny* is quite rolling and even hilly, being, in fact, in the foothills of the mountains and thus not so well suited to cotton growing. Land not suitable for the cultivation of cotton and, hence, available and used for corn and truck products was consequently far more abundant near *Ny* than near *In*.

b) Contrast in market conditions.—Conditions affecting the market for farm produce from the two sections were quite different in some important respects. The village of *Ny* is itself more isolated than the village of *In* and is not near any important community. The nearest railway station is a mile away and is surrounded by only about a dozen houses, including three small stores. Seneca, the nearest town of any size (population 1,313 in 1910), is some 4 miles from *Ny*, and Greenville, the nearest city (population 15,741 in 1910), is about 40 miles distant. Seneca exports comparatively little produce and hence its market is limited to local needs which are not sufficient to absorb all the miscellaneous farm products of the vicinity. *Ny* is thus a competitor for such produce as the adjacent farm territory affords. The village itself has been in existence without much change in size for about 25 years, and we found that some of the sellers of farm produce had been visiting it regularly for over 10 years. On the other hand, *In* mill village is almost on the outskirts of the town of Inman (population 474 in 1910), which is on the railroad connecting Spartanburg, S.C., with Asheville, N.C. The demands of the Inman market for farm products are far from being confined to securing sufficient supplies for the needs of its townspeople, since several resident buyers purchase the surplus produce of the adjacent territory and ship it to Spartanburg. Since Spartanburg (population 17,517 in 1910) is but 13 miles distant along a good highway, buyers from that city cover the territory around *In* village fairly thoroughly, and farmers having produce to market often take it to the city when they go there to avail themselves of Spartanburg's superior shopping advantages. The position of *In* village appears, therefore, to be distinctly disadvantageous with respect to farm produce since it must compete for this not only with the town of Inman but, more important, also with the city of Spartanburg. So far as could be ascertained in 1916, no regular trade with near-by farms had been established, and, as has been pointed out, such casual trade as existed was only that afforded by occasional visits of hucksters who, after making the rounds in the town of Inman, had unsold remnants of produce.

4) *Home-provided foods.*—Specific inquiries were made of all mill workers' households regarding their possession of cows, poultry, and gardens and, as far as practicable, regarding their importance particularly during the spring of 1916. Different proportions of the households in the two villages were found to have such sources of food supplies.

a) Milch cows.—There was but little difference in the proportion of households in either village owning productive cows during the spring of 1916, the percentage being 17.2 for *Ny* and 23.3 for *In* among households having less than the average income. Such difference as existed in this respect was in favor of *In*. But it should be noted in this connection that 33.3 per cent of the *In* households had no fresh-milk supply at all during the 15-day period for which household supply records were kept, as against only 8 per cent of the *Ny* households (see Table XIV). This difference in distrbbution was caused by the larger proportion of *Ny* households that purchased milk from hucksters, since, as shown in Table XII, 51 per cent of *Ny* households purchased fresh milk from hucksters as against 4.5 per cent of *In* households.

b) Swine.—Slaughtering of hogs is done in autumn and winter. This is a general practice and prevailed in *Ny* as well as in *In*. Home-produced pork did not figure in the spring food supply of mill workers' households in either village, except in the form of cured and salt meat. Of the *Ny* households, 17 per cent slaughtered home-raised hogs as compared with 33.3 per cent of *In* households. All of these households slaughtered their hogs before February 1, 1916, the majority in either village slaughtering before Christmas, 1915. Of the *Ny* households, 11 per cent cured home-slaughtered meat, as compared with 29 per cent of *In* households; but very little of this meat was on hand for use in the late spring. Inquiries of households slaughtering swine revealed the fact that in less than 5 per cent of such households were there any supplies of home-cured pork on hand on May 16, 1916, these being principally salt pork. The home-produced pork, therefore, did not appear to enter in significant degree into the spring food supply of the households in either village.

c) Poultry.—Inquiries of households having less than the average income showed that 40 per cent of the *Ny* households and 25 per cent of the *In* households either did own poultry during the winter and spring months ending May 30, 1916, or were owning poultry at the time of the canvass (from June 1 to June 10, 1916). The average number of poultry consumed per household during the preceding year was 22 in *Ny* and 8 in *In*. The per cent of *Ny* households reporting that they had had radishes, lettuce, or English peas, only about one-third of the *In* households reported that two per cent of *Ny* households reported a fairly regular supply of eggs from home-owned hens as against 21 per cent of *In* households. It appears that the advantage in the supplies of home-produced poultry and eggs during the preceding winter and spring lay distinctly with *Ny* households.

d) Gardens.—Home gardens were much more generally found in the village of *In* than in *Ny*. Nearly 92 per cent of the *In* households had gardens planted on June 1, 1916, as against less than 23 per cent of *Ny* households. The opportunity afforded by suitable garden space was decidedly better in *In* than in *Ny*; practically every home in *In* had a good-sized garden plot, whereas many of the *Ny* households had no suitable space at all.

It was quite evident, however, that home gardens contributed but very slightly, if at all, to the food supply of households in either village during the spring of 1916. With the exception of an occasional ("rare" is perhaps a more accurate term) "mess" or dish of greens, a very little lettuce, and a few young onions, the gardens had yielded no supplies during 1916 up to about June 1. Not until after June 15 did garden produce become abundant, a condition that was somewhat contrary to the expectation of the authors, who had anticipated finding considerably earlier garden production in this section. The principal reason for this tardiness appears to be the fact that gardens in mill villages are usually planted later than gardens elsewhere in this section. Difficulty in getting the ground prepared early enough, owing in part to the fact that the long hours of work in the mill leave no available daylight for gardening until well along in the spring, lack of initiative in making other preparations, and possibly other causes, apparently almost preclude good early spring gardens in most of the mill villages studied, including *Ny* and *In*, although climatic conditions ordinarily are such that gardens can be made to yield supplies of early varieties of vegetables during May and even in April. Aside from a half dozen households reporting that they had had radishes, lettuce, or English peas, only about one-third of the *In* households reported that they had had greens or young onions even occasionally and in small quantities before this date. In *Ny* the proportion was even less.

Summing up the principal differences in availability of food supplies during the spring of 1916 as between *Ny* and *In*, it may be said that 1) supplies of fresh milk, butter, green vegetables, and fresh fruit were available to a greater degree (better distributed among the households) in *Ny* than in *In*, because, in the farm territory adjacent to *Ny*, there was a larger production of these articles of food and because *Ny* occupied a more advantageous location as a market for such products, and 2) that a supply of fresh

meat was available to a greater degree in *Ny* than in *In* because of
the existence of a fresh-meat market in *Ny* all the year around. In
practically all other respects the availability of food supplies appeared to be generally similar in the two villages.

The conditions outlined above are reflected in a comparison of
the total food supplies during the 15-day period May 16–30, 1916,
of households in *Ny* and *In*. In this comparison (Tables XIII and
XIV) in order to eliminate as far as practicable the influence of
differences in economic status, only those households with less
than the average of incomes[20] have been considered.

In Table XIII is shown the average quantity of each article of
food for all the households considered. Inasmuch as an "average"
affords no idea of the vitally important factor of distribution, we
have prepared Table XIV in which are shown the percentages of
the households in each village which had various quantities of
each article of food, such quantities being expressed in terms of
the average for all households in order to shorten the statistical
presentation. The two tables should be considered together in
comparing the supplies of any article of food.

This comparison indicates that during the 15-day period, May
16–30, 1916, 1) supplies of fresh meat, fresh milk, green vegetables, and fresh fruit were more abundant (i.e., better distributed)
in *Ny* than in *In* households; 2) supplies of cured and canned
meats, salt pork, butter, flour, lard, and lard substitutes, and dried
peas and beans in *Ny* households were quite similar to those in *In*
households; and 3) supplies of eggs, corn meal, Irish potatoes, and
most canned goods were more abundant in *In* than in *Ny* households. Other differences in the supplies of articles of food occurring either rarely or in small quantities are indicated.

From the foregoing considerations it clearly appears that the
character of the household food supply in the two villages was
considerably influenced by the availability of certain foods, notably fresh meats, fresh milk, green vegetables, and fresh fruits, all
of which were relatively less abundant or less equally distributed

[20]The average half-month family income per adult male unit for all households
in *Ny* and *In* was $7.90. Hence all households with such incomes under $8 were
considered.

TABLE XIII   Approximate average daily supply of various foods in households of cotton-mill operatives during the 15-day period May 16–30, 1916, compared for the villages of Ny and In, South Carolina

[All households considered have incomes of less than the average of the total households of both villages (less than $8 per adult male unit during the 15-day period).]

Article of food	AVERAGE SUPPLY PER ADULT MALE UNIT IN GRAMS PER DAY		Ratio of supply of In to Ny households
	Ny[a]	In[b]	
Fresh meats	34	7	0.21
Cured lean meats	24	20	.83
Canned meats	19	17	.89
Eggs	34	50	1.47
Fresh milk	426	457	1.07
Preserved milk	1	3	3.00
Butter	26	30	1.15
Cheese	3	([c])	. . . . .
Dried peas and beans	32	25	.78
Canned peas and beans	2	4	2.00
Wheat flour	358	358	1.00
Wheat bread, cakes, and crackers	13	18	1.38
Corn meal	139	180	1.30
Grits	4	2	.50
Canned corn	3	6	2.00
Rice	4	5	1.25
Salt pork	54	53	.98
Lard and lard substitutes	41	40	.98
Green string beans	11	1	.09
Canned string beans	1	4	4.00
Green vegetables	88	46	.52
Canned vegetables	36	36	1.00
Fresh fruits	40	20	.50
Dried fruits	12	8	.67
Canned fruits	10	20	2.00
Irish potatoes	34	60	1.76
Raw sweet potatoes	0	0	. . . . .
Canned sweet potatoes	5	3	.60
Sugar	46	39	.85
Sirup	17	17	1.00
Jellies and jams	3	9	3.00
All other foods (cost in cents)	2	1	.50

[a]48 households composed of 210.3 adult male units. Data were available for the following number of adult male units for the foods specified: Salt pork and dried fruits, 206.2; Irish potatoes, 205.7; wheat flour, 160.2; corn meal, 204.0.
[b]67 households composed of 287.4 adult male units. Data were available for the following number of adult male units for the foods specified: Fresh milk and butter, 257.4.
[c]Less than 0.5 gram.

in In than in Ny. It is clear also that these differences in the food supply of Ny and In households are quite similar to the differences which, as already reported, we found to exist in the food supply of nonpellagrous and of pellagrous households.[21]

We have here, therefore, a striking and significant correspondence between the differences in the availability of certain foods

[21]Goldberger, Wheeler, and Sydenstricker, 1918; also 1920a.

TABLE XIV Percentages of cotton-mill operatives' households having supplies of various articles of food in different quantities per adult male unit per day, compared for the mill villages of Ny and In, South Carolina

[All households considered have incomes of less than the average for the two villages.]

Article of food	Village	Average daily supply per adult male unit	None	Some, but less than one-third of the average of all households	One-third or more, but less than the average of all households	The average or more than the average of all households
		Grams				
Fresh meats	Ny	34	31.2	6.2	16.7	45.8
	In	7	67.2	10.4	13.4	9.0
Cured lean meats	Ny	24	37.5	4.2	27.1	31.2
	In	20	46.3	6.0	14.9	32.8
Canned meats	Ny	19	22.9	10.4	37.5	29.2
	In	17	35.8	3.0	31.3	29.9
Eggs	Ny	34	31.2	4.2	31.2	33.3
	In	59	7.5	6.0	26.9	59.7
Fresh milk	Ny	426	8.3	10.4	45.8	35.4
	In	457	33.3	0.0	30.2	36.5
Preserved milk	Ny	1	87.5	2.1	2.1	8.3
	In	3	73.6	1.5	1.5	22.4
Butter	Ny	26	16.7	10.4	33.3	39.6
	In	30	14.9	16.4	21.4	46.3
Cheese	Ny	3	87.5	2.1	0.0	10.4
	In	(a)	97.0	0.0	0.0	3.0
Dried peas and beans	Ny	32	25.0	14.6	20.8	39.6
	In	25	32.8	7.5	29.9	29.9
Canned peas and beans	Ny	2	83.3	0.0	0.0	16.7
	In	4	85.1	0.0	0.0	14.9
Wheat flour	Ny	358	6.2	0.0	43.7	29.2
	In	358	18.5	3.1	32.3	46.2
Wheat bread, cakes and crackers	Ny	13	18.7	12.5	33.3	35.4
	In	18	25.4	6.0	22.4	46.3
Cornmeal	Ny	139	29.8	4.3	29.8	36.2
	In	180	20.9	0.0	17.9	61.2
Grits	Ny	4	87.5	0.0	0.0	12.5
	In	2	95.6	0.0	0.0	4.5
Rice	Ny	4	75.0	0.0	0.0	25.0
	In	5	70.2	0.0	0.0	29.9
Salt pork	Ny	54	4.3	4.3	57.2	34.0
	In	53	10.4	0.0	41.8	47.8
Lard and lard substitutes	Ny	41	6.2	4.2	52.1	37.5
	In	40	10.4	3.0	37.3	49.3
Green string beans	Ny	11	68.7	0.0	0.0	31.2
	In	1	100.0	0.0	0.0	0.0
Canned string beans	Ny	1	97.9	0.0	0.0	2.1
	In	4	89.5	0.0	0.0	10.5
Green vegetables (bought)	Ny	88	14.6	12.5	39.6	33.3
	In	46	22.7	16.7	37.9	22.7
Other canned vegetables	Ny	36	29.2	2.1	22.9	45.8
	In	36	26.9	7.5	28.4	37.3
Fresh fruits	Ny	40	25.0	10.4	20.8	43.7
	In	20	43.9	9.1	28.8	18.2
Dried fruits	Ny	12	53.2	0.0	17.0	29.8
	In	8	70.2	1.5	6.0	22.4
Canned fruits	Ny	10	66.7	0.0	2.1	31.2
	In	20	56.7	0.0	1.5	41.8
Irish potatoes	Ny	34	45.8	4.2	20.8	29.2
	In	60	53.7	3.0	3.0	40.3
Fresh sweet potatoes	Ny	0	0.0	0.0	0.0	0.0
	In	0	0.0	0.0	0.0	0.0
Canned sweet potatoes	Ny	5	81.2	0.0	0.0	18.7
	In	3	88.1	0.0	0.0	11.9
Sugar	Ny	46	10.4	4.2	45.8	39.6
	In	39	9.0	9.0	43.3	38.8
Sirup	Ny	17	68.7	0.0	2.1	29.2
	In	17	64.2	0.0	0.0	35.8
Jellies and jams	Ny	3	70.2	0.0	4.3	25.5
	In	9	40.3	1.5	0.0	58.2

a Less than 0.5 gram.

(and thus, it is permissible to assume, in the character of the diet) in the two villages, on the one hand, and the difference with respect to the incidence of pellagra among their households on the other. Since between these two villages no other differences to which significance could properly be attached were disclosed by our study, the conclusion would seem to be warranted that the difference in the availability of food supplies above summarized was the outstanding determining factor in relation to the marked difference in the incidence of the disease.

Thus, of all the factors we have studied in relation to differences in pellagra incidence among our villages, the factor of food availability is the only one in connection with which significant evidence of such relationship was found. The conclusion would, therefore, seem to be warranted that in this factor we have the explanation for the differences among the villages studied in the incidence of the disease, so far as this incidence was a reflection of community conditions.[22]

IV. Discussion

From the data presented in the foregoing pages it is evident that a variety of factors of an economic nature, through their effect on the character of the household diet, had an important influence on the incidence of pellagra in the communities studied. Among

[22] If such factor as food availability operated to effect the rate of pellagra incidence in our villages, then it may be reasonably expected that in the locality with exceptionally unfavorable conditions of food availability, family income would be less efficient as a protective factor than in other similar localities with better conditions of food availability. With a view of testing this we prepared the following table, in which the pellagra incidence rate for each of our income classes of *In* village in which, we believed food availability conditions were least favorable, is compared with that of a group of five villages in which conditions in respect to food availability are believed to have been better. It may be seen that (1) the incidence rate in those income groups in which a significant number of cases occurred was decidedly higher in *In* village; and (2) that the curve of incidence shows a highly suggestive tendency to extend to a higher plane of income in *In* village than in the group of five villages. The indications thus afforded would,

these factors family income and food availability stand out most conspicuously.

As has been seen, the data presented reveal a very marked inverse correlation between family income and the incidence of the disease. When it is recalled that the range of income enjoyed by our families was small (see pp. 275, 278), that the amount of income of even the highest of our income classes was actually quite low (but few had annual incomes of over $1,000), the reduction of incidence to the point of practical disappearance of the disease in this income class is all the more striking and significant. It would seem quite impressively to indicate that the occasional occurrence of the disease in well-to-do individuals must be regarded as a relatively quite exceptional occurrence, and that the explanation of such occurrence must be sought in circumstances of a special or exceptional character.

Cases in the well-to-do, instances of which have been observed repeatedly since the time of Strambio (1796), are of more than ordinary interest because of the perplexity and confusion to which they tend to give rise with respect to the etiology of the disease. Favorable economic status of the individual tends to create the presumption that diet can have little or no etiological significance, since there can be no question of the ability of such

---

therefore, appear to be consistent with and to bear out the assumption which the table was prepared to test.

Pellagra incidence according to family income in In mill village compared with that in a group of five[a] other mill villages of South Carolina during 1916

[Rate per 1,000 of population classified according to a half-month's family income per adult male unit in May or June, 1916. Only definite cases of pellagra with onset after a residence of not less than 30 days in specified village or in a member of group considered.]

Income group	NUMBER OF PERSONS		NUMBER OF PELLAGRINS		RATE PER 1,000 OF POPULATION	
	In	Five other villages	In	Five other villages	In	Five other villages
All incomes	651	2,785	43	53	66	10
Under $6	266	856	27	29	102	34
$6–$7.99	167	730	10	15	60	21
$8–$9.99	118	506	5	6	42	12
$10–$13.99	74	499	1	2	14	4
$14 and over	26	194	0	1	0	5

[a]Village Ny not considered, no pellagra, as above restricted, having occurred in 1916.

individual to provide himself with a liberal diet. Natural as this presumption may be under the circumstances, it nevertheless involves danger of serious error. This results from the implied assumptions that because of financial ability, not only was a satisfactory diet available, but that such was also consumed. Even granting what is not necessarily the case, that financial ability to provide may be assumed to be invariably synonymous with the actual provision of a good diet[23] and that a liberal diet was actually available to the individual, it by no means follows that such diet was in fact consumed. For such assumption would totally ignore the existence of individual likes and dislikes, more or less marked examples of which may be observed at almost any family table.

A great variety of causes may operate to bring about individual peculiarities of taste with respect to food. They may have their origin in the seemingly inherent human prejudice against the new and untried food or dish; they may date from some disagreeable experience associated with a particular food; they may arise as the result of ill-advised, self-imposed, or professionally directed dietary restrictions in the treatment of digestive disturbances, kidney disease, etc.; they may originate as a fad; and in the insane they may arise because of some delusion such as the fear of poisoning, etc.

The individual peculiarities of taste which may thus arise have a significance in relation to pellagra that has been but little appreciated until recently (Goldberger, 1914 and 1916). In much the greater proportion of a moderate number of cases in well-to-do individuals with a good diet presumably available, coming under our observation, a significant eccentricity in diet could readily be determined (unpublished observations). Vedder (1916, pp. 157–160) and Roberts (1920) have reported observations of a similar character. It is of interest to note also that analogous facts

[23]In this connection the following from Roussel (1866, pp. 430–431) is of interest: "Almost all the individual histories, found in the literature of pellagra in the well-to-do, are remarkable because of this constant fact * * * namely, that because of some misfortune or by reason of some unwholesome trait (mauvaises habitudes), such as avarice, these well-to-do or wealthy pellagrins subsisted exactly as did the poor pellagrins about them."

have been recorded in connection with beriberi (see Vedder, 1913, pp. 154, 156, 171, 180, 184). Therefore, in seeking to explain cases of pellagra in individuals believed to have a good diet available, this factor must be given due consideration.

With conditions (including labor supply) in the cotton-milling industry substantially stable, family income may, in general, be expected to fluctuate but little from year to year. With conditions unsettled, family income may either fall or rise very considerably; a depression, accompanied by increasing unemployment and, possibly, reductions in wage rates will be reflected in a reduced family income, while industrial prosperity, with a diminution of unemployment and, possibly, increased wage rates, will be reflected in larger family income. In the former event we may have a diminution in family income to the point of inability to provide the family with a proper diet, with a consequent danger of the development of pellagra and thus with a more or less marked rise in the incidence rate of the disease. In the latter event we have the opposite effects, with a tendency to a reduction in or practical disappearance of the disease. In this we have, we believe, an illustration of the manner of operation of one of the most powerful factors in relation to the endemic and epidemic prevalence of the disease. Through its effect on diet, economic status is also an important element in, if not the entire explanation of, the oft repeated observation of the occurrence of a marked increase in the incidence or the development of an epidemic of the disease following on crop failure[24] (Weiss, 1914, p. 327) or other cause of "hard times," as was actually observed in the United States in 1915, following depression consequent on the outbreak of the World War in 1914, and as there is some reason to fear may again be observed in the spring of 1921 if the present depression, especially in the price of cotton and cotton-textile manufacturing, continues.

At this juncture it may be well to point out that family income should always be considered in connection with living (food) costs if confusion and error are to be avoided. It is the purchasing

[24]It should not be forgotten that overproduction, by glutting the market, may affect family income (of the farmer) as disastrously as may crop failure.

power of family income that is significant and not necessarily its absolute amount.

Although economic status (as typified by family income) is, ordinarily, perhaps the most important factor (particularly in industrial communities) in relation to fluctuation of incidence of pellagra in different years,[25] marked changes in food availability conceivably play a similar role (particularly in agricultural communities). The reported occurrence, in some localities, of a sharp increase in the prevalence of the disease following an epizootic among swine or cattle (Niederman, Konrad, and Farkas, 1898) or after the loss of these through floods, we believe, is to be explained, in part, at least, in this manner.

The very great importance of food availability in relation to pellagra prevalence seems heretofore not to have been very clearly recognized. Under some circumstances, as we have shown, this factor may operate notably to affect the character of the diet and thus the incidence of the disease. Our data dealt with differences in availability between localities of relatively small area, but it is readily conceivable that analogous differences may exist between areas of great extent such as there is reason to believe actually is the case between the northern and southern parts of the United States. This difference is probably an important factor (together with the well-known difference in dietary habit, Sydenstricker, 1915) in the notable inequality in the incidence of the disease in these two sections of the country.

The results of the present study clearly suggest fundamental lines along which efforts looking to the eradication of the disease should be directed, namely, 1) economic, by improvement of economic status (income), and 2) food availability, by improvement in availability of food supplies.

Measures for improving the economic status of those people most subject to the disease, are in the main, outside of the sanitarian's sphere and but little subject to his influence. While much the same may be said to apply to the conditions of food availability, this field is more easily accessible, both directly and

[25]We hope to consider the relation of economic status to the course of the disease from year to year in a separate paper.

indirectly, to his activities and influence. Thus, for instance, by avoiding ill-considered regulations governing milk production he can, negatively at least, favor an adequate supply of this invaluable food. Furthermore, he can and should aid in improving the conditions of food availability by lending his powerful influence in support of and, by cooperating with, the agencies at work in this field, in their efforts to stimulate milk production (particularly through cow ownership) and to induce the farmer to adopt a suitable system of crop diversification.

And in this connection it may perhaps be remarked that certain preliminary observations have created in our minds a rather strong suspicion that the single-crop system as practiced in at least some parts of our southern States, by reason of apparently unfavorable conditions of food supply and of other conditions of an economic character bound up therein, will be found indirectly responsible for much of the pellagra morbidity and mortality with which local agricultural labor is annually afflicted.

Although considerable study will be required to determine definitely the factors responsible for the high incidence of the disease in the rural areas in question, it would, nevertheless, seem to be the part of wisdom to make an earnest effort to improve conditions in the ways suggested above.

V. Summary and Conclusions

1. In the present paper are reported the results of the part of the pellagra study of cotton-mill villages, during 1916, dealing with the relation of conditions of an economic nature to the incidence of pellagra. It is the first reported study in which the degree of the long-recognized association between poverty and pellagra incidence is measured in a definite, purely objective manner.

2. The study was made among the white mill operatives' households in seven typical cotton-mill villages of South Carolina. Pellagra incidence was determined by a systematic, biweekly, house-to-house canvass and search for cases, only active cases being considered. Information relating to household

food supply, family income, etc., was secured by enumerators for a sample section of the period April 16 to June 15, assumed to be representative of the season during which the factors favoring the production of pellagra were assumed to be most effective.

3. Family income was made the basis of classification according to economic status, the Atwater scale for food requirements being used for computing the size of families in comparing their incomes.

4. In general, pellagra incidence was found to vary inversely according to family income. As the income fell, the incidence of the disease rose and showed an increasing tendency to affect members of the same family; as the income rose, incidence fell, being reduced almost to the point of practical disappearance in the highest of our income classes, although the income enjoyed by this class was comparatively quite low.

5. The inverse correlation between pellagra incidence and family income depended on the unfavorable effect of low income on the character of the diet; but family income was not the sole factor determining the character of the household diet.

6. Differences in incidence among households of the same income class are attributable to the operation of such factors as tend to determine the amount and proportion of family income available for the purchase of food, the intelligence and ability of the housewife in utilizing the available family income, and to the differences among households with respect to availability of food supplies from such sources as home-owned cows, poultry, gardens, etc.

7. Differences in incidence among villages whose constituent households are economically similar, are attributable to differences among them in availability of food supplies resulting from differences (a) in the character of the local markets, (b) in the produce from adjacent farm territory, and (c) in marketing conditions.

8. The most potent factors influencing pellagra incidence in the villages studied were (a) low family income, and (b) unfavorable conditions regarding the availability of food supplies, suggesting that under the conditions obtaining in some of these villages

in the spring of 1916 many families were without sufficient income to enable them to procure an adequate diet, and that improvement in food availability (particularly milk and fresh meat) is urgently needed in such localities.

Acknowledgments

We desire to express our grateful appreciation of the valuable cooperation accorded us by the medical practitioners, mill officials, and families of the mill operatives in the locations studied. We are indebted also to Statistician W. I. King, United States Public Health Service, for helpful criticisms and suggestions and assistance in the preparation of some of the tables.

VI. References

1915. Atwater, W. O., Principles of Nutrition and Nutritive Value of Food: U.S. Dept. of Agric., Farmers' Bull. No. 1042, 1915, p. 33.

1903. V. Babes, Ueber Pellagra in Rumanien: Wien Med. Presse, 1903, vol. 44, pp. 1184, 1239.

1890. Berger, L., Pellagra: Wiener Klinik Wien, 1890, vol. 16, pp. 161–179.

1919. Boyd and Lelean, Report of a Committee of Enquiry Regarding the Prevalence of Pellagra Among Turkish Prisoners of War. Alexandria, Egypt, 1919. Also Jour. Roy. Army Med. Corps, 1919, vol. 33, p. 426 et al.

1870. Calmarza, J. B., Memoria sobre La Pelagra, Madrid, 1870.

1870. Casal, Obra Postuma del Dr. Casal Publicada en 1762: Corresp. Med., Madrid, 1870, vol. 5, p. 78.

1910. Gaumer, Geo. F., Pellagra in Yucatan: Trans. Nat'l. Conf. on Pellagra, Columbia, S.C., 1910, pp. 101–107.

1914. Goldberger, Jos., The Cause and Prevention of Pellagra: Pub. Health Reports, Washington, D.C., Sept. 11, 1914, vol. 29, pp. 2351–2357. Also Reprint No. 218 from Pub. Health Reports.

1916. ——, Pellagra—Causation and a Method of Prevention: Jour. Am. Med. Assn. Feb. 12, 1916, vol. 66, pp. 471–476.

1918. Goldberger, Wheeler, and Sydenstricker, A Study of the Diet of Nonpellagrous and of Pellagrous Households, etc.: Jour. Am. Med. Assn., Sept. 21, 1918, vol. 71, p. 944–949.

1920a. ——, ——, and ——, A Study of the Relation of Diet to Pellagra Incidence in Seven Textile-Mill Communities of South Carolina in 1916: Pub. Health Reports, Washington, D.C., Mar. 19, 1920, vol. 35, pp. 648–713.

1920b. ——, ——, and ——, Pellagra Incidence in Relation to Sex, Age, Season, Occupation, and "Disabling Sickness" in Seven Cotton-Mill Villages of South Carolina during 1916: Pub. Health Reports, Washington, D.C., July 9, 1920, vol. 35, pp. 1650–1664.

1920c. ——, ——, and ——, A Study of the Relation of Factors of a Sanitary Character to Pellagra Incidence in Seven Cotton-Mill Villages of South Carolina in 1916: Pub. Health Reports, Washington, D.C., July 16, 1920, vol. 35, pp. 1701–1714.

1829. Hameau, Note sur une maladie peu connue observée dans les environs de la teste (Gironde): Jour. de Med. Prat. (etc.) de la Soc. Roy. de Med. de Bordeaux, 1829, vol. 1, pp. 310–314.

1820. Holland, Henry, On the Pellagra, A Disease Prevailing in Lombardy: Med. Chir. Trans., London, 1820, vol. 8, pp. 313–346.

1903. Huertas, F., La Pelagra en España: Arch Latin. de Med. y de Biol., Madrid, Oct. 20, 1903, vol. 1, pp. 9–15.

1917. Jobling and Peterson, The Epidemiology of Pellagra in Nashville, Tennesee, II: Jour. Infec. Dis., August, 1917, vol. 21, pp. 109–131.

1846. Lalesque, Actes de l'Acad. Roy d. Sc. (etc.) de Bordeaux, 1846, p. 421.

1907. Manning, C. J., Report on Certain Cases of Psilosis Pigmentosa Which Have Recently Occurred at the Lunatic Asylum. Barbadoes, 1907.

1898. Niederman, Konrad, and Farkas, A Report on Pellagra in Transylvania (abstract), Lancet, London, July 16, 1898, vol. 2, p. 164.

1899. Von Probizer, Die Pellagra: Die Heilkunde, Wien, December, 1899, vol. 4, pp. 139–142.

1920. Roberts, S. R., Types and Treatment of Pellagra: Jour. Amer. Med. Assn., July 3, 1920, vol. 75, pp. 21–25.

1894. V. Rosen, H., Ueber die Pellagra in Russland, Petersburg, Med. Wchnschrft. 1894, n. F. Vol. 11, pp. 21–23.

1845. Roussel, Th., La Pellagre, Paris, 1845.

1866. ——, Traité de la Pellagre, etc., Paris, 1866.

1903. Sandwith, F. M., How to Prevent the Spread of Pellagra in Egypt: Lancet, London, March 14, 1903, vol. 1, p. 723.

1913. Siler and Garrison, An Intensive Study of the Epidemiology of Pellagra: Am. J. Med. Sc., Philadelphia, July and August, 1913, vol. 146.

1909. Sofer, T., Die Pellagra in Oesterreich und ihre Bekampfung als Volkskrankheit: Therap. Monatshefte, April, 1909, vol. 23, pp. 216, 219.

1796. Strambio, G., Abhandlungen ueber das Pellagra, Leipzig, 1796.

1915. Sydenstricker, Edgar, The Prevalence of Pellagra—Its Possible Relation to the Rise in the Cost of Food: Pub. Health Reports, Washington, D.C., October 22, 1915. Also Reprint No. 308 from Pub. Health Reports.

1919. Sydenstricker, Wheeler, and Goldberger, Disabling Sickness Among the Population of Seven Cotton-Mill Villages of South Carolina in Relation to Family Income: Pub. Health Reports, Washington, D.C., November 22, 1918, vol. 33, pp. 2038–2051.

1913. Vedder, E. B., Beriberi, New York, 1913.
1916. ——, Dietary Deficiency as the Etiological Factor in Pellagra: Arch. Int. Med., August, 1916, vol. 18, pp. 137–172.
1914. Weiss, Ettore, Die Pellagrä in Südtirol und Die staatliche Bekämpfungsaktion. Das Osterreichische Sanitätswesen, Wien, May 7, 1914, vol. 26, pp. 309–331.
1919. White, R. G., Report on an Outbreak of Pellagra Among Armenian Refugees at Port Said, 1916–1917. Cairo, Egypt, 1919.

2

The Incidence of Influenza
Among Persons of
Different Economic Status
During the Epidemic of 1918[1]

EDGAR SYDENSTRICKER

Perhaps no observation during the great influenza epidemic of 1918–1919 was more common than the familiar comment that "the flu hit the rich and the poor alike." Apparently there was ample ground for a belief in the impartiality of the disease. Its widespread prevalence throughout the country, the frequency with which households in every social class were attacked, and the fact that prominent persons in every community were struck down, were among the outstanding, undeniable experiences in the epidemic. A certain consolation seemed to be afforded by the

[1]From the office of statistical investigation, United States Public Health Service. Acknowledgment is made to Miss Mary H. Louden, under whose immediate supervision the tabulations presented in this paper were made.

The data used in this paper were collected by special surveys of influenza in a number of localities by the United States Public Health Service under the general direction of Surg. W. H. Frost and the writer. Partial presentation of the results of these surveys have already been made in the Public Health Reports, as follows:

Influenza in Maryland: Preliminary Statistics for Certain Localities, by W. H. Frost and Edgar Sydenstricker. Public Health Reports, vol. 34, No. 11, Mar. 14, 1919.

The Epidemiology of Influenza, by W. H. Frost. Journal Am. Med. Association, vol. 73, No. 5, Aug. 2, 1919. Reprinted in Public Health Reports, vol. 34, No. 33, Aug. 15, 1919.

Statistics of Influenza Morbidity, with special reference to certain factors in case incidence and case fatality, by W. H. Frost. Public Health Reports, vol. 35, No. 11, Mar. 12, 1920.

thought that the pestilence was democratic, even in so dreadful a sense, in its behavior.

Like many conclusions based on general impressions, this observation was true only in part. Epidemic influenza undoubtedly was very prevalent among all classes of persons and its mortality toll was levied from the wealthy as well as from the poor. But when the generalization was subjected to the closer analysis afforded by actual records of influenza incidence in 1918 in enumerated populations, the interesting indication appeared that there were marked and consistent differences in its incidence—with respect both to morbidity and to mortality— among persons of different economic status. An association between the incidence of epidemic influenza and economic condition was manifested. Apparently the lower the economic level the higher was the attack rate. This relationship was found to persist even after allowance had been made for the influence of the factors of color, sex, and age, and certain other conditions.

Character of the Data

The scope and method of the special influenza surveys by the Public Health Service have been discussed in previous publications, but so far as they relate to the particular series of data presented here, a brief explanation may be made.

The surveys were made in 10 cities ranging in population from 20,000 to 500,000 and in several smaller cities and rural areas in Maryland. The data here presented are only for nine urban localities with a population of 25,000 and over, and relate to slightly over 100,000 individuals. The information was collected by intelligent enumerators working under careful supervision and with detailed instructions. In each locality a house-to-house canvass was made of not less than 10 areas which were selected in such a way as to include fairly representative samples of different parts of the locality as well as of different classes of the population. The size of the sample populations canvassed in each locality is shown in the detailed tables presented in this report.

Regarding each individual in the population canvassed the enumerators recorded the name, color, sex, and age at last birthday; and whether sick or not sick since September 1, 1918, from influenza, pneumonia, or indefinitely diagnosed illness suspected to be influenza.

Regarding each case of sickness, the facts recorded were the nature of the illness (i.e., whether influenza, pneumonia, or "doubtful"), date of onset, duration, and date of death, if death occurred. The statement of the informant as to the occurrence of sickness was accepted, although the informant was questioned as to what diagnosis the attending physician had made, if a physician was in attendance. While three "types" of sickness were recorded, namely "influenza," "pneumonia," and "doubtful," various analyses of the data strongly suggest that cases recorded as any of the three types properly can be considered, for practical purposes, as epidemic influenza. For example, the chronological curve of "doubtful" cases was very similar to the curves for "influenza" and "pneumonia."

Regarding each household, the enumerators recorded the number of rooms occupied by the household and the economic status of the family. The actual economic classification was made by the enumerators themselves. Each enumerator was instructed to record at the time of her visit to the household her impression of its economic condition in one of four categories—"well-to-do," "moderate," "poor," "very poor." The enumerators were local persons of average intelligence and education. They were purposely given no standards for comparison or more detailed instructions on this point, the intention being to have them record their own impressions naturally and according to their own standards. It was believed also that if not less than four possible categories were allowed them in which to place the families visited, the families classified in the two extremes would permit sufficient contrast.

The results appear to justify the soundness of these assumptions. The distribution of the populations in the various economic classes suggested by the terms employed, the differences in the distribution according to age of persons within each economic class, the distinct and fairly regular differences in influenza incidence among the several classes, as well as other internal evidences, suggest that although the method was crude, a classification was made that was sufficiently accurate for finding out whether or not a differential incidence did occur.

Influenza Incidence Among Persons of Different Economic Status

Morbidity.—A somewhat detailed tabulation showing the number of persons, the number of cases, and the rates in each economic class, subdivided according to broad age groupings, is given in Table I.

Since the morbidity rate from influenza varies among persons of different sexes and ages, and since the distribution of persons according to sex and age varies in the different economic classes, it is necessary to make allowance for the influence of these factors in comparing the morbidity rates for the several economic classes. The factor of sex was found in trial tabulations to be so inconsiderable that adjustments for sex were regarded as an unnecessary

TABLE I Incidence of epidemic influenza in 1918 among white persons of different ages classified according to the general economic condition of the households surveyed in nine localities

Age group	RATE PER 1,000				NUMBER OF PERSONS CANVASSED				NUMBER OF INFLUENZA CASES			
	Well-to-do	Mod-erate	Poor	Very poor	Well-to-do	Mod-erate	Poor	Very poor	Well-to-do	Mod-erate	Poor	Very poor
ALL LOCALITIES												
All ages	232	264	330	372	9,550	55,784	25,356	3,988	2,211	14,751	8,376	1,486
Under 15 years	308	330	374	408	2,129	14,862	9,291	1,695	656	4,910	3,474	692
15–24	297	297	335	374	1,494	9,704	4,412	672	443	2,878	1,480	251
25–44	248	277	347	370	3,244	19,153	7,388	1,060	804	5,303	2,565	392
45 and over	115	138	201	269	2,683	12,065	4,265	561	308	1,660	857	151
NEW LONDON, CONN.												
All ages	170	164	280	257	271	4,727	2,442	175	46	776	562	45
Under 15 years	229	186	228	211	48	1,033	975	95	11	196	222	20
15–24	167	183	220	250	30	875	400	20	5	160	88	5
25–44	239	185	270	370	92	1,576	725	46	22	291	196	17
45 and over	79	105	164	214	101	1,223	342	14	8	129	56	3

TABLE I Incidence of epidemic influenza in 1918 among white persons of different ages classified according to the general economic condition of the households surveyed in nine localities—*Continued*

Age group	RATE PER 1,000				NUMBER OF PERSONS CANVASSED				NUMBER OF INFLUENZA CASES			
	Well-to-do	Moderate	Poor	Very poor	Well-to-do	Moderate	Poor	Very poor	Well-to-do	Moderate	Poor	Very poor
BALTIMORE, MD.												
All ages	187	252	312	379	2,786	14,585	8,612	1,400	520	3,670	2,685	530
Under 15 years	285	323	364	422	509	3,765	3,003	602	145	1,215	1,093	254
15–24	261	300	318	347	417	2,528	1,594	239	109	757	506	83
25–44	195	265	332	389	912	4,823	2,456	342	178	1,278	816	133
45 and over	93	121	173	276	948	3,469	1,559	217	88	420	270	60
AUGUSTA, GA.												
All ages	335	404	524	343	358	633	1,203	35	120	256	630	12
Under 15 years	432	476	623	273	118	185	390	11	51	88	243	3
15–24	257	436	504	500	70	110	230	4	18	48	116	2
25–44	374	429	505	445	91	212	327	9	34	91	165	4
45 and over	215	230	414	273	79	126	256	11	17	29	106	3
MACON, GA.												
All ages	222	195	270	301	1,023	2,998	1,142	614	229	584	309	185
Under 15 years	311	263	316	303	264	699	395	221	82	184	125	67
15–24	250	192	266	310	148	667	244	126	37	128	65	39
25–44	234	202	266	307	384	1,046	319	176	90	211	85	54
45 and over	88	104	185	275	227	586	184	91	20	61	34	25
DES MOINES, IOWA												
All ages	204	238	262	279	505	3,801	907	165	103	904	238	46
Under 15 years	294	312	270	352	102	1,091	356	54	30	340	96	19
15–24	257	217	326	242	70	632	135	33	18	137	44	8
25–44	252	252	262	245	155	1,227	244	49	39	309	64	12
45 and over	90	139	198	241	178	851	172	29	16	118	34	7
LOUISVILLE, KY.												
All ages	81	157	217	380	726	6,519	2,106	376	59	1,026	456	143
Under 15 years	128	236	272	422	148	1,738	817	187	19	411	222	79
15–24	97	158	193	450	113	1,085	353	60	11	171	68	27
25–44	94	148	223	313	223	2,162	583	83	21	320	130	26
45 and over	33	81	102	239	242	1,534	353	46	8	124	36	11
LITTLE ROCK, ARK.												
All ages	291	356	435	427	574	4,939	1,254	89	167	1,756	545	38
Under 15 years	419	421	508	500	117	1,460	488	42	49	615	248	21
15–24	310	368	465	286	100	832	200	14	31	306	93	4
25–44	295	360	419	458	224	1,873	403	24	66	674	169	11
45 and over	158	208	215	222	133	774	163	9	21	161	35	2
SAN ANTONIO, TEX.												
All ages	500	532	571	605	1,217	6,677	3,160	466	609	3,553	1,805	282
Under 15 years	511	575	614	655	311	2,042	1,248	200	159	1,175	766	131
15–24	623	602	593	687	257	1,283	550	83	160	772	326	57
25–44	516	557	581	548	397	2,240	937	126	205	1,247	544	69
45 and over	337	323	398	439	252	1,112	425	57	85	359	169	25
SAN FRANCISCO, CALIF.												
All ages	171	204	253	307	2,090	10,905	4,530	668	358	2,226	1,146	205
Under 15 years	215	242	284	346	512	2,829	1,619	283	110	686	459	98
15–24	187	236	246	280	289	1,692	706	93	54	399	174	26
25–44	195	221	284	322	766	3,994	1,394	205	149	882	396	66
45 and over	86	108	144	172	523	2,390	811	87	45	259	117	15

TABLE II   1918 Influenza morbidity rate (adjusted for age)[1] per 1,000 white persons of different economic status in nine localities in which special surveys were made

ECONOMIC STATUS OF HOUSEHOLD

Locality	Well-to-do	Moderate	Poor	Very poor
All localities	252	272	326	364
New London	192	170	227	266
Baltimore	218	263	309	370
Augusta	339	408	526	[2]
Macon	234	201	267	300
Des Moines	236	243	265	278
Louisville	94	166	210	361
Little Rock	312	352	418	[2]
San Antonio	502	527	559	589
San Francisco	179	209	250	293

[1]The "standard population" used was the total population of the United States in 1910.   [2]Insufficient data.

refinement. The factor of age, however, was more important.[1] Therefore in the table presented below the rates for the various economic classes were adjusted to a standard age distribution, that of the continental United States in 1910 being used.

While the number of persons classified as "very poor" and as "well-to-do"—the two extremes of the economic scale—are relatively small, the relationship between economic status and influenza incidence is fairly regular, not only for the nine localities taken together, but for each of the localities. The ratio of the rate for the "very poor" to that for the "well-to-do" is 1.3 to 1.0 for the nine localities as a group, but it varies considerably in the different localities. The nature of the data did not permit of analyses in sufficient detail to suggest the reasons for this variation.

Mortality.—The same relation is shown when the mortality rates from influenza and pneumonia (all forms) are compared for

[1]In the following tabulation is shown the distribution of persons in each economic class according to broad age groups.

TABLE IIA   Distribution of the white population included in special surveys of the 1918 influenza epidemic according to age for each of the general economic classes

PERCENTAGE IN SPECIFIED GROUPS

Economic status of household	All ages	Under 15 years	15–24 years	25–44 years	45 years and over
All classes	100.0	29.6	17.2	32.6	20.7
Well-to-do	100.0	22.3	15.7	34.0	28.1
Moderate	100.0	26.6	17.4	34.3	21.6
Poor	100.0	36.6	17.4	29.1	16.8
Very poor	100.0	42.5	16.9	26.6	14.1

It will be noted that the proportion of the population in the younger age groups regularly increases as we descend in the economic scale, and vice versa. The dif-ferences in morbidity rates among persons of different ages in the several economic classes is discussed later.

persons in the different economic classes. After making allowance
for differences in the age distribution, it was found that the death
rate was the same in the two highest classes, was over 33 per cent
greater in the class denoted as "poor," and was nearly three times
as high among persons classified as "very poor." The rates are
shown in the following table:

TABLE III   Mortality from influenza and
pneumonia during the epidemic of 1918
among white persons included in surveys
made in nine localities classified according
to the general economic condition
of the household

Economic status of household	Rate per 1,000 persons (adjusted for age)[1]
Well-to-do	3.8
Moderate	3.8
Poor	5.2
Very poor	10.0

[1]The "standard population" used was the total population
of the United States in 1910.

That the higher mortality in the economically less favored
classes was not due entirely to a higher incidence, but that the
fatality of cases among "poor" and "very poor" persons was higher
than among the "well-to-do" and those in "moderate" circumstances was clearly shown when the case fatality rate, after making
allowances for differences in age distribution, was computed for
each economic class. This is exhibited in the following table:

TABLE IV   Case fatality of influenza in
the epidemic of 1918 among white persons
included in surveys made in nine localities
classified according to the general
economic condition of the household

Economic status of household	Rate per 100 cases (adjusted for age)[1]
Well-to-do	1.5
Moderate	1.5
Poor	1.7
Very poor	2.8

[1]The "standard population" used was the total
population of the United States in 1910.

It will be noted that the case fatality rate was nearly twice as great among the "very poor" as among the "well-to-do" and those classified as in "moderate" circumstances.

The Effects of Certain Specific Conditions

What specific conditions included under the term "economic status" were responsible for these differences in influenza incidence?

The discovery of an association of relatively high influenza incidence with poor economic condition does not, by any means, invest poor economic condition with causal significance. It points to the probability that the incidence of the disease is influenced by one or more of the many factors that are themselves bound up, causally or otherwise, with the economic status of a population. Whether or not an inheritance of feeble resistance to influenza or to secondary complicating infections goes with incapacity to earn a good living; what effects upon resistance to the disease a continued unfavorable environment may have; what increase in the chance for infection is brought about by the conditions under which members of the poorer households work and live; what differences in the medical and other care of patients in the poorer and richer households may have prevailed and the effect of such differences upon the fatality of the disease—these are only some of the questions which the existence of a statistical correlation does not specifically answer. The correlation merely suggests that some of these conditions may have a bearing on the question.

The specific conditions that may be involved probably are not only numerous but are so intertwined that even a very intensive investigation of a very much larger exposure could give only partial and incomplete answers to the epidemiological questions that present themselves. The present study, therefore, can not be considered as carrying our inquiry much further than the rough determinations presented above. On one or two points, however, some rather definite evidence is given, and suggestive evidence is afforded on other points.

TABLE V   Proportion of total households in which one or more persons were attacked by influenza during the epidemic of 1918 in selected areas in nine localities in which special surveys were made

Locality	PER CENT OF TOTAL HOUSEHOLDS AFFECTED WITH INFLUENZA FOR EACH ECONOMIC CLASS[1]			
	Well-to-do	Moderate	Poor	Very poor
New London	43	37	41	59
Baltimore	42	48	54	61
Augusta	46	63	70	72
Macon	41	39	42	56
Des Moines	52	46	47	43
Louisville	21	30	39	51
Little Rock	50	57	59	77
San Antonio	96	99	95	94
San Francisco	36	41	44	46

[1]Adjusted to a standard distribution of households according to size. Adjustment for sex and age indicated that differences in sex and age composition of households did not affect the rates materially.

1. A comparison of the proportion of households in which at least one case of influenza occurred, for the different economic classes, shows that the *introduction* of the disease tended to be relatively more frequent in the poorer than in the richer households.

In making this comparison, obviously it is necessary to make allowance for the possible influence of (a) differences among the various economic classes in the sex and age composition of members of the households, and (b) differences among the various economic classes in the size of the households. It was found that differences in sex and age of members of the household affected the morbidity rates only slightly while differences in the size of the households appreciably affected the result in some instances. Accordingly, for each locality the percentages of households attacked were weighted according to a standard size distribution of households. The resulting attack rates per 100 households are shown in Table V.

Although the rates do not always vary greatly and some of the groups do not comprise large populations, the indication is fairly consistent in seven of the nine localities.[1] Obviously, if an association existed between the incidence of influenza and economic

[1]One of the two localities for which this indication does not appear was San Antonio, in which practically all (98 per cent) of the households were attacked. The other was Des Moines; I am unable to suggest any explanation from the data for this exception.

status, some effect of this association in the selection of house-holds by the disease might be expected, other things being equal. But to what extent this selection was due to greater opportunity for infection, or reflects less resistance to infection on the part of persons composing the poorer households, or is the result of other factors, are also questions that can not be answered definitely by our data.

2. On the other hand, a much more marked correlation is evident between economic status and influenza incidence in households after the disease had been introduced, as the follow-ing table shows:

TABLE VI   Influenza attack rate during the 1918 epidemic in white households of different economic status[1] in Baltimore

Economic status	Attack rate per 1,000 persons in households in which one or more cases occurred
All classes	475
Well-to-do	390
Moderate	455
Poor	506
Very poor	577

[1]The rates for the different economic classes have been ad-justed to a standard age distribution, the "standard population" used being the total population of the United States in 1910.

Here it is seen that in affected households, comparable from the points of view of size and sex and age composition, the in-fluenza attack rate manifests an association with economic status similar to that already shown by the influenza morbidity rate among persons constituting the entire population of each economic class. The ratio of the attack rates in affected households to the total morbidity rates in the various economic classes man-ifests no great nor consistent differences, the ratios being as fol-lows: "Well-to-do," 1.55:1; "moderate," 1.67:1; "poor," 1.55:1; "very poor," 1.56:1.

From the two foregoing indications yielded by these data the observation may be made that economic status, or, more precisely, some condition or conditions of which economic status is an

index, was a relatively unimportant determinant of the extent to
which the disease spread in a community but was of considerable
importance as a determinant of the morbidity rate within the
households attacked, and thus presumably among persons definitely exposed to an active case of the disease at all of its stages.
That factors other than those associated with economic status
were far more powerful in the spread of the epidemic within the
community is clearly evident from the wide variation in the proportions of households attacked as well as in the morbidity rates in
the nine localities surveyed, as the following table shows:

**TABLE VII   A comparison of the proportion of households attacked by
influenza and the influenza morbidity rate per 1,000 persons for nine localities
in which special surveys of 1918 were made**

Locality	Per cent of households attacked[1]	Morbidity rate per 1,000 persons[2]
New London	39	185
Baltimore	50	246
Augusta	63	341
Macon	42	213
Des Moines	46	231
Louisville	32	150
Little Rock	57	359
San Antonio	98	535
San Francisco	41	215

[1]Weighted for size of household.   [2]Adjusted to age distribution of the population in the United States in 1910.

In fact, there is a very close correlation between the percentages of households attacked and the morbidity rates,[1] and this
correlation persists for each economic class. (Tables II and V.) On
the other hand, the attack rates in affected households did not vary
greatly in the nine localities. Thus in San Antonio where 98 per
cent of the households were affected, the attack rate within these
households was 548 per 1,000 persons, whereas in Baltimore,
where only 50 per cent of the households were affected, the attack
rate within these households was 475 per 1,000.

These indications naturally lead us to such consideration of
possible intra-household factors as the data may afford.

3. The only information bearing upon intra-household factors
that was obtained related to "crowding." The data on this point

[1]Although only nine observations are available, their values when plotted in a
correlation diagram fall practically on a straight line, and, considering the number,
are well distributed (r = 0.79 ± 0.08).

**TABLE VIII   1918 influenza morbidity rate per 1,000 white persons
classified according to degree of household "crowding" in nine localities[1]**

	NUMBER OF PERSONS PER ROOM		
Locality	*1 or less*	*More than 1 but not over 2*	*More than 2*
All localities	265	328	405
New London	175	219	304
Baltimore	267	323	242
Augusta	386	564	(2)
Macon	202	249	323
Des Moines	240	251	(2)
Louisville	284	202	280
Little Rock	318	412	408
San Antonio	522	545	619
San Francisco	199	260	257

[1]The rates for the different classes have been adjusted to a single age distribution, the "standard population" used being the total population of the United States in 1910. [2]Insufficient data.

were the number of persons and the number of rooms occupied in each household. The individuals thus could be classified according to the number of persons per room. Obviously, "crowding," as expressed by "persons per room," is a very crude index of the opportunity for contact among persons living in households, but upon the assumption that such contact generally would be more close and frequent in crowded households than in households where, say, there were two rooms per person, it was thought worth while to compute the influenza morbidity rate for different groups living under different degrees of crowding. These rates are given in Table VIII, adjusted to a standard age distribution.

Taking the nine localities together, a quite definite association of household congestion and influenza is suggested. This, however, might be nothing more than a reflection of economic status. In fact, the actual distribution of the individuals in each economic class according to "persons per room" shows quite clearly that a much larger proportion of individuals were members of relatively congested households in the poorer classes than in the classes denoted as "well-to-do" and as in "moderate" circumstances. The differences in distribution are shown in Table IX.

A more detailed analysis of the data, therefore, was necessary in which the influenza morbidity rate among persons living in households of different degrees of household "congestion" could be compared for each economic class; or, to state it in another way, the influenza morbidity rate among persons in different economic

TABLE IX   Relation of over-crowding to economic status in white households included in special influenza surveys of 1918 in four localities

Economic status of household	Total number of persons in the households visited	NUMBER OF PERSONS PER ROOM		
		One or less	More than 1 but not over 2	More than 2
		NUMBER OF PERSONS		
Well-to-do	6,575	6,115	446	14
Moderate	36,764	27,789	8,732	243
Poor	17,398	9,240	7,273	880
Very poor	2,583	860	1,377	346
		PER CENT OF TOTAL NUMBER OF PERSONS		
Well-to-do	100.0	93.0	6.8	0.2
Moderate	100.0	75.6	23.7	.7
Poor	100.0	53.1	41.8	5.1
Very poor	100.0	33.3	53.3	13.4

classes could be compared for various degrees of household "congestion." In such an analysis economic status thus would be used as an index of all environmental and other conditions in order to single out with greater distinctness the influence of one of these conditions, namely, household congestion. Obviously those households in which no cases occurred have no bearing on the question of intra-household incidence and should be excluded. It was not practicable to tabulate the entire mass of data in such detail, but the experience of San Antonio, where an extensive survey was made and where 98 per cent of the households had one or more cases, conformed to the requirements of the desired analysis.

The San Antonio data afford no clear-cut evidence that the mere fact of household crowding, as measured by the ratio "persons per room," was associated with the incidence of influenza. This indication is at variance with W. Vaughn's[1] observation in Boston that crowded families were more apt to have multiple cases of influenza in the 1918 epidemic, but "crowding" in Boston might be a quite different thing from "crowding" in San Antonio. On the other hand, it is in accordance with the findings of various British investigators.[2] Although some doubt may be entertained as to the efficiency of household congestion as an index of the degree of effective contact between a case and susceptible persons, which is the datum desired, it seems to be clear that the

TABLE X   1918 influenza morbidity rate among white persons surveyed in San Antonio and classified according to degree of household crowding and economic status

Economic status of household	ATTACK RATE PER 1,000 IN HOUSEHOLD WITH NUMBER OF PERSONS PER ROOM AS FOLLOWS:[1]		
	One or less	More than 1 but not more than 2	More than 2
Well-to-do	504	514	([2])
Moderate	525	533	570
Poor	562	561	650
Very poor	542	619	603

[1]Adjusted to the age distribution of the population of the United States in 1910 and excluding persons in households that were not affected by influenza in the epidemic of 1918.
[2]Insufficient data.

association between influenza incidence and economic status persists within each "persons per room" class. This suggests the conclusion that household congestion, although a concomitant of poverty, is not per se the determining factor in establishing the association of economic status and influenza in 1918.

Influenza Incidence Among Persons of Different Economic Status and Age

Morbidity.—A comparison of the influenza morbidity and of case fatality rates at different ages among persons of different economic status throws some light on the relative importance of some of the various conditions included under the term "economic status" as factors in determining incidence and lethal rates. It has been necessary in presenting the various tabulations incident to this analysis of our material, to make combinations of the four economic classes into two, and of the ages into a few broad age groups, especially when mortality from influenza is brought into consideration, since the number of deaths is too small for minute subdivision. Even with these combinations the data are too scanty to place the results entirely beyond the influence of errors arising from chance, but the general indications seem to be fairly clear.

When the morbidity rate at different ages is compared for

persons classified as "well-to-do" and in "moderate" circumstances and for persons classified as "poor" and "very poor," it is
seen that the higher incidence among members of the poorer
households prevailed at all ages. This is shown in the following
table, in which the rates are given for 5-year age groups and for
broader age groups, and in Figure 1.

Aside from the fact of a persistently higher level of influenza
morbidity among persons classified as "poor" and "very poor,"
there is an interesting—and possibly significant—tendency toward a relatively higher morbidity rate in the older ages among
persons classified as "poor" and "very poor" than among those
classified as "well-to-do" and in "moderate" circumstances. This
is conveniently expressed in the ratio at each specified age of the
morbidity rate for the poorer class to that for the higher economic
class. The series of ratios (see Table XI) exhibit a tendency to
become greater in the adult ages, reaching their maximum in old
age. The ratio for children under five years of age is also relatively
high.

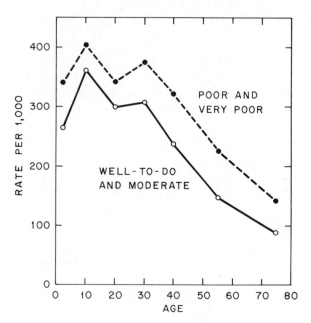

Figure 1   Age incidence of influenza in the epidemic of
1918 among persons of different economic status.

TABLE XI   Incidence of epidemic influenza in 1918 in each age group among white persons, classified according to the general economic condition of the household, in nine localities where surveys were made

Age group	RATE PER 1,000 WHITE PERSONS IN HOUSE-HOLDS CLASSIFIED AS—		Ratio of (B) to (A)
	Well-to-do and moderate (A)	Poor and very poor (B)	
Under 5	262	339	1.29
5–9	370	412	1.11
10–14	350	390	1.11
15–19	303	349	1.15
20–24	290	331	1.14
25–29	310	378	1.22
30–34	299	375	1.25
35–39	261	348	1.33
40–44	205	281	1.38
45–49	178	245	1.37
50–54	137	237	1.73
55–59	130	197	1.51
60–64	108	190	1.76
65 and over	87	142	1.63
Under 5	262	339	1.29
5–14	360	401	1.11
15–24	297	340	1.15
25–34	305	376	1.23
35–44	235	318	1.35
45–64	145	224	1.54
65 and over	87	142	1.63

The suggestion is afforded, therefore, that in the poorer households either the resistance to attack on the part of infants and older adults was lower, or the opportunity for their infection was greater, or both conditions obtained. In this connection, a similar comparison of the attack rates in households affected is of interest. The tabulations include only the Baltimore survey, but the number of persons is sufficiently large (15,513) to yield a fairly regular series of rates, as shown in the table following.

TABLE XII   Influenza attack rate in the epidemic of 1918 in each specified age group among white persons in affected households of different economic status, in areas canvassed in Baltimore

Age group	ATTACK RATE PER 1,000 PERSONS IN HOUSE-HOLDS CLASSIFIED AS—		Ratio of (B) to (A)
	Well-to-do and moderate (A)	Poor and very poor (B)	
Under 5	452	522	1.15
5–14	547	585	1.08
15–24	491	522	1.14
25–34	535	601	1.12
35–44	375	489	1.31
45–64	278	388	1.39
65 and over	186	333	1.79

Upon the assumption that all of the individuals in these households were definitely exposed, perhaps frequently, to the disease,
the hypothesis that the susceptibility to attack among young children and older adults was greater in poorer households than in
households economically better off would seem to be
strengthened.

Case fatality.—A similar comparison of the fatality of influenza at different ages among persons of relatively poor
economic condition with that among persons in moderate and
well-to-do circumstances, is given in the following table and in
Figure 2.

If the curves were parallel, the conclusion would be admissi-
ble that the influences connoted by the term "economic status"
operated with equal force at all ages. But the curves are not
parallel. As shown in the ratios given in Table XIII, the case
fatality rate among poorer persons is distinctly higher than among
persons economically better off in three age groups, viz, under 5
years, 15–34, and 45 and over.

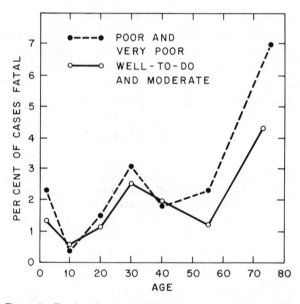

Figure 2   Fatality of cases of influenza in the epidemic of 1918
according to age among persons of different economic status.

TABLE XIII   Fatality at each age group of cases of influenza in the epidemic of 1918, classified according to the general economic condition of the households affected

Age group	PER CENT OF CASES FATAL IN HOUSEHOLDS CLASSIFIED AS—		Ratio of (B) to (A)
	Well-to-do and moderate (A)	Poor and very poor (B)	
Under 5	1.4	2.3	1.64
5–14	.5	.4	.80
15–24	1.2	1.5	1.25
25–34	2.6	3.1	1.19
35–44	1.9	1.8	.95
45–64	1.2	2.4	2.00
65 and over	4.3	7.0	1.63

What interpretation can be made of these differences, assuming that the sample is sufficiently large to warrant their serious consideration? Since so many conditions unobserved in the course of the survey may have been involved, a definite conclusion is unwarranted. The definitely greater fatality in the older persons in the lower economic classes than in the higher economic classes suggest that their resistance, for some reason associated with their economic status, was lowered. This suggestion is upon the rather broad but generally favored hypothesis that the mortality rate among a given group of persons of middle age or over is usually a fair indication of their resistance to the effects of disease when compared with that of a standard or normal group. The greater fatality among poorer children under 5 years of age and among poorer adults under 30 or 35 years of age does not fit in with this hypothesis so well. While unfavorable heredity conceivably might be assigned as an important cause of the high fatality rate from influenza among young children in the poorer classes, other factors can not be left out of consideration. Among these factors should be included that of medical and nursing care, in which respect the poor were usually at a disadvantage. The strain on parents who were themselves attacked at the same time as their children must have been more severe among the poor than among the well-to-do, particularly in view of the fact that the families of the poor more frequently were larger and composed of younger children than those classed as economically better off. But we can only speculate as to the various conditions that possibly or probably might have been involved. The circumstances at the time of the epidemic were such that more detailed data were not obtainable for a sufficiently large sample of our population.

References

[1]Vaughn, Warren: A Detailed Review of the Epidemiology of Influenza, Monograph No. 1, American Journal of Hygiene, Baltimore, 1921.
[2]Ministry of Health (Great Britain): Report on Influenza, 1918–1919, Chap. VIII.

Preceding Papers on the Epidemiology of Influenza

Preceding papers from the office of statistical investigations dealing with various phases of the epidemiology of influenza are listed below:

Mortality from Influenza and Pneumonia in 50 Large Cities of the United States, 1910–1929. By S. D. Collins, W. H. Frost, Mary Gover, and Edgar Sydenstricker. Public Health Reports, Vol. 45, No. 39, Sept. 26, 1930. (Reprint 1415.)

Influenza-Pneumonia Mortality in a Group of about 95 Cities in the United States, 1920–1929. By S. D. Collins. Public Health Reports, Vol. 45, No. 8, February 21, 1930. (Reprint 1355.)

The Influenza Epidemic of 1926. Public Health Reports, August 20, 1926. (Reprint 1104.)

Variations in Case Fatality During the Influenza Epidemic of 1918. By Edgar Sydenstricker. Public Health Reports, September 9, 1920. (Reprint 692.)

Statistics of Influenza Morbidity. By W. H. Frost. Public Health Reports, March 12, 1920. (Reprint 586.)

Difficulties in Computing Civil Death Rates for 1918. By Edgar Sydenstricker and Mary L. King. Public Health Reports, February 13, 1920. (Reprint 583.)

The Epidemiology of Influenza. By W. H. Frost. Public Health Reports, August 15, 1919. (Reprint 550.)

Epidemic Influenza in Foreign Countries. By W. H. Frost and Edgar Sydenstricker. Public Health Reports, June 20, 1919. (Reprint 537.)

Influenza in Maryland. By W. H. Frost and Edgar Sydenstricker. Public Health Reports, March 14, 1919. (Reprint No. 510.)

A Comparison of the Mortality Rates by Weeks During the Influenza Epidemic of 1889–90 and during the Primary Stage of the Influenza Epidemic of 1918 in 12 Cities in the United States. Public Health Reports, January 31, 1919. (Reprint 502.)

Preliminary Statistics of the Influenza Epidemic. By Edgar Sydenstricker. Public Health Reports, Vol. 33, No. 52, December 27, 1918.

Public Health Reports
January 23, 1931

3

Effect of a Whooping Cough Epidemic Upon the Size of the Nonimmune Group in an Urban Community

EDGAR SYDENSTRICKER

The extent to which an uncontrolled epidemic of an infectious disease spreads in human populations under different environments is a matter of practical importance to the sanitarian whenever any attempt at control is made. It cannot be settled easily, however, for many factors are involved. The etiology of the specific disease; the period of its infectivity; the opportunity for effective contact between susceptible individuals and infectious cases or carriers, which is subject to so many and so varied circumstances; the proportion of the population already immune—these are only some of the most essential facts required by the epidemiologist in considering the problem for a given type of community. He is faced by a complexity of conditions, so intricately related and so difficult to evaluate in exact terms, that very precise measurements of an epidemic's behavior are well-nigh impossible. Even if he arrives at a successful answer for one population group, he cannot assume its accuracy for other groups or communities.

Precision beyond certain general limits, however, is neither always necessary nor profitable, and much can be learned from observing epidemics in populations of different general types, provided reasonably complete records of histories of previous attacks and of current cases are secured. In the course of the morbidity study in Hagerstown, Maryland,[1] the opportunity was presented of observing certain epidemiological phases of whooping cough with a greater degree of accuracy and completeness than is ordinarily possible from routine records of cases reported in compliance with regulations for disease notification. This opportunity was afforded by reason of three conditions:

1. A population of over 7,000 persons was "under observation" for incidence of sickness for twenty-eight consecutive months. Each household was visited by a competent staff or field assistants at intervals of six to eight weeks in order to obtain a record from responsible informants (usually the housewife) of cases of sickness and attacks of communicable diseases. The diagnosis of cases attended by physicians (of whooping cough, such cases were 49 per cent of the total recorded) were reviewed by the physicians themselves.

2. At the initial visit to each household a careful effort was made to ascertain for each individual enumerated the age at which he had previously been attacked by whooping cough as well as by other infectious diseases. Similar information was obtained for new persons coming into the observed population during the ensuing twenty-eight months. We had, therefore, a record, although admittedly neither absolutely accurate nor complete, of those persons who had a history of clinically obvious attacks previous to December 1, 1921, and of those who had no such history.

3. A record was obtained of all births, deaths, and of migration of persons from and into the group during the period.

For the purpose of this particular study another rather interesting and favorable condition was found to exist. For about twenty months prior to December 1, 1921, no unusual prevalence of

[1]A series of reports dealing with the Hagerstown morbidity study has been published in various issues of the United States *Public Health Reports*. The reader is referred especially to the following: Sydenstricker, Edgar: The Incidence of Various Diseases According to Age. Study No. VIII. United States *Public Health Reports*, May 11, 1928. Reprint No. 1227.

Sydenstricker, Edgar, and Hedrich, A. W.: Completeness of Reporting of Measles, Whooping Cough, and Chickenpox at Different Ages. Supplement to Study II. United States *Public Health Reports*, June 28, 1929. Reprint No. 1294.

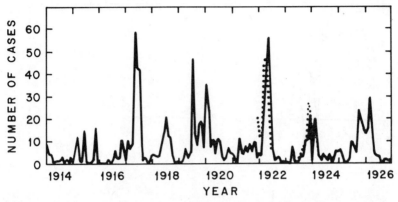

Figure 1   Cases of whooping cough in Washington County, Maryland, *reported* to the State Health Department, 1914–1926, and cases *recorded* in an observed population in Hagerstown, Maryland, December 1, 1921 to March 31, 1924.

whooping cough had occurred in Hagerstown, a fact evidenced by our own record of previous attacks in the observed population and by the records of the Maryland State Department of Health. Almost immediately after the study was begun, an outbreak of the disease occurred. In fact, two outbreaks apparently took place, one in December, 1921 - July, 1922, and another in September, 1923 - March, 1924, but they occurred in different parts of the City and, taken together, constituted a fairly widespread epidemic over the entire area in which the observed population resided. It is proper, therefore, to regard them as a single epidemic.

In the present communication it is proposed to present such data as we were able to collect during the twenty-eight-month period that relate more particularly to the effect of the outbreak of whooping cough upon the size of the "susceptible" moiety of the population so observed, in the hope of throwing some light upon the relation of immunity to the magnitude of recurring epidemic outbreaks in a typical small urban community. Hagerstown, in 1921, had a total population of about 30,000. The group observed comprised a little less than one-fourth of this total and was from areas inhabited only by white residents.

In Figure 1 the position of the outbreak is shown in relation to the chronology of the disease from 1914 through 1926 in Washing-

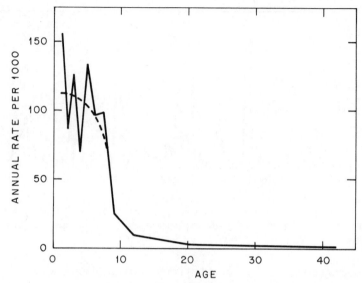

Figure 2   Incidence of whooping cough among persons of different ages in a white population group in Hagerstown, Maryland, December 1, 1921, to March 31, 1924.

ton County, Maryland, of which Hagerstown is the principal center.[2] The seasonal distribution of cases in the observed population also is portrayed in Figure 1. A total of 374 cases was recorded as incident during the twenty-eight-month period, or at an annual rate of 27.8 per 1,000 years of life observed.

The incidence of whooping cough according to age upon the total observed population is shown in Figure 2 for the period of twenty-eight months. The concentration of cases among persons under five years of age, the sharp drop in incidence upon persons five–nine years old, and the low rate after fifteen years of age at once suggest that an immunity, increasing with age, existed at the beginning of the period of observation. This indication is con-

[2]The data for Washington County, with a total population of about 65,000 are cases *reported* to the State Health Department. The dotted line in Figure I shows the cases *recorded* for the population observed. The fact that the latter are approximately equal to the numbers for the entire County is due principally, of course, to more complete records in the observed population. Notification of whooping cough in Hagerstown was about 15 per cent of the incident cases. The chronological picture for Washington County, however, seems fairly similar to that for Hagerstown.

TABLE I   History of whooping cough among white persons at different ages up to fifteen years as of December, 1921, in Hagerstown, Maryland

Age in Years	PERCENTAGES		NUMBERS		
	Having Had Prior Attack	Not Having Had Prior Attack	Total Considered	Having Had Prior Attack	Not Having Had Prior Attack
Total—15	49	51	1,891	928	963
Under 1	5	95	131	6	125
1	6	94	125	7	118
2	15	85	124	18	106
3	22	78	109	24	85
4	37	63	169	62	107
5	40	60	139	55	84
6	49	51	150	74	76
7	64	36	118	75	43
8	65	35	150	97	53
9	72	28	125	90	35
10	77	23	116	89	27
11	72	28	113	81	32
12	77	23	108	83	25
13	76	24	106	80	26
14	81	19	108	87	21

firmed by the records of persons at each age for whom positive histories of whooping cough were obtained as of December 1, 1921, upon the assumption that an attack of the disease usually confers immunity. The percentages at each age with positive history are given in Table I and are plotted in Figure 3. The logistic curve fitted by Collins[3] to similar data for whooping cough from various sources, including that obtained in the Hagerstown study, is also shown. The Hagerstown percentages fall closely on Collins' curve.*

Now if the histories of previous attacks of whooping cough could be assumed to afford a complete and accurate record of all of the persons immune to the disease on December 1, 1921, it would be easy to determine how much of the remaining susceptible human material was "exhausted" before an epidemic "burned itself out." The facts that in an urban population the percentage of persons with positive histories of whooping cough practically reaches its asymptote at about fifteen years of age, and that this asymptote is approximately 75 per cent constitute unmistakable evidence that such an assumption is not sufficiently precise. On

[3]Collins, Selwyn D.: Age Incidence of the Common Communicable Diseases of Children. United States *Public Health Reports*, April 5, 1929. Reprint No. 1275.

*[The equation for this curve was: $y = 77 \{1 - \exp(-.05383 - .01334x - .02703x^2)\}$ where y = percentage of persons who have had an attack of whooping cough and x = age in years. ED.]

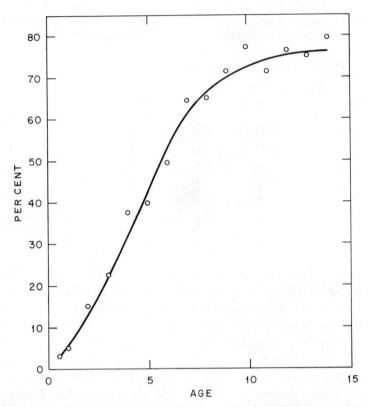

Figure 3   Percentage of the observed population at different ages who had had attacks of whooping cough prior to December 1, 1921. (Smooth line from Collins, *see* footnote page 337.)

the contrary, it is obvious that 25 per cent of the population over fifteen years of age possessed an immunity not accounted for by histories[4] of clinically obvious attacks. The question then arises:

[4]It is realized that some of the persons *with* positive histories of whooping cough are still susceptible since second attacks do occur. The proportion of persons suffering clinically obvious multiple attacks is not large, however. In the outbreaks under consideration only 20 of the 363 cases under fifteen years of age were among persons reported to have a previous attack. Assuming this record to be absolutely correct, the immunity conferred by an attack of whooping cough is high, only 1.7 of total persons under fifteen having suffered a second attack during this period. Or, assuming the immunity conferred to be 100 per cent, the error in the record is relatively slight, being only 5.5 per cent.

TABLE II   Attack rate of whooping cough among white persons of different ages *without* previous history of whooping cough and resident in households attacked by the disease in 1922 and 1923, Hagerstown, Maryland

Age	NUMBER OF		PER CENT	
	Persons	Cases	Attacked	Not Attacked
Total under 15	**441**	**356**	**81**	**19**
Under 6 months	6	3	50	50
6 months—1 year	15	14	93	7
1 year	12	11	92	8
2 years	59	55	93	7
3 "	41	39	95	5
4 "	49	42	86	14
5 "	48	42	88	12
6 "	55	46	84	16
7 "	45	37	82	18
8 "	43	31	72	28
9 "	20	14	70	30
10 "	18	11	61	39
11 "	13	8	62	38
12 "	9	1	11	89
13 "	4	1	25	75
14 "	4	1	25	75

at what ages did the individuals comprising this 25 per cent of the population acquire immunity to the disease?

A satisfactory answer would be afforded if the experiment could be tried of taking a statistically adequate number of persons at different ages who had no history of clinically obvious whooping cough, exposing them sufficiently to active cases when such cases were at a fully infectious stage, and observing the number of such persons attacked by the disease as the result of the exposure. Such an experiment is, of course, impracticable, but we can approximate it by ascertaining the attack rate of whooping cough among persons of different ages *without histories of the disease but residing in households that were attacked* during the outbreaks under consideration. This has been done in Table II. It will be noted that the proportion of such persons attacked (i.e., for whom clinically obvious cases were recorded) was over 90 per cent at ages six months to four years, and thereafter declined to approximately 25 per cent at ages thirteen and fourteen. The numbers are too small to yield dependable results for any one year of age, but the resulting curve (Figure 4) of the percentages of persons presumably exposed to cases in the same households but *not* attacked at least suggests that the proportion of the population which has acquired an immunity without suffering clinically ob-

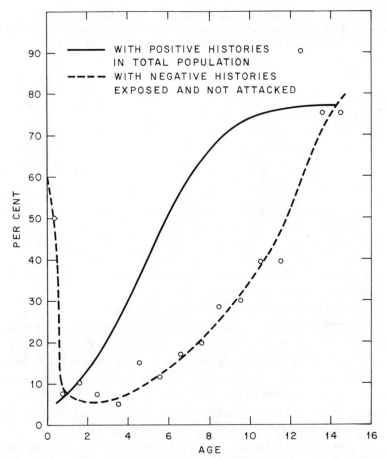

Figure 4   Percentage of population with positive histories of whooping cough and percentage of those with negative histories who were not attacked when exposed to familial cases.

vious attack rises rapidly with age (after the first six months of life) to a point which approximates the 25 per cent for whom no history of previous attack is ordinarily given. The further suggestion is afforded that the percentage of persons acquiring an immunity without any clinically obvious or remembered attack does not rise with age at the same rate at which the percentage of persons with clinically obvious attacks rises with age; the curve of the former, as depicted in Figure 4, lags considerably behind that of the latter. Obviously, the older the child the greater is the likelihood of exposure to the disease in some previous epidemic and of a subclinical attack which conferred immunity. It may also be that attacks of the disease tend to be milder and more frequently "subclinical" as age advances.

Whatever may be the value of these indications at different ages, the point with which this discussion is particularly concerned is the gross proportion of the population under fifteen years of age which was immune to whooping cough at the beginning of the period of observation. Of 441 persons without any history of whooping cough (i.e., attacks that were remembered by the informants) and then presumably exposed to it through familial or other effective contact, 356 persons contracted the disease and 85 did not. These 85 persons may be assumed to have either acquired an immunity previous to the epidemic, or to have suffered subclinical attacks during its course.

Applying the percentages at each age obtained in our "experiment" to the number of persons of corresponding ages who were recorded as having no history of the disease on December 1, 1921, it may be estimated that a maximum of 195, or 20.6 per cent, of the 963 persons under fifteen years of age without a history of a previous attack actually possessed immunity. Subtracting, this leaves 768 persons who may be assumed to have been susceptible at that time, which is 41 per cent of the entire population in the age group under fifteen years. The method of estimation obviously is rough and the estimate itself must be regarded as only an approximation to the actual number of nonimmune persons. It is, however, more accurate for this purpose than the number of persons recorded as not having had a previous attack.

Starting with these 768 persons[5] on December 1, 1921, it is now possible to estimate the effect of the ensuing outbreaks upon the size of the "susceptible" population. In making the necessary computations, the following facts were taken into account: 1)

[5] If practically 100 per cent of this urban population over fifteen years of age was no longer susceptible to whooping cough, these 768 persons constituted nearly all of the nonimmune in the group observed.

TABLE III   Variations in the number and percentage of a population group under fifteen years of age who were nonimmune to whooping cough and who would have been nonimmune if no epidemic had occurred during twenty-eight months, December 1, 1921 to March 31, 1924, in Hagerstown, Maryland

Date	Population under Fifteen Years	TOTAL SUSCEPTIBLES UNDER FIFTEEN YEARS		SUSCEPTIBLES IF NO EPIDEMIC HAD OCCURRED	
		Number	Per Cent	Number	Per Cent
1921, Dec. 1	1,891	768	41	768	41
1922, June 1	1,894	634	33	822	43
1922, Dec. 1	1,878	653	35	863	46
1923, June 1	1,869	695	37	906	48
1923, Dec. 1	1,858	667	36	940	51
1924, Mar. 31	1,834	611	33	949	52

births, 2) deaths, 3) persons reaching the age of fifteen years, 4) persons actually attacked by the disease in clinically obvious forms, and 5) persons acquiring an immunity without clinically obvious attacks, during the twenty-eight month period. Emigration and immigration of individuals from and into families constituted a negligible factor and were disregarded. Births were added to the susceptible group,[6] but persons dying, persons attacked by the disease, persons presumably acquiring an immunity during the epidemic (estimated upon the ratio of one to five clinically definite cases), and susceptible persons reaching the age of fifteen, were subtracted.[7] The computations were made as of several dates in the twenty-eight months, as shown in Table III, and the variations in the proportion of the entire population under fifteen years of age which remained susceptible are plotted in Figure 5.

[6]Strict accuracy would demand that persons born into the population should not be added to the susceptible group until after some period of possible "natural" immunity had elapsed. The data were inadequate for a determination of such a period or to ascertain whether or not it existed.

[7]Calculation of susceptible population under fifteen years of age at successive dates.[1]

Date	Number of Susceptibles Under Fifteen Years of Age	Add Births	SUBTRACT			Net + or −
			Deaths	⁶/₅ Cases	Fifteen Years Old	
1921, December	768	109	9	210	5	−115
1922, December	653	100	18	63	5	+ 14
1923, December	667	18	8	65	1	− 56
1924, March	611					

[1]To calculate susceptibles in case no epidemic had occurred, do not use the figures in column headed ⁶/₅ cases, i.e., persons who had the disease and an additional 20 per cent who acquired immunity without a clinically obvious attack.

   With a full realization of the necessarily crude procedure in
making these approximations and of the caution that must be
exercised in drawing too precise conclusions, the following observations may be ventured:

   1. The proportion of the *total* population in a typical small
urban community (as judged from a sample of nearly one-fourth of
the total) which was nonimmune to whooping cough after an
interepidemic interval of about twenty months was about 10 per
cent. Of persons under fifteen years of age, the percentage
nonimmune was about 40.

   2. After an outbreak of the disease which immediately began in
December, 1921, was acute for four months, and affected only
certain areas, the proportion of the population under fifteen years
of age which was nonimmune declined to 35 per cent in De-

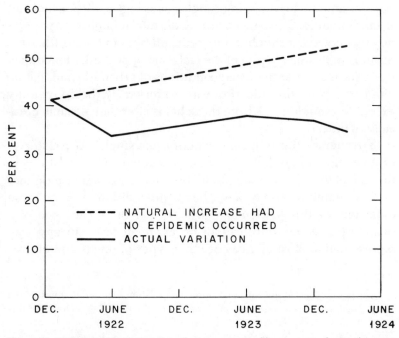

Figure 5   Variation in the proportion of persons under fifteen years of age who were
nonimmune to whooping cough during twenty-eight months, December 1, 1921 to
March 31, 1924, in Hagerstown, Maryland.

cember, 1922. Had this outbreak not occurred, the percentage of nonimmunes under fifteen years of age in the families actually observed would have risen to 46 on the assumption that no new immunity had been conferred on the older children[8] and that the infants added by birth were susceptible.

3. After a second outbreak, beginning in August, 1923, and lasting through March, 1924, and affecting chiefly the areas not attacked in 1921–1922, the proportion of nonimmunes in the general population was further reduced to about 8 per cent and of the group under fifteen years of age to 33 per cent.

Our inquiry thus may be regarded as an approach to the observation—admittedly incomplete—of a single epidemic in a series of epidemics of whooping cough that occur more or less periodically in a small urban community. So regarded, it indicates that when the proportion of total children under fifteen years of age nonimmune to whooping cough was as high as 40 per cent and an epidemic of the disease occurred, the total nonimmune population was not exhausted but only reduced by about one-fifth. This result is indicated in spite of the facts that opportunity for contact was afforded under the usual conditions of urban life and that no effort to control the infection was exercised by the community except to exclude cases from the schools after they became clinically manifest.

To reiterate, this is but one experience, a single "case history," as it were, of an epidemic of whooping cough. The variations in the size of the nonimmune population in prior or later epidemics in this community may have been quite different from those indicated for this particular outbreak, and the experience of a small urban community cannot be assumed to be in any way representative of rural areas or other types of towns and cities.

---

[8]The possibility that some of our observed population acquired immunity from carriers or from cases outside the city could not, of course, be explored in this study.

Milbank Memorial Fund Quarterly
October, 1932

4

The Declining
Death Rate from Tuberculosis
EDGAR SYDENSTRICKER

I

Perhaps the most direct introduction to the topic you have assigned me is afforded by a telescopic glance at the course of
mortality from pulmonary tuberculosis over the longest period for
which, so far as I am aware, any kind of continuous statistical
record of the disease exists. This is for London from 1631 to the
present.[1] (Figure 1) If this record is to be depended upon at
all—and it is accurate enough for a distant view—it shows two
very interesting facts: 1) that during the eighteenth century there
was an increase in the phthisis death rate until it reached the
extraordinary height of nearly 700 deaths annually per 100,000
population; 2) that shortly before 1800 the phthisis death rate
began to decrease rapidly, the decline continuing without any
great interruption until the present time. The phenomenon in
general may be said to have occurred in all civilized countries.
From records beginning with 1812 for Boston, New York City and
Philadelphia compiled by Hoffman[2] and for Baltimore compiled
by Howard,[3] and other records for shorter periods, it is quite
evident that the trend of tuberculosis mortality in this country has
been downward since at least the beginning of the nineteenth
century.

To what factors may we ascribe this decline of the tuberculosis
death rate in the last 150 years?

"It is so easy, and, to most people, so pleasant," as Greenwood[4] has remarked, "to blame others and to assign cut and dried reasons for the infinitely complex phenomena of human life" that we are apt to avoid taking into account what he has termed "uncontrollable conditions" and to give entire or undue credit to efforts to control, forgetting that an analysis of the causal factors involved in any social phenomenon "offers problems the solution of which is hardly easier than Hercules' cleansing of the Augean stables." Hoffman,[2] addressing this organization fourteen years ago, asserted that the statistics he presented for the three American cities for 1812–1912 "prove conclusively that the deliberate, thoroughly intelligent, and nation-wide campaign against tuberculosis on the principle of its being an infectious disease and transmissible from man to man, has been successful beyond reasonable expectations." More recently Pearl[5] drew what has been construed by some to be a deadly parallel between the rate of decrease during the period 1900–1918 in mortality from tuberculosis and certain other diseases against which more or less vigorous campaigns have been waged, and the rate of decrease during the same period in mortality from certain "non-controlled causes of death" with the indication that the course of the two groups of diseases are not dissimilar, and affording the implication, apparently, that some varieties of public health effort have had no appreciable results. Although some of us may not agree with Pearl's method of attacking the problem, we surely can have no quarrel with his comment:

> If they (the comparisons referred to above) may serve to drive sharply home into the mind that it is only the tyro or the reckless propagandist long ago a stranger to truth who will venture to assert that a declining death rate in and of itself marks the successful result of human effort, I shall be abundantly satisfied.

I have cited these two examples from the great volume of interpretations and conclusions extant with the purpose of permitting the utter futility to expose itself of evaluating statistically with any degree of precision the part played by the anti-tuberculosis campaign or any other *specific* factor or condition in the reduction of the tuberculosis death rate during the past century or even in the last generation. I am quite aware that at least some of you, who are engaged in the forefront of the battle with the disease, will be in violent disagreement with this. It is but natural for you to ask: Does this mean that we shall *never* be able to know whether or not the organized campaign against the disease has had any effect upon its prevalence? Surely we can not deny the evidence of our own senses, of our daily experience, of a multitude of individual histories, that anti-tuberculosis work, as it is generally conducted now, does contribute to the prevention of the disease, to arresting its progress in active cases, and to prolonging the lives of many persons. Must such facts as these be disregarded by the cold–blooded statistician?

II

The question of measuring the results of the anti-tuberculosis movement will be clarified a good deal if we consider, although very briefly, first, what are the requirements for reasonably accurate measurement, and, second, how far these requirements are met or can be met by the information available. The principles underlying the measurement of social efforts are, I take it, identi-

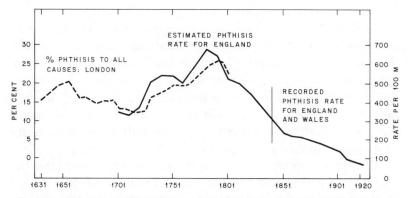

Figure 1   The course of phthisis mortality in London and England, 1631–1920.

cal with those underlying all scientific experimentation; and scientific experimentation, whether it be the analysis of previous or existing conditions by statistical technique or by the deliberate manipulation of future conditions, postulates a comparison of events that occur when the specific factor, which we wish to measure, acts with varying degrees of force, with events that occur when it is absent, all other relevant conditions being unchanged or, if changed, being themselves capable of evaluation.[6] Now, it is painfully evident that our *past* records of anti-tuberculosis work, of tuberculosis prevalence, and of the important conditions possibly directly and indirectly concerned, do not afford even an adequate approach to a scientific analysis of the factors involved in the course of tuberculosis mortality. We may as well face that fact and seek more suitable methods in our attempt to portray the factors that have operated for or against the result which undoubtedly has occurred and in which we are so interested.

This does not mean that the force of various important factors and of deliberate efforts to reduce the prevalence or the fatality of tuberculosis can not be measured. It *can* be measured provided we are willing to take enough pains to set up an experiment with its necessary "controls," watch developments as they occur, record our observations accurately, and analyze the results, using human population groups for our purpose and maintaining a long enough period of observation. This is the only way, I venture to assert, whereby we can measure *scientifically* the results of anti-tuberculosis work.

In the assignment given me, I must of necessity, therefore, relinquish the task of the analytical statistician and frankly assume the rôle of the historian who, with such understanding of the nature of the events as he may have, employs deductive rather than inductive processes in reaching a conclusion. I shall present no statistics except those which assist in description and narration; even the graphs I shall show you will be used more for pictorial illustrations than for analysis.

With this purpose in mind, the thesis may be proposed that *the decline in the tuberculosis death rate ought to be viewed primarily as a social development.* There is nothing novel in this view, of course: it is the well established attitude of the social historian when he "looks at" the increase in automobiles, the decrease in the birth rate, or any of the many interesting phases of human history. Nor is there anything *new* in the way we shall go about an inquiry along these lines.

III

Let us put down first as a basic and established fact that any condition which appreciably affects the opportunity for the transmission of the disease from person to person or which affects the physiological resistance of the individual is a factor to be taken into account epidemiologically and historically. Now what are some of these conditions which conceivably might have influenced the chronological behavior of the disease?[7]

It has been suggested that our population has been, as Bushnell puts it, gradually "tubercularized," a development which has contributed to a declining fatality of the disease, if not a decrease in its prevalence. Reasonable as this hypothesis is, its soundness has yet to be tested.

The view is also held by some that the virulence of the bacillus has diminished. Again we have an hypothesis that has not been subjected to scientific test. Some evidence at least does not support it. For example, when the bacillus is transplanted from populations long affected with the disease to populations among whom the disease has not existed, its virulence apparently is quite strong; whether or not it is as great as it was a thousand years ago, we do not know.

It has been argued that the factor of inheritance as manifested by a net survival of individuals who possess constitutional resistance to tuberculosis over and above keeping alive, by social artifices, individuals who are not resistant to it and whose progeny presumably are more or less not resistant, has contributed to the decrease in the death rate from tuberculosis. The hypotheses involved in this suggestion are subject to so much question and the information we need is so scanty that it seems futile to speculate upon the role of heredity in the phenomenon before us.

Certain biological phases of our topic have been discussed adequately and brilliantly by Professor Jennings[8] and I shall not refer to the factor of heredity except with respect to the possible influence of the changing racial composition of our population and of the change in "industrial selection" of constitutional types of individuals.

Lastly, there is the opposing fact, namely that the death rate from tuberculosis among peoples that are "tubercularized," and among whom the virulence of the organism has had opportunity to be weakened, is extremely sensitive to variations in that set of conditions which we classify vaguely as "environmental." That is to say, regardless of the force of any or all other factors, environmental conditions still appear as a major factor.

The interrelation of the many conditions that are connoted under the very general term by which we designate these general factors is so complicated that no clear-cut analysis, even by the historian's method, is feasible. Certainly it is impossible in a mere essay to attempt even a presentation of the interrelationships. What I would like to do in the short time at my disposal is to refer briefly first to the possible effects of racial changes and of changes in industrial selection; second, to some of the evidence of environmental and occupational conditions; and third, to the nature of public health activities and its possible influence.

IV

In view of the indication of a higher tuberculosis death rate among certain foreign born groups, particularly persons of Irish extraction, the inference has been drawn by some that race *per se* is a major determinant of tuberculosis mortality in this country and that, since we have had successive waves of immigration from different countries, it has been a considerable factor in determining the course of the death rate. In an important sense this inference seems to be warranted but not, I believe, to the extent it has been emphasized.[9] The data made available in the extremely valuable studies by Dublin and Baker[10] upon the mortality of foreign race stocks in 1910, a time of industrial activity before the

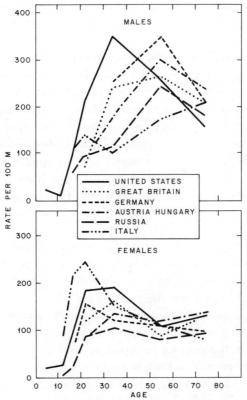

Figure 2   Tuberculosis mortality by nativity. New York
and Pennsylvania, 1910. (Dublin and Baker)

recent movement in this country to improve working conditions
had born fruit, are illuminating on this point. If we plot the sex-age
curves for populations of different nativities (Figure 2) we can not
fail to be impressed by two striking facts: 1) that the mortality of
males of each nativity differs from that of females of the same
nativity in the same way as in the case of native born, thus indicating that *occupation*, in its broad sense, more than race is the
determining factor in the adult male rate; 2) that, contrasted with
the age curve of the tuberculosis death rates among immigrants
from northern Europe and native born, the tuberculosis mortality
among southern and southeastern male immigrants is actually low

in the younger adult ages but rises sharply in the older adult ages, thus again indicating the effect of occupation after residence in this country for some time.

Collis,[11] in common with other writers upon this subject, has singled out occupation from other environmental conditions as a major specific factor in tuberculosis mortality. There can be no question as to the soundness of this view. So much has been said on the influence of occupation that no attempt will be made to review it here. Abundant evidence has established the fact that certain dusts, for example, bring about a pulmonary condition favorable to the tubercle and that work which breaks down physiological resistance is conducive to the disease. There are, however, two observations bearing upon this phase of our topic that may be offered.

The first observation is that the magnitude of the factor of industrial work—not necessarily any specific occupational hazard—in determining the tuberculosis death rate in the later adult ages has not been fully realized. The death rates in the lighter occupations, although generally high among the working populations, do not rise in the older adult ages to nearly the extent that they do in the heavier occupations and in those occupations which have a specific hazard, in spite of a selection of apparently sturdier individuals by these heavier and more hazardous industries.

The second observation is that before placing upon occupation all of the responsibility for an unfavorable tuberculosis death rate, it is proper to take into account the physical character of the workers themselves *before* the effect of occupation can make itself felt. A physical selection of workers by industry must and does result in a concentration of physically less resistant individuals in certain occupations and of the physically robust in other occupations. What happens to these workers afterwards, provided they stay in these occupations, is another matter. But it is entirely reasonable to expect a higher tuberculosis death rate in certain occupations than in others solely because these occupations are recruited from the ranks of the physically less robust and resistant. Fortunately it is not necessary to leave this assumption as an hypothesis. If we use the mortality rate for the younger adult

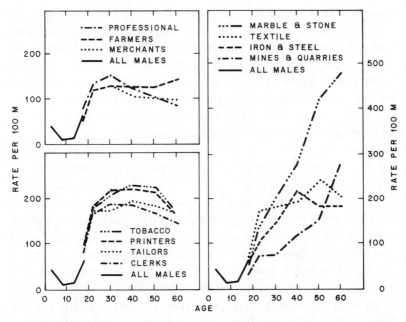

Figure 3   Tuberculosis mortality among males by occupational groups. United States, 1908–1909.

ages—from 20 to 29—instead of the rate for the total adult ages, we find not only from English experience but also from American mortality experience that the tuberculosis death rate at those ages is higher in the more sedentary occupations than in the heavy. (Figure 3). This can be interpreted, I believe, as showing definitely that, since we are dealing with the tuberculosis death rate at *entrance* or *very soon after entrance* into occupation, it is not the lighter occupations which are responsible for the relatively high rate but the type of individuals who, because of their physical inheritance or acquired physical condition or both, choose or gravitate into these occupations.

V

One effect of this industrial selection apparently may be seen in certain differentiations and changes in the composition of population groups. In the course of an inquiry[12] in the Office of

Statistical Investigations of the United States Public Health Service into the reasons why the tuberculosis death rate is so much higher in some localities than in others, we found that they could not be entirely explained by differences in sex, age, race, specific occupational hazard, climate, or economic status. Some other factor or factors obviously were present. Among them seemed to be this factor of *selection*. The evidence is too voluminous and the method of study is too detailed to be presented in a short paper, but the apparent findings were as follows: That the physique of the young adult male population, as expressed by various indices of robustness and build which were based on physical measurements of considerable samples upon entrance into the army in 1917 and 1918, was inversely correlated with the general physical character of the predominant occupation in the large cities. In other words, cities with a relatively large proportion of persons employed in heavy industries such as steel manufacturing, had relatively large proportions of physically robust young men; and cities with a relatively large proportion employed in light industries, such as trade and clerical, had relatively large proportions of less robust young men. The tuberculosis death rate among young adult males employed in light occupations, as we have seen, is considerably higher than that among young adult males employed in heavy occupations. The tuberculosis rate among the more "robust," as shown by Army and other anthropometrical studies, is significantly less than that among the less "robust." A considerable volume of data collected by us has shown statistically what may be generally expected, that under modern conditions of easy migration workers tend to change jobs until they find work that they can bear; the labor turnover, for example, is high in an arduous or irritating occupation, but a proportion of workers are found suited to the work and remain. After allowing for differences in race, climate, and several other factors, we found that the net correlation between the tuberculosis death rate among young adult males in the large cities and the mean index of robustness for young adult males in the same cities was statistically significant.

In this sense, therefore, physical inheritance probably does play a part in determining the tuberculosis death rate of a population. As the type of industry, measured by its physical demands upon the worker, changes in a given locality, it may be expected to affect the tuberculosis rate *to some extent.* Obviously, to the extent that this is true, the tuberculosis problem in one place is more serious than in another. Obviously also, as the physical requirements of factory work are lessened, so the strain upon the less robust is lightened. Whether or not our population contains a larger proportion of these physical weaklings than it did a century ago is a question upon which no adequate information is available.

VI

Whether changes in environment have affected the tuberculosis death rate more by diminishing the amount of infection or more by increasing the power of resistance or more by lessening the force of conditions that break down resistance, it is, of course, impossible to say. The probabilities are that they have operated in all these ways and certainly in the manner last mentioned. The influence of environment, in its broad sense, is clearly reflected in the age-curves of tuberculosis mortality. In an accompanying diagram (Figure 4) I have plotted the age-specific death rates from phthisis in England and Wales for 1910–12 beginning with the age-period 15–19 for broad occupational, or rather socio-economic, populations. Here it is seen that the rates for professional and salaried persons, skilled labor, and unskilled labor groups are almost identical in the age period 15–19 but that they diverge widely thereafter, the rates being much higher in the unskilled labor group than in the skilled labor group and the rates for both of these groups being higher than for the professional and salaried group. Similarly in the United States, the age curves for rural and urban and wage-earning populations, as plotted in Figure 5, exhibit differences which reflect the influence of environment to such an extent that the bundle of conditions which we connote under that term appears distinctly as the major factor. A study of the age curves of urban and rural populations in the

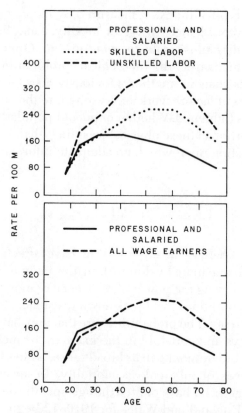

Figure 4   Death rate from phthisis in certain occupational groups, England and Wales, 1910–12.

different states, which is too detailed to present here, point to the same conclusion.

Frankel,[13] in a recent address before this Association, referred in some detail to the extraordinarily interesting and unpremeditated experiment which occurred at the close of the world war when the German people, affected by lack of nutritious diet, by strain and by other unfavorable conditions, were in striking contrast to the American people not so affected and in fact more than usually favored. The tuberculosis death rate in both populations had been steadily declining for generations, but at this juncture in Germany it not only ceased to decline but rose sharply and continued on a relatively high level for several years until economic

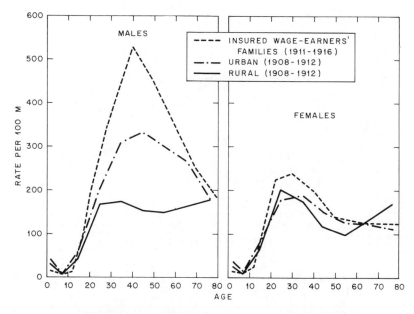

Figure 5   Mortality from pulmonary tuberculosis, 1908–1912 among rural, urban, and wage earning groups.

conditions were improved; in the United States, on the other hand, the decline in the tuberculosis death rate was accelerated.

If we had suitable data, a direct correlation between periods of arrested or rising tuberculosis incidence in certain groups and periods of economic depression, and the obverse, doubtless could be found for the United States. We have made a preliminary attempt to do this with such records as are available. The result is not statistically demonstrable but it may be of sufficient interest to portray it graphically. In the upper section of Figure 6 the annual mortality rates for tuberculosis in Massachusetts have been plotted for 1857–1923 and a smooth curve has been drawn through the points. The annual deviations from the smooth line, which we may call the trend, have been magnified in the lower section of Figure 6 and it is evident that a series of rises and falls, each lasting several years, occurred about the trend, here shown as a horizontal line. For graphical purposes a smooth line has been drawn through these deviations and a picture of a wave-like varia-

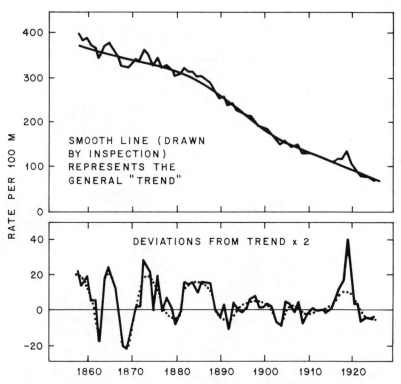

Figure 6   Mortality from pulmonary tuberculosis, 1857–1926 in Massachusetts.

tion is the result. In the upper section of Figure 7 have been plotted the annual deviations from an index of "normal" business activity in the United States for the same period. (A dotted line showing annual variations in unemployment in Massachusetts in the years for which unemployment records were available clearly exhibits an inverse relationship to business activity.) These deviations from "normal" in business activity also present the picture of wave-like variations so familiar to economic students, the troughs of the waves indicating periods of economic financial depressions. Now if we place these two series of waves in juxtaposition, as has been done in the lower section of Figure 7, and allow for a "lag," as reasonably we should do, the resulting sketch (I shall not call it by a name denoting any greater precision) portrays in a very

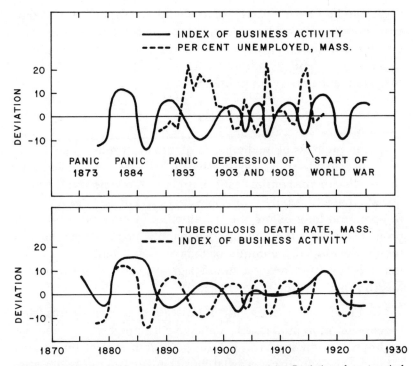

Figure 7   Mortality from tuberculosis and industrial activity. Deviations from trend of death rate in Massachusetts compared with deviations of business activity from estimated normal.

interesting fashion, even with crude data, a fairly regular inverse historical relation between industrial activity and tuberculosis mortality.

Out of all the discussion of the association between tuberculosis incidence and poverty it is perfectly clear to those who are engaged in anti-tuberculosis work that among persons who are below a certain economic level and having similar inheritance of physiological resistance, relatively slight further depressions of economic status will be reflected in increased tuberculosis incidence and mortality unless poverty is compensated by some special protection from those conditions that lower resistance. In fact, our measures for the prevention of tuberculosis consist, in effect, largely of alterations in the environment of those who are threatened with the disease, of removing conditions that accompany poverty and replacing them with conditions that constitute economic well-being, with of course relatively greater emphasis upon those specific conditions which lessen the opportunity for infection and strengthen pulmonary resistance.

VII

If the progress of medicine, in its broadest sense, be considered in true historical perspective, it will be evident even to those who are most enthusiastic over the achievements of the last decade that anti-tuberculosis measures of no mean potency were in operation long before the recollection of most of us. We are prone to overlook their importance in our concentration upon the highly developed technique of today. In substantiation of this reminder I venture to quote from a page of a Massachusetts annual health report written 60 years ago:[14]

> From some causes, or combination of causes, deaths from consumption in Massachusetts have diminished . . . , and the improvement seems to be still going on. It is of the utmost importance to discover what these causes are; but here statistics fail us, and we are left to conjecture. Our own belief is that they are to be found *in the advance of medical science,* which has given to physicians a better knowledge of the nature of the disease, derived from pathology; a better mode of treatment, derived from the careful observation of cases, and from modern discoveries in chemistry and physiology; and a greatly improved acquaintance with the means by which consumption may be avoided by those predisposed to it by inheritance, derived from all these sources combined.
>
> This knowledge is becoming diffused among the people, so that all intelligent persons now know more about the prevention of consumption than the wisest physicians knew fifty years ago.
>
> Fresh air by day and by night, strong and nourishing food, dry soil on which to live, sunlight, and warm clothing, are the means of saving many lives which would have been

hopelessly lost in the preceding generation. If our conjectures are correct this improvement may be expected to continue, and everybody can help to make it greater. Ventilate the school-rooms, and the workshops, and the stores, and the houses; in cold weather let the air, comfortably and equally warmed, be generously supplied from without in a constantly flowing current. Let those who can provide it in their homes remember that an open fire, which sends two-thirds of the heat up the chimney, furnishes the best ventilation for a room of moderate size which the ingenuity of man has yet devised, and that the heat escaping by the flue is the price to be paid for it. Let in the sunlight, and never mind the carpets: better they should fade than the health of the family. When a man proposes to build a dwelling in a swamp warn him of his danger.

I submit that this is pretty sound anti-tuberculosis doctrine today. The historian who arbitrarily marks the beginning of the "modern" campaign against the disease at 1890 or 1900 with the mischievous idea of "proving" that the death rate from tuber-culosis declined as rapidly before as it did after, may with consid-erable profit study the public health documents and medical writings of even earlier days than sixty years ago. It ought to be evident to any one who has mastered the simplest elements of history that no social habit, such as the protection of public health, bound up as it is in the evolution of several basic sciences, in the revolution of political and social ideals and economic standards, and in the development of industrial processes, is started sud-denly by the passing of a resolution or by an executive command or even by a scientist's discovery.

VIII

With the certainty that all of these factors—and probably many more—are involved in the decline of the tuberculosis death rate, let us take another telescopic glance and indulge in a brief retro-spect. For pictorial purposes I have chosen the course of the tu-berculosis death rate in Baltimore since 1812, the date being ex-

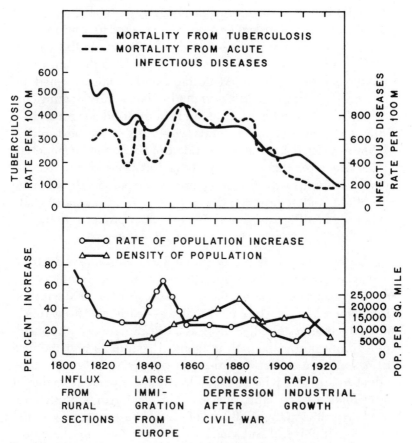

Figure 8   The course of tuberculosis mortality in Baltimore, 1812–1925.

tracted from Howard.[3] The general course of tuberculosis mortality has been plotted in Figure 8 together with certain other facts.

   In the decade 1800–1810 the population of Baltimore increased very rapidly, the augmentation being from adjacent rural
sections and Europe. The tuberculosis death rate was extraordinarily high, even if we allow for considerable inclusions of other
causes under this title. From 1810 to 1840 was a period of greatly
diminished population growth, no marked increase in density of
population, a decline in the death rate from the disease, and in
general by economic progress and prosperity. In the decade

1840–1850, however, a great immigration from Europe occurred, chiefly of economically unfortunate families, which resulted in a marked increase of population density. This was accompanied by an aggravation of insanitary conditions, as is evidenced by the greatly increased incidence of infectious diseases. It is true that the high incidence of these diseases was due partly to the introduction of yellow fever and diphtheria, but they are grouped together for the reason that, whether they included one disease or another, they reflect the existence of conditions that were favorable to the spread of disease. The period 1840–1880 was marked not only by these conditions but also by economic conditions that were distinctly unfavorable to the health of a large portion of the urban population.

It is hard for us in this era to realize the conditions of life in our rapidly growing cities in the middle of the nineteenth century. Our forefathers boasted of democracy, but there was a wide social gap between those who had been financially endowed by preceding generations and the professional and trade groups, on the one hand, and the working classes, on the other hand, that we in this day can scarcely appreciate. All lacked most of the knowledge of hygiene which now is taken for granted, but the wage earner and his family were relatively more ignorant. Their hours of work were unbelievably long; houses were insanitary and crowded; food was less varied. Today we bemoan the passing of the handcrafts and of the artisan who was an artist; yet there are some things which compensate for the monotony of specialization. The son of the tailor, the grinder, the printer, the blacksmith had less choice of a vocation then than now. He was apprenticed to his trade whether he was physically suited to it or not.

Between 1880 and 1890 the tuberculosis death rate as well as the death rate from acute infectious diseases began to decline rapidly. The tuberculosis rate continued to decline for a decade; then its rate of decrease slackened during a period of accelerated industrial expansion. This period, near the end of the nineteenth and in the first decade of the twentieth century was another time in which health was sacrificed to ideals of business success. But with this difference from the period preceding: that a strong movement, partly within the ranks of the workers and partly composed of a vigorous humanitarian contingent of thinkers, was started to ameliorate the economic, working, and living conditions of the wage-earning population. Even those of us who are not beyond middle age can recall this awakening, the insistence of this protest against what was termed "industrial slavery." By 1910 the public's conception of the "rights of the workingman" had changed notably. The employer, who had by that time become the gigantic corporation, discovered an "enlightened selfishness." Wages were increased slowly, hours of work reduced gradually, the homes of wage earners were opened to altruistic inquiry, investigation after investigation followed, and by 1915 the popular idea of what ought to be and could be a reasonable standard of life had undergone a radical revision. This was followed by the marvelous improvement in the economic status and the life of the wage earner made possible by the extraordinary prosperity after the first financial shock of the World War.

The effect of this combination of factors upon the tuberculosis death rate may be indicated more precisely by examining the specific sex-age curves at decennial intervals in Massachusetts from 1870 to 1920, which is shown in the accompanying chart (Figure 9). If we compare the *rate of decline* in the mortalities of the two sexes at different ages, the interesting fact is brought out that the male rates, especially in the ages 30–69, declined much more slowly than the corresponding female rates, thus suggesting the hindering influence of those factors which bore more directly upon adult males than upon females. The greatest divergences in the rates was about 1910. Since that time, the decrease in the rate for males of working ages has been even greater than in the rates for other ages of the same sex and for females. The same result is evidenced in the sex-age curves for a larger area, as shown in Figure 10. For 1905 and 1915 the age curves for males, particularly in the wage earning ages, were almost identical; in 1925, the curve had shown an extraordinary decline from either 1915 or 1905, whereas the curve for females exhibited a fairly consistent drop at each decade.

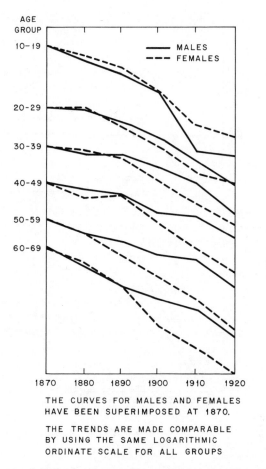

Figure 9   The rate of decline in tuberculosis mortality among males and females in Massachusetts, 1870–1920.

IX

The decline of the tuberculosis death rate is so merged into the current of our social, economic and scientific history that it has become indistinguishable from other forces which have made up the evolution of modern social ideals and the industrial revolution. The reduction of mortality from the disease undoubtedly has

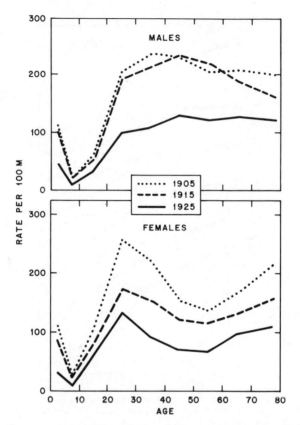

Figure 10 Sex-age curves of tuberculosis mortality, 1908, 1915, and 1925. Mean of rates for N.Y., Conn., Ind., and Mich.

been helped by some of the very conditions attending the urbanization of the population that were concomitant with conditions which anti-tuberculosis efforts tried to ameliorate. Such a net result, for example, may be a tubercularization of city people. It has been helped by the development of public health administration, particularly by the control of infectious diseases and by the efforts to lessen infant mortality. It has been helped by the emergence of new standards of living, of humane as well as efficient conditions of labor, of ideals of play and recreation, of an esthetic as well as an utilitarian emphasis upon physical health. On the other hand, directed as the anti-tuberculosis movement must be against poverty, overcrowding, ignorance, and insanitary environment in order fully to attain its aim, it has contributed to this betterment of mankind in more ways than the reduction of tuberculosis infection, the prevention of active cases, the arresting of the disease in affected persons, the prolongation of the lives of serious cases and the promotion of general as well as personal hygiene. It was in the vanguard of public health work in its earlier years along with efforts to control the visitation of dreadful epidemics and it has proved to be the leader in the modern movement of preventive medicine.

Except by scientifically, coldly planned and delicately conducted experiments in populations of human beings, we shall not be able to evaluate accurately the *specific* public health effort which we call anti-tuberculosis work. Until that is done, it seems to me that we ought to be satisfied with a real and vitally important participation in the forces that are guiding and making mankind to progress.

Notes and References

1. This record is based on Bills of Mortality in London from 1631 down to the beginning of death registration in 1838, and after 1838 on the vital statistics of England and Wales. Brownlee who first presented in his "Investigation into the Epidemiology of Phthisis in Great Britain and Ireland," a series of proportionate mortalities computed from the statistics afforded by these Bills of Mortality, was fully aware of their diagnostic shortcomings, but after a careful review of the medical writings and an examination of the original documents came to the conclusion that, taken in perspective rather than in detail, the ratios reflected roughly the real course of the disease as manifested in mortality. In the accompanying graph I have used Brownlee's ratios until the beginning of the nineteenth century, and have plotted the indicated tuberculosis mortality rate at successive periods from 1801 to 1838, using the gross death rates for England and Wales when available and applying the proportions due to phthisis for London. The two curves—for proportionate mortality in London and for the phthisis rate in England and Wales—roughly parallel each other for the period. From 1838 the recorded phthisis rate for England and Wales is plotted.

   This record is a rough one, it is true, but in general the main variations in the curve seem to reflect the actual changes in the phthisis rate.

   It may be of interest to note also that in Vienna the tuberculosis mortality

rate rose from 5.3 per 1,000 in 1752–4 to 8.6 in 1867–70, thereafter showing a
steady decline (S. Peller: Ztchr. f. Hyg. u. Infektions–Krankh., 1920, xix, 227.)
and that in Sweden, as Greenwood has shown, there was an increase in
phthisis mortality from 1751–60 (at least) until 1821–30 (Journ. Royal Stat.
Soc. July, 1924, p. 520).

2. Hoffman, F. L.: The decline in the tuberculosis death rate, 1871–1912. Transactions of the Ninth Annual Meeting (1913), National Association for the Study and Prevention of Tuberculosis, pp. 114; 130–135.

3. Howard, William Travis, Jr.: Public health administration and the natural history of disease in Baltimore, Md. 1797–1920.

4. Greenwood, M.: The vital statistics of Sweden and England and Wales: An essay in international comparison. Jour. Royal Stat. Soc. July, 1924, p. 527. The remark quoted does not, of course, suggest the value of Dr. Greenwood's inquiry which will repay careful study by those who are seeking methods for scientific comparisons of mortality rates among different populations.

5. Pearl, Raymond: The biology of death. Scientific Monthly, September, 1921, pp. 196–200.

6. Sydenstricker, Edgar: The measurement of public health work—An introductory discussion. Reprinted from the annual report of the Milbank Memorial Fund, 1926.

7. It is important to have clearly in mind just what the *death* rate from a disease actually means. We assume, of course, that the deaths are recorded with *reasonable* accuracy and that this classification, so far as tuberculosis is concerned, is also reasonably accurate or at least that it follows a fairly constant procedure over the period under consideration. We know that this record has serious lacunae and that their classification possesses serious faults but we have reason to believe that they are trustworthy enough for general purposes. Of more importance is the consideration that the death rate from a given disease measures neither (a) the incidence of infection if it be an infectious disease, nor (b) the prevalence of the disease since the *fatality rate* may vary 1) according to natural or acquired resistance of the persons affected 2) care of the case and 3) the severity of the infection or reactivation which in turn may depend (a) the amount of dosage and (b) environmental conditions affecting resistance, etc. At best, a specific mortality rate is an expression of the *net* effect of a disease upon a population n terms of loss of human life.

8. Jennings, H. S.: Public health progress and race progress—are they incompatible? Proceedings of the 23rd Annual Meeting of the National Tuberculosis Association, 1927.

9. The high mortality among the Irish, which has been commented upon since the days they first began their conquest of Boston, has come to be regarded as an Irish characteristic. It may be; but our conclusions on this point ought to be tempered, at best, by two considerations of no little significance: 1) that Irish immigrants have come mainly from rural areas in their own land into the heart of our urban centers where they quickly mingled with our population and

were peculiarly unfortunate in their economic condition and 2) that the later tuberculosis death rate among the Irish where they are removed from the extremely unfavorable environmental conditions under which they first lived, is not far above that of native born Americans.

10. Dublin, Louis I., and Baker: Mortality of race stocks in New York and Pennsylvania, volume 17, No. 129, March 1921—Statistical Quarterly Publication of the American Statistical Association.

11. Collis, Edgar L.: (Report on Tuberculosis–Silicosis as revised by the Correspondence Committee on Industrial Hygiene of the International Labor Office) International Labor Office, Brochure No. 62. Geneva, 1926.

12. Sydenstricker, Edgar and Gover, Mary: Data presented at the Society of Hygiene, Johns Hopkins University, to be published.

13. Frankel, Lee L.: The evidence of intensive anti-tuberculosis effort upon the death rate. Proceedings of the 17th Annual Meeting, National Tuberculosis Association, 1921.

14. Twenty-sixth Report to the Legislature of Massachusetts, 1867.

5

The Decline
in the Tuberculosis Death Rate
in Cattaraugus County
EDGAR SYDENSTRICKER

During the past five years a public anti-tuberculosis program has
been developed in Cattaraugus County, New York, by the Board
of Health of that County, that, according to the judgment of competent critics, embodies and practices modern principles and
procedures of tuberculosis prevention, relief and cure.

During the same period and in the same area all five annual
death rates from tuberculosis have been lower than the rates as
predicted from the experience of the previous twenty-two years.
For each of the last three years the tuberculosis death rate has
been lower than in any year of its previous recorded history which
goes back as far as 1900. Furthermore these three successive low
rates constitute an event which has not been paralleled in this area
since 1900.

To most persons, especially to those who are conversant with
the modern anti-tuberculosis program, this decline will appear as
a result due in large measure to the development of an efficient
public health administration in Cattaraugus County, more particularly of its anti-tuberculosis work. For, the prolongation of the
lives of tuberculous individuals, the prevention of new cases, and
the arresting of incipient cases, by modern methods of controlling
the disease, are well established facts in the experience of those
who are intimately engaged in these activities. But to the coldly
scientific mind, accustomed to caution and trained in the habit of

doubt, any conclusion as to a causal relationship between the two series of events should rest on more complete evidence and should be established by more elaborate methods of appraisal. The situation may be likened to that in which the laboratory worker finds himself. He may be honestly convinced of the soundness of his hypothesis and of the accuracy of his results but at the same time he realizes that his work must stand the test of scientific scrutiny not only for his own intellectual satisfaction but also in order that it may be established in other critical minds.

In a sense, therefore, the tuberculosis experience of Cattaraugus County, as well as that of any area or population group, may be regarded as an "experiment" in that it requires the application of the principles and the methods of scientific experimentation in measuring results of a specific factor especially when that factor has been deliberately introduced in order to bring about a definite result.*

The measurement of the results of anti-tuberculosis efforts, however, is not an easy task. We are accustomed to attempt it in terms of mortality, although we realize, or ought to realize, that a death rate is a poor index of what we are trying to evaluate. It is a faulty statistic for the reason that it may indicate on the one hand the prevalence of the disease, and on the other hand its fatality. It measures neither the one nor the other accurately. Furthermore, the annual number of deaths is so small in an area the size of Cattaraugus County as to be subject to wide variation from fortuitous circumstances. Again, it is a poor measure because the greatest emphasis in an anti-tuberculosis program is on preventing the disease, and on arresting it in those persons in whom the tubercle has been activated; the tuberculosis death rate can therefore measure only a fraction of the full force of the campaign. Moreover, in the measurement of anti-tuberculosis efforts we observe the effects of various preventive and curative activities upon a stream of many continuous cases, each of which has its own course over a period of time. From this point of view the measurement of anti-tuberculosis work in adolescent and adult ages

*Annual Report, Milbank Memorial Fund, 1926, Part II: The Measurement of the Results of Public Health Work.

should be by different methods from those by which we measure an effort to prevent a definite event, such as a case of diphtheria or a death from measles. For the anti-tuberculosis campaign is not an effort directed toward a single objective; its objectives are several, each calling for a different kind of activity. It includes efforts to prevent incipient tuberculosis, to prevent the development of incipient cases into more serious stages; to arrest active cases, and to relieve cases in very advanced stages, and so far as possible to prolong their lives also. Obviously any single measure is inadequate for evaluating precisely the complete results of so varied a program.

In reviewing the experience thus far of Cattaraugus County, therefore, it is essential to keep in mind that the mortality rate for a period as short as three years, or even as five years, can reflect the results of specifically those anti-tuberculosis activities which affect the prolongation of lives of tuberculous individuals. In other words, the tuberculosis mortality rate in so limited a period can measure, and with a fair degree of definiteness, the effect of public health efforts upon the *fatality* of active cases only, rather than the activities that seek to prevent incipient cases or new "active" cases.

With the limitations set before us by these necessary definitions, it is proper to examine the tuberculosis death rates of Cattaraugus County from at least two points of view: (a) the statistical significance of the decline in the gross rate, and (b) the nature of the decline as indicated by the changes in the rates among persons of different ages. Other analyses of the mortality record will be made later when further experience is available, and the case and morbidity data are now being studied for the purpose of ascertaining more precisely the results of other kinds of anti-tuberculosis activities.

So far as we know, no marked change in the ordinary conditions that affect the tuberculosis death rate, other than those which were generally prevalent and common to similar communities, has occurred in Cattaraugus County in the five years 1923–1927. Provisionally at least, therefore, we are warranted in assuming that the only factor of major importance, so far as possible effects upon the tuberculosis death rate are concerned, was the development of a modern anti-tuberculosis administration during this period.

Now in judging of the statistical significance of the decline in the tuberculosis death rate in Cattaraugus County in 1925–1927, we have so far attempted to answer three questions: 1) Could any of these low rates have been a variation arising solely from the small numbers involved, since only about 30 deaths have occurred in each of the three years? 2) Do these three rates constitute a unique occurrence judging by past variations in the tuberculosis rates in Cattaraugus County itself? 3) Is the Cattaraugus County experience of the past three years unique in comparison with generally similar areas in the same period.

The data for Cattaraugus County are given in the accompanying table (Table I) together with certain explanations as to the sources of the statistics used and certain corrections and eliminations made in order to render the statistics as comparable as possible throughout the period covered.

In applying any one of these tests, it is necessary to ascertain as accurately as possible what the trend of the tuberculosis death rate was in Cattaraugus prior to 1923, as well as in other counties with which comparisons were made. For Cattaraugus County it was found that the tuberculosis death rate since 1900 had been practically on a level* with annual variations above and below this level which is indicated by the straight line on the accompanying chart (Figure 1). The experience of Cattaraugus was unusual in this respect. For in twelve other counties with whose tuberculosis mortality rates a comparison is made later in this report, the mortality was higher at the beginning of the period and a definite decline is shown since 1900. Why Cattaraugus has had such a favorable rate, we are unable to say until certain inquiries now under way may afford some explanation. But, feeling assured that the mortality record is reasonably accurate, this fact need not concern us here except in a respect which may be stated as follows: The intensive anti-tuberculosis work in Cattaraugus County was undertaken in an area where the death rate from the disease was already relatively low and had been on a low level for some

---

*A straight line fitted to the rates for 1900–1922 showed that the slope (value of b) was -0.33 ± 0.09 per 100,000 per year.

TABLE I   Mortality from tuberculosis in Cattaraugus County, 1900-1927

In the following table are given the data upon which the tuberculosis mortality rates for Cattaraugus County for 1900–1927 are based. The deaths of Indians are excluded for the reasons that it is believed that registration of deaths among Indians on the reservation situated in the County has been incomplete and that the Indian population has not been included in the health activities of the County. The Indian population has been deducted in the manner stated in a footnote. Deaths of non-residents in the J. N. Adam Memorial Hospital at Perrysburg, which is primarily an institution for residents of Buffalo, have been excluded, but no other correction for residence of decedents has been made.

	POPULATION				DEATHS			
Year	Total (1)	Exclusive of Indians (2)	Indians (3)	Non-residents (4)	Total Indians and non-residents	Total (5)	Net including Indians and non-residents	Death rate per 100,000
1900	65,645	64,645	3		3	57	54	83.5
1901	65,673	64,673	3		3	49	46	71.1
1902	65,701	64,701	3		3	41	38	58.7
1903	65,729	64,729	3		3	37	34	52.5
1904	65,757	64,757	3		3	50	47	72.6
1905	65,785	64,785	3		3	48	45	69.5
1906	65,813	64,813	3		3	58	55	83.9
1907	65,841	64,841	3		3	61	58	89.4
1908	65,869	64,869	3		3	63	60	92.5
1909	65,897	64,897	3		3	43	40	61.6
1910	66,035	65,035	3		3	61	58	89.2
1911	66,592	65,592	3		3	53	50	76.2
1912	67,148	66,148	3		3	46	43	65.0
1913	67,705	66,705	3	1	4	56	52	77.9
1914	68,262	67,262	3	1	4	59	55	81.8
1915	68,818	67,818	3	2	5	39	34	50.1
1916	69,375	68,375	0	5	5	53	48	70.2
1917	69,932	68,932	3	4	7	54	47	68.2
1918	70,488	69,488	1	3	4	57	53	76.3
1919	71,045	70,045	4	4	8	48	40	57.1
1920	71,546	70,546	4	7	11	52	41	58.1
1921	72,000	71,000	2	4	6	58	52	73.2
1922	72,453	71,453	3	15	18	66	48	67.2
1923	72,907	71,907	3	9	12	61	49	68.1
1924	73,360	72,360	4	14	18	64	46	63.6
1925	73,814	72,814	2	14	16	49	33	45.3
1926	74,267	73,267	5	25	30	62	32	43.7
1927	74,720	73,720	3	25	28	59	31	42.1

(1) Population estimates on following basis: Period 1900–1920, on Federal censuses; 1920–1925, on Federal census of 1920 and State census of 1925.

(2) Assumed deduction of Indian population: 1,000 annually. Census enumeration showed the Indian population to be 1104 in 1900, 1013 in 1910 and 1162 in 1920 (XX Census Volume III: 678).

(3) For period 1900–1915, number of deaths of Indians estimated at 3 annually.

(4) Non-residents dying at the J. N. Adam Memorial Hospital in Perrysburg.

(5) Mortality data from the following sources: Period 1900–1914 from U. S. Mortality Statistics: 1915–1924, from New York State Department of Health; 1925–1927, from Cattaraugus County Department of Health.

years, and the further reduction of the death rate under such conditions becomes an experiment of unusual interest. Now, if no change in the trend of tuberculosis mortality had occurred subsequent to 1922, we would expect the value of this level to be about 67† per 100,000 in 1925–1927. As a matter of fact, the actual rates (45.3, 43.7 and 42.1) were from 34 to 37 per cent below the expected trend values.

†66.8 ± 6.4 for 1926, using .67449 of $\sqrt{\dfrac{pq}{n}}$ where n = estimated population as of July 1, 1926.

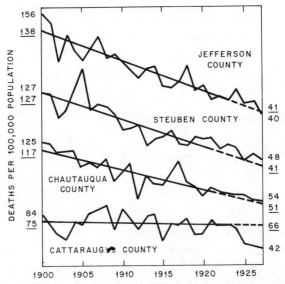

Figure 1   Deaths from tuberculosis, all forms, in Cattaraugus County and in three other counties in New York State, per 100,000 population, 1900–1927. The straight lines indicate the trend of the death rate based on the period 1900–1922.

Applying the first test, the probability that rates in three successive years as far below the trend values as the observed deviations would occur, as a result of fluctuations due to small numbers, is about 4 in a million. So that the decline can not be ascribed to these "chance" fluctuations.

Applying the second method, the probability that rates in three successive years as far below the trend values as the observed deviations would occur, using the annual deviations in the period 1900–1922 as the basis, is about 1 in 100,000.* In other words, if we can apply the theory of probability to such a problem as this, and assuming the independence of the events considered (and, statistically speaking, they may be so assumed), the occurrence of three rates as low as these for 1925–1927 may be judged as constituting a distinctly unique event.

Applying the third method we have used very roughly as

*The value of *sigma* of annual deviations from the trend of the rates per 100,000 in 1900–1922 is 11.34.

TABLE II   Mortality from tuberculosis (all forms) at different ages in
Cattaraugus County in 1916-1924 and 1925-1927

[*Indian deaths and non-residents dying at the
J. N. Adam Memorial Hospital are excluded.*]

Age	Rate per 100,000		Total number of deaths		Population estimated July 1	
	1916-24	1925-27	1916-24	1925-27	1920	1926
All ages	67.1	43.7	426	96	70,546	73,267
0–4	14.5	14.5	9	3	6,913	6,887
5–9	15.0	0	9	0	6,673	7,143
10–19	35.3	12.5	40	5	12,577	13,342
20–29	129.3	59.0	127	19	10,912	10,741
30–39	121.1	78.8	110	25	10,095	10,580
40–49	61.6	66.6	47	18	8,478	9,005
50–59	65.3	42.1	41	9	6,977	7,122
60–69	53.4	51.7	23	8	4,790	5,158
70 & over	67.4	81.1	19	8	3,131	3,290
Unknown			1	1		

"controls," twelve other counties in New York State, namely, Otsego, Ontario, Delaware, Fulton, Chenango, Columbia, Herkimer, Montgomery, Tompkins, Steuben, Chautauqua and Jefferson. A preliminary selection of these counties was made on the grounds that they were generally comparable with Cattaraugus in that they did not contain any cities with a population of 50,000 or over, had established a county tuberculosis sanitorium during the period of consideration (1900–1927), do not constitute or contain a suburban area, and included no State institutions or large private sanatoria. The annual variations were considered in the same way as those for Cattaraugus County. On the accompanying diagram three of them have been plotted as illustrations (Figure 1). A preliminary analysis indicates that the rates for 1925, 1926 and 1927 in these twelve counties were either above or not significantly below the expected rate for these years.*

The latter comparison has not been carried to the point of completion by any means. In order that more precise and complete comparisons will be possible, it is expected to refine them and to continue them in ensuing years, to study the comparability, in important respects, of these counties, as well as possibly other

---

*For Tompkins County each of the tuberculosis death rates as recorded for 1924–1927 was below the trend value but the difference in each instance was not statistically significant. Taking the four successive rates together, however, an apparently significant change is indicated.

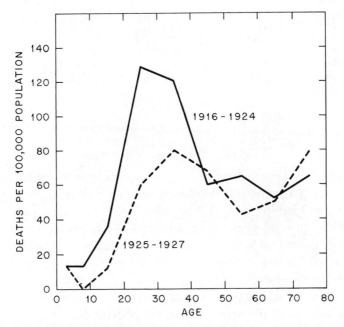

Figure 2   Deaths from tuberculosis, all forms, by age groups in Cattaraugus County, per 100,000 population, in 1916–1924 and 1925–1927.

areas, with Cattaraugus; and to obtain data on the character and volume of the anti-tuberculosis work in some of the counties generally comparable in other relevant respects with Cattaraugus County.

Of greater significance, in the writer's opinion, than the results of purely statistical tests, such as the first two employed in the foregoing paragraphs, is the fact that the decrease in the Cattaraugus County tuberculosis death rate has taken place in the younger ages. This fact is clearly indicated by the accompanying table and diagram (Table II and Figure 2) which compare the mean annual rates for 1916–1924 with those for 1925–1927 at different ages. The actual changes in the rates, as well as the relative changes, were as shown in the accompanying table (Table III).

The rate among children under 5 years of age shows no

**TABLE III   Changes in the mean annual
tuberculosis death rate by age groups in
Cattaraugus County 1916-1924 over
1925-1927**

Age group	Actual change in rate per 100,000	Relative change per cent
Under 5	0	0
5–9	−15.0	−100
10–19	−22.8	− 64
20–29	−70.3	− 54
30–39	−42.3	− 35
40–49	+ 5.0	+ 8
50–59	−23.1	− 35
60–69	− 1.7	− 3
70 and over	+13.7	+ 20

change, but it was already low in comparison with other areas,* the largest number of deaths in any year during the period 1916–1927 having been 3. The decreases in the succeeding age periods up to 40 years were considerable and were consistent. This is in contrast to the absence of such changes in the older age periods (40 years and over). If we make a division of the ages in three groups—under 5 years, 5 to 40 years, and 40 years and over—which is roughly characteristic of the ways the disease manifests itself in different periods of life, the decline in the tuberculosis rate in 1925–1927 was confined to the ages of later childhood, adolescence, and young adults, the decrease amounting to about 50 per cent of the mean rate for the previous nine years, and being in itself statistically significant.†

*For example: the 1924 rate among white persons under 5 years of age in the registration states of 1920 was 38 per 100,000; the 1925 rate among all persons under 5 years of age in New York State (exclusive of New York City) was 40 per 100,000.

†Since the downward trend of tuberculosis mortality for all ages in the period 1916–1922 was of negligible importance, and since no definite trend was indicated for the rates at any age, the comparison made above seems justifiable. The difference in the mean rates for the ages 5–39 years is 8 times its probable error, as shown below:

MEAN ANNUAL RATE PER 100,000

Age group	1916–1924	1925–1927	Difference
0–4	14.5	14.5	0.0
5–39	78.9±3.1	39.1±3.8	39.8±4.9
40+	61.8±3.7	58.3±6.0	3.5±7.0

It may be stated that most of the differences in the mean rates for the more refined age groups in the ages 5–39 are also statistically significant when judged according to their ratios to their probable errors, and that the age distributions of the deaths in the two periods (using the quinquennial and decennial divisions) are significantly different when the Chi Square test is applied.

Milbank Memorial Fund Quarterly Bulletin April, 1928

A Bibliography of the Writings of

Edgar Sydenstricker

Compiled by Richard V. Kasius

1914 School History of Virginia. (With A. L. Burger) Lynchburg, Dulaney-Boatwright Co., 1914.

1915 A Brief History of Taxation in Virginia. Richmond, The Legislative Reference Bureau of Virginia, 1915.

The Prevalence of Pellagra. Its Possible Relation to the Rise in the Cost of Food. Public Health Reports, 1915, 30: 3132 – 3147.

1916 Health Insurance, Its Relation to the Public Health. (With B. S. Warren) Treasury Department, U.S. Public Health Service, Public Health Bulletin No. 76. Washington, Government Printing Office, 1916.

Collective Bargaining in the Anthracite Coal Industry. Bureau of Labor Statistics, U.S. Department of Labor, Bulletin 191. Washington, Government Printing Office, 1916.

The Settlement of Disputes Under Agreements in the Anthracite Industry. Journal of Political Economy, 1916, 24:254–283.

Statistics of Disabiity. A Compilation of Some of the Data Available in the United States. (With B. S. Warren) Public Health Reports, 1916, 31: 989 – 999.

Health of Garment Wrokers. The Relation of Economic Status to Health. (With B. S. Warren) Public Health Reports, 1916, 31: 1298 – 1305.

1917 Conditions of Labor in American Industries, a Summarization of the Results of Recent Investigations. (With W. J. Lauck) New York, Funk and Wagnalls Co., 1917.

1918 Morbidity Statistics of War Industries Needed. (With B. S. Warren) Public Health Reports, 1918, 33: 127 – 132.

A Study of the Diet of Nonpellagrous and of Pellagrous Households in Textile Mill Communities in South Carolina in 1916. (With J. Goldberger and G. A. Wheeler) Journal of the American Medical Association, 1918, 71: 944 – 949.

Disabling Sickness Among the Population of Seven Cotton Mill Villages of South Carolina in Relation to Family Income. (With G. A. Wheeler and J. Goldberger) Public Health Reports, 1918, 33: 2038 – 2051.

Preliminary Statistics of the Influenza Epidemic. Public Health Reports, 1918, 33: 2305 – 2321.

The Relation of Wages to the Public Health. (With B. S. Warren) American Journal of Public Health, 1918, 8: 883 – 887.

1919   Economic Pressure as a Factor in Venereal Disease. In: Proceedings of the National Conference of Social Work, 46th Annual Session, June 1 – 8, 1919. Chicago, National Conference of Social Work, 208 – 211.

Influenza in Maryland. Preliminary Statistics of Certain Localities. (With W. H. Frost) Public Health Reports, 1919, 34: 491 – 504.

Health Insurance, the Medical Profession, and the Public Health. Including the Results of a Study of Sickness Expectancy. (With B. S. Warren) Public Health Reports, 1919, 34: 775 – 789.

Epidemic Influenza in Foreign Countries. (With W. H. Frost) Public Health Reports, 1919, 34, 1361 – 1376.

1920   Difficulties in Computing Civil Death Rates for 1918, with Especial Reference to Epidemic Influenza. (With M. L. King) Public Health Reports, 1920, 35: 330 – 344.

A Study of the Relation of Diet to Pellagra Incidence in Seven Textile-Mill Communities of South Carolina in 1916. (With J. Goldberger and G. A. Wheeler) Public Health Reports, 1920, 35: 648 – 713.

Pellagra Incidence in Relation to Sex, Age, Season, Occupation, and "Disabling Sickness" in Seven Cotton-Mill Villages of South Carolina During 1916. (With J. Goldberger and G. A. Wheeler) Public Health Reports, 1920, 35: 1650 – 1664.

A Study of the Relation of Factors of a Sanitary Character to Pellagra Incidence in Seven Cotton-Mill Villages of South Carolina in 1916. (With J. Goldberger, G. A. Wheeler and R. E. Tarbett) Public Health Reports, 1920, 35: 1701 – 1714.

Some Possibilities in the Statistical Analysis of Case Reports of Venereal Diseases. (With C. C. Pierce) Public Health Reports, 1920, 35: 2046 – 2055.

A Study of the Relation of Family Income and Other Economic Factors to Pellagra Incidence in Seven Cotton-Mill Villages of South Carolina in 1916. (With J. Goldberger and G. A. Wheeler) Public Health Reports, 1920, 35: 2673 – 2714.

A Method of Classifying Families According to Incomes in Studies of Disease Prevalence. (With W. I. King) Public Health Reports, 1920, 35: 2829 – 2846.

Venereal Disease Incidence at Different Ages. A Tabulation of 8,413 Case Reports in Indiana. (With M. L. King) Public Health Reports, 1920, 35: 3091–3107.

Review of: Special Tables of Mortality from Influenza in Indiana, Kansas, and Piladelphia, Pa., September 1–December 1, 1918 (Washington, 1920). Quarterly Publication of the American Statistical Association, 1920, 17: 522 – 523.

1921 Industrial Establishment Disability Records as a Source of Morbidity Statistics. (With D. K. Brundage) Quarterly Publication of the American Statistical Association, 1921, 17: 584 – 598.

The Classification of the Population According to Income. (With W. I. King) Journal of Political Economy, 1921, 29: 571 – 591.

The Measurement of the Relative Economic Status of Families. (With W. I. King) Quarterly Publication of the American Statistical Association, 1921, 17: 842 – 857.

Variations in Case Fatality During the Influenza Epidemic of 1918. Public Health Reports, 1921, 36: 2201 – 2210.

1922 Sickness Records in Preventive Work. The Nation's Health, 1922, 4: 485 – 488.

Heights and Weights of School Children. A Study of the Heights and Weights of 14,335 Native White School Children in Maryland, Virginia, and North and South Carolina. (With T. Clark and S. D. Collins) Public Health Reports, 1922, 37: 1185 – 1205.

Mortality from Pulmonary Tuberculosis in Recent Years. The Variation in Its Course During the War and Its Decline Since 1918. (With R. H. Britten) Public Health Reports, 1922, 37: 2843 – 2858.

1923 Weight and Height as an Index of Nutrition. Weight and Height Measurements of 9,973 Children Classified upon Medical Examination as "Excellent," "Good," "Fair," or "Poor" in Nutrition as Judged from Clinical Evidence. (With T. Clark and S. D. Collins) Public Health Reports, 1923, 38: 39 – 58.

Indices of Nutrition. The Application of Certain Standards of Nutrition to 506 Native White Children Without Physical Defects and with "Good" or "Excellent" Nutrition as Judged from Clinical Evidence. (With T. Clark and S. D. Collins) Public Health Reports, 1923, 38: 1239 – 1270.

1924 The New Baldwin-Wood Weight-Height-Age Tables as an Index of Nutrition. The Application of the Baldwin-Wood Standard of Nutrition to 506 Native White Children Without Physical Defects and with "Good" or "Excellent" Nutrition as Judged from Clinical Evidence. (With T. Clark and S. D. Collins) Public Health Reports, 1924, 39: 518 – 525.

Disabling Sickness in Cotton Mill Communities of South Carolina in 1917. A Study of Sickness Prevalence and Absenteeism, As Recorded in Repeated Canvasses, in Relation to Seasonal Variation, Duration, Sex, Age, and Family Income. (With D. Wiehl) Public Health Reports, 1924, 39: 1417 – 1443.

A Study of the Incidence of Disabling Sickness in a South Carolina Cotton Mill Village in 1918. Based on Records of a Continuous Canvass of Households during the Period March 1 to November 30, 1918. (With D. Wiehl) Public Health Reports, 1924, 39: 1723 – 1738.

The Income Cycle in the Life of the Wage-Earner. (With W. I. King and D. Wiehl) Public Health Reports, 1924, 39: 2133 – 2140.

The Epidemic Outbreak in Japan. Public Health Reports, 1924, 39: 3125 – 3129.

The Outlook for International Vital Statistics. American Journal of Public Health, 1924, 14: 832 – 838.

Review of: I. S. Falk: Principles of Vital Statistics (Philadelphia, 1923). Journal of the American Statistical Association, 1924, 19: 420 – 421.

1925   Population Statistics of Foreign Countries. Journal of the American Statistical Association, 1925, 20: 80 – 89.

The Incidence of Illness in a General Population Group. General Results of a Morbidity Study from December 1, 1921, through March 31, 1924, in Hagerstown, Md. Public Health Reports, 1925, 40: 279 – 291.

A Brief Review of Vital Statistics. American Journal of Public Health, 1925, 15: 1086 – 1089.

1926   Studies in Regard to the Lighting of Post Offices, Made by the United States Public Health Service. (With J. E. Ives) Journal of Industrial Hygiene, 1926, 8: 232 – 248.

A Study of Illness in a General Population Group. Hagerstown Morbidity Studies No. I: The Method of Study and General Results. Public Health Reports, 1926, 41: 2069 – 2088.

The Reporting of Notifiable Diseases in a Typical Small City. Hagerstown Morbidity Studies No. II. Public Health Reports, 1926, 41: 2186 – 2191.

Review of: R. Pearl: The Biology of Population Growth (New York, 1925). Science, 1926, N.S. 64: 42 – 44.

1927   The Measurement of Results of Public Health Work. An Introductory Discussion. In: Milbank Memorial Fund Report for the Year Ended December 31, 1926. New York, Milbank Memorial Fund, 27 – 60.

The Declining Death Rate from Tuberculosis. In: Transactions of the Twenty-Third Annual Meeting. New York, National Tuberculosis Association, 1927, 102 – 124.

Epidemiological Study of Minor Respiratory Diseases. Progress Report II: Based on Records for Families of Medical Officers of the Army, Navy, and Public Health Service and of Members of Several University Faculties. (With J. G. Townsend) Public Health Reports, 1927, 42: 99 – 121.

The Extent of Medical and Hospital Service in A Typical Small City. Hagerstown Morbidity Studies No. III. Public Health Reports, 1927, 42: 121 – 131.

The Age Curve of Illness. Hagerstown Morbidity Studies No. IV. Public Health Reports, 1927, 42: 1565–1576.

A Comparison of the Incidence of Illness and Death. 1) By Cause and 2) By Age of Persons Affected. Hagerstown Morbidity Studies No. V. Public Health Reports, 1927, 42: 1689 – 1701.

The Illness Rate Among Males and Females. Hagerstown Morbidity Studies No. VI. Public Health Reports, 1927, 42: 1939 – 1957.

Pellagra in the Mississippi Flood Area. Report of an Inquiry Relating to the Prevalence of Pellagra in the Area Affected by the Overflow of the Mississippi and its Tributaries in Tennessee, Arkansas, Mississippi, and Louisiana in the Spring of 1927. (With J. Goldberger) Public Health Reports, 1927, 42: 2706 – 2725.

1928   Introduction to: Mortality Among Negroes in the United States. Treasury Department, U.S. Public Health Service, Public Health Bulletin No. 174. Washington, Government Printing Office, 1928, 1 – 2.

Introduction to: An Epidemiological and Statistical Study of Tonsillitis. Treasury Department, U.S. Public Health Service, Public Health Bulletin No. 175. Washington, Government Printing Office, 1928, 1 – 3.

The Statistician's Place in Public Health Work. Journal of the American Statistical Association, 1928, 23: 115 – 120.

The Statistical Evaluation of the Results of Social Experiments in Public Health. Journal of the American Statistical Association, Proceedings Supplement, 1928, 23: 155 – 165.

Is Diphtheria Still Declining? The Survey, 1928, 61: 77 – 78.

The Prevalence of Ill Health. Bulletin of the New York Academy of Medicine, 1928, 4: 191 – 215.

The Decline in the Tuberculosis Death Rate in Cattaraugus County. Milbank Memorial Fund Quarterly Bulletin, 1928, 6:41 – 50.

The Causes of Illness at Different Ages. Hagerstown Morbidity Studies No. VII. Public Health Reports, 1928, 43: 1067 – 1074.

The Incidence of Various Diseases According to Age. Hagerstown Morbidity Studies No. VIII. Public Health Reports, 1928, 43: 1124 – 1156.

Sex Differences in the Incidence of Certain Diseases at Different Ages. Hagerstown Morbidity Studies No. IX. Public Health Reports, 1928, 43: 1259 – 1276.

Review of: Sir Arthur Newsholme: Health Problems in Organized Society — Studies in Social Aspects of Public Health (London, 1927). Journal of the American Statistical Association, 1928, 23: 462 – 463.

1929   Tuberculosis Among Relatively Neglected Groups. In: Transactions of the Twenty-Fifth Annual Meeting. New York, National Tuberculosis Association, 1929, 262 – 274.

A Study of Endemic Pellagra in Some Cotton-Mill Villages of South Carolina, (With J. Goldberger, G. A. Wheeler and W. I. King) Treasury Department, U.S. Public Health Service, Hygienic Laboratory Bulletin No. 153. Washington, Government Printing Office, 1929.

The Trend of Tuberculosis Mortality in Rural and Urban Areas. American Review of Tuberculosis, 1929, 19: 461 – 482.

Completeness of Reporting of Measles, Whooping Cough, and Chicken Pox at Different Ages. Hagerstown Morbidity Studies: Supplement to Study No. II. (With A. W. Hedrich) Public Health Reports, 1929, 44: 1537–1543.

Economic Status and the Incidence of Illness. Hagerstown Morbidity Studies No. X: Gross and Specific Illness Rates by Age and Cause Among Persons Classified According to Family Economic Status. Public Health Reports, 1929, 44:1821 – 1833.

Differential Fertility According to Economic Status. Hagerstown Morbidity Studies No. XI: Live Birth and Still Birth Rates Among Married Women of Different Ages Classified According to Family Economic Condition. Public Health Reports, 1929, 44: 2101 – 2106.

1930   The Proposed Public Health Program for Ting Hsien, China, of the Chinese National Association of the Mass Education Movement in Collaboration with the Milbank Memorial Fund. Ting Hsien, 1930.

The Physical Impairments of Adult Life. General Results of a Statistical Study of Medical Examinations by the Life Extension Institute of 100,924 White Male Life Insurance Policy Holders Since 1921. (With R. H. Britten) American Journal of Hygiene, 1930, 11: 73 – 94.

The Physical Impairments of Adult Life. Prevalence at Different Ages, Based on Medical Examinations by the Life Extension Institute of 100, 924 White Male Life Insurance Policy Holders Since 1921. (With R. H. Britten) American Journal of Hygiene, 1930, 11: 95 – 135.

Differential Fertility According to Social Class. A Study of 69, 620 Native White Married Women Under 45 Years of Age Based Upon the United States Census Returns of 1910. (With F. W. Notestein) Journal of the American Statistical Association, 1930, 25: 9 – 32.

Physical Impairments and Occupational Class. Differential Rates Based Upon Medical Examinations of 100,924 Native-Born, Adult-White Insured Males. (With R. H. Britten) Public Health Reports, 1930, 45: 1927 – 1962.

Mortality from Influenza and Pneumonia in 50 Large Cities of the United States, 1910 – 1929. (With S. D. Collins, W. H. Frost and M. Gover) Public Health Reports, 1930, 45: 2277 – 2328.

1931   Age Incidence of Communicable Diseases in a Rural Population. (With S. D. Collins) Public Health Reports, 1931, 46: 100–113.

The Incidence of Influenza Among Persons of Different Economic Status During the Epidemic of 1918. Public Health Reports, 1931, 46'; 154 – 170.

Some Results of Tuberculosis Administration in Cattaraugus County, New York. (With J. Downes) Tubercle, 1931, 12: 1 – 17.

Some Results of Tuberculosis Administration in Cattaraugus County, New York. (With J. Downes) American Review of Tuberculosis, 1931, 23: 183 – 206.

1932	Statement. In: Medical Care for the American People, The Final Report of the Committee on the Costs of Medical Care. Chicago, The University of Chicago Press, 1932, 201.

A Study of the Fertility of Native White Women in a Rural Area of Western New York. Milbank Memorial Fund Quarterly Bulletin, 1932, 10: 17–32.

Statistics of Morbidity. Milbank Memorial Fund Quarterly Bulletin, 1932, 10: 101 – 119.

Effect of a Whooping Cough Epidemic Upon the Size of the Nonimmune Group in an Urban Community. Milbank Memorial Fund Quarterly Bulletin, 1932, 10: 302 – 314.

1933	Health and Environment. New York, McGraw-Hill Book Company, Inc., 1933.

Morbidity. In: Encyclopaedia of the Social Sciences, Vol. 11., ed. E. R. A. Seligman. New York, Macmillan Co., 1933, 3–7.

The Vitality of the American People. In: Recent Social Trends in the United States, Report of the President's Research Committee on Social Trends, Vol. I. New York, McGraw-Hill Book Company, Inc., 1933, 602 – 660.

Statistical Study of Arteriosclerosis. In: Arteriosclerosis, A Survey of the Problem, ed. E. V. Cowdrey. New York, Macmillan Co., 1933, 131–151.

Health and Nutrition in the Depression. In: Minutes of the 59th Meeting of the New Jersey Health and Sanitary Association, Nov. 24 – 25, 1933.

Why State Medicine is Necessary. Forum. 1933. 90: 47–51.

The Prevalence of Tuberculosis Infection in a Rural Community in New York State. (With J. Downes) Milbank Memorial Fund Quarterly Bulletin, 1933, 11: 221 – 232.

Health and the Depression. Milbank Memorial Fund Quarterly Bulletin, 1933, 11: 273 – 280.

Sickness and the Economic Depression. Preliminary Report on Illness in Families of Wage Earners in Birmingham, Detroit, and Pittsburgh. (With G. St. J. Perrott and S. D. Collins) Public Health Reports, 1933, 48: 1251 – 1264.

1934	A Study of Standards for Health Insurance. In: Social Security in the United States 1934. New York, American Association for Social Security, Inc., 79–88.

Changes in Family Income and Rental During the Economic Depression. (With G. St. J. Perrott) Journal of the American Statistical Association, Proceedings Supplement, 1934, 29: 43 – 46.

How Unemployment Affects Illness and Hospital Care. (With G. St. J. Perrott) Modern Hospital, 1934, 42: 41 – 44.

Group Medicine or Health Insurance. Which Comes First? American Labor Legislation Review, 1934, 24: 79 – 86.

What is Health Insurance–And Will it Work? Literary Digest, July 7, 1934. 118: 15.

Effect of Low Income on Health. (With G. St. J. Perrott) Journal of Home Economics, 1934, 26: 512.

Some Recent Studies on Differential Fertility in the United States. (With F. W. Notestein) Bulletin of the International Institute of Statistics, 1934, 28: 82 – 92.

Medical Practice and Public Needs. Transactions of the College of Physicians of Philadelphia, 1934, Series 4, 2: 21 – 30.

Sickness and the New Poor. Income and Health for 7500 Families, 1929 – 1933. Survey Graphic, 1934, 23: 160 – 162, 208.

Medical Care During the Depression. A Preliminary Report Upon a Survey of Wage-earning Families in Seven Large Cities. (With G. St. J. Perrott and S. D. Collins) Milbank Memorial Fund Quarterly, 1934, 12: 99 – 114.

Sickness, Unemployment, and Differential Fertility. (With G. St. J. Perrott) Milbank Memorial Fund Quarterly, 1934, 12: 126 – 133.

Health in the New Deal. Annals of the American Academy of Political and Social Science, 1934, 176: 131 – 137.

1935 The Changing Concept of Public Health. Milbank Memorial Fund Quarterly, 1935, 13: 301 – 310.

Health Insurance and the Public Health. Proceedings of the Academy of Political Science, 1935, 16: 284 – 292.

Causal and Selective Factors in Sickness. (With G. St. J. Perrott) American Journal of Sociology, 1935, 40: 804 – 812.

The Economics of Medical Care. Virginia Medical Monthly, 1935, 61: 574 – 579.

Annotation on: Causal and Selective Factors in Sickness. Milbank Memorial Fund Quarterly, 1935, 13: 286 – 289.

Annotation on: The Efficacy of the School Medical Examination. Milbank Memorial Fund Quarterly, 1935, 13: 391 – 392.

1936 Next Steps in Public Health. In: The Next Steps in Public Health, Proceedings of the Fourteenth Annual Conference of the Milbank Memorial Fund. New York, Milbank Memorial Fund, 1936, 13 – 33.

Economy in Public Health. Milbank Memorial Fund Quarterly, 1936, 14: 3 – 12.

Health Under the Social Security Act. Social Service Review, 1936, 10: 12 – 22.

Public Health Provisions of the Social Security Act. Law and Contemporary Problems, 1936, 3: 263 – 270.

Building a Nation's Health. Independent Woman, 1936, 15: 69, 93 – 94.

Whooping Cough in Surveyed Communities. (With R. E. Wheeler) American Journal of Public Health, 1936, 26: 576 – 585.

Annotation on: Surgeon General's Report on Health and Depression Study. Milbank Memorial Fund Quarterly, 1936, 14: 205 – 208.